A Flourishing Yin

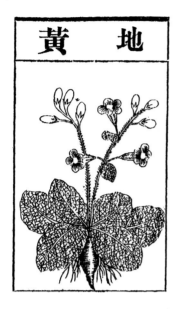

A Flourishing Yin

Gender in China's Medical
History, 960–1665

Charlotte Furth

UNIVERSITY OF CALIFORNIA PRESS

Berkeley / Los Angeles / London

University of California Press
Berkeley and Los Angeles, California

University of California Press, Ltd.
London, England

© 1999 by
The Regents of the University of California

Library of Congress Cataloging-in-Publication Data

Furth, Charlotte.
     A flourishing yin : gender in China's medical history, 960–1665 /
Charlotte Furth.
          p.   cm.
     "A Philip E. Lilienthal book."
     Includes bibliographic references and index.
     ISBN 978-0-520-20829-2 (pbk. : alk. paper)
          1. Medicine, Chinese—History.   2. Women—Health and
hygiene—China—History.   3. Body,   Human—Social   aspects—
China—History.   4. Yin-yang.   5. Sex role—China—History.
6. Obstetrics—Social aspects—China—History   I. Title.
          [DNLM: 1. History of Medicine—China.   2. Women.
3. Women's Health—China.   WZ 70 JC6 F99f 1998]
     R602.F87   1998
     610'.951—dc21
     DNLM/DLC
     for Library of Congress   97-38116

Printed in the United States of America
10   09
12   11   10   9   8   7   6   5
The paper used in this publication is both acid-free and totally
chlorine-free (TCF). It meets the minimum requirements of
ANSI/ NISO Z39.48-1992 (R 1997) (*Permanence of Paper*). ♾

Dedicated to the memory
of my dear husband
MONTGOMERY FURTH (1933–1991)

Contents

Illustrations

Acknowledgments

In writing this book I accumulated debts of gratitude over the years. They begin with a group of scholars many of whom I have never met. These are the specialists who over the last two generations in the People's Republic of China have labored to provide the research tools for serious scholarship on the history of Chinese medicine. Many of their works were collaborative projects under the guidance of staff of the China Academy of Traditional Chinese Medicine in Beijing, together with other regional academies of Chinese medicine in Shanghai, Guangzhou, Anhui, and elsewhere. Scholars associated with these institutes, many of them anonymous, compiled the massive bibliography of surviving medical texts in Chinese libraries under the direction of Xue Qinglu. They produced the multivolume *Encyclopedic Dictionary of Chinese Medicine* (*Zhongyi da cidian*) under the direction of Ma Jixing, Ma Kanwen, Li Jingwei, Yu Ying'ao, and Cai Jingfeng. Other valuable works have been the biographical dictionaries compiled by He Shixi, Li Jingwei, and Li Yun; the concordance to the *Huangdi neijing* edited by Ren Yingqiu; Ma Jixing's history of medical publishing; Chen Bangxian's documentary collection of medical passages from the twenty-six dynastic histories; Guo Aiqun's documentary collection of medical sections references in representative local histories; and the massive *Zhong yao da cidian* of the Jiangsu New Medical Academy, which combines historical, botanical, and pharmacological data on China's huge repertory of materia medica.

Beyond reference works, I have benefited from the accumulated critical scholarship of these and others in China who also supervised the republication of medical classics—both in photolithographed versions and in new critical editions. Here I am particularly indebted to Yu Ying'ao and his associates, whose edition of Chen Ziming's classic *Furen da quan liang fang* gave me a reconstruction of its Song textuality. I have also benefited from many works of historical scholarship, among which Ma Dazheng's history of *fuke, Zhongguo fuchanke fazhan shi*, in particular stands out, combining as it does the insights of a clinician and those of a scholar. A more complete listing of these works will be found in the bibliography, but those dry entries do not communicate the importance of their contribution. This scholarship, a byproduct of the Chinese government's desire to promote Chinese medicine as a living clinical practice, has largely been produced under the most meager material conditions. Without it, it would have been impossible for an outsider like myself to gain the basic orientation in the enormous literature of Chinese medical history that any serious research requires.

The personal list of individuals and institutions who have helped me is a very long one, stretching back fifteen years now. Among them I want to express my especial gratitude to Nathan Sivin, who has been generous with his time as an informal teacher, supporter, and critic from the time I first thought of taking up the study of Chinese medicine. My friends and fellow explorers of China's medical history, Francesca Bray, Judith Farquhar, and Angela Ki-che Leung, have always been there with stimulation, advice, critical suggestions, encouragement, and comradeship. Dorothy Ko has been an acute, finely tuned sounding board for theoretical and historical issues of gender history in China. Judith Zeitlin and Ellen Widmer have guided me through the gardens of Chinese belles lettres. Martha Tocco has been an invaluable first outside reader, insisting that my text reach out to audiences beyond the sphere of initiates of classical Chinese history and medicine.

Over a decade or more institutions on three continents welcomed me. Professor Ch'en Kuang-ho and the faculty and staff of the Chung-t'ai I-chuan of Dakang, Taichung, Taiwan were hosts to my daughter and myself for a summer of field research in the summer of 1985. Professor Ch'en Shu-yueh and her team of nursing students were my collaborators there in a highly educational exploration of the gynecological uses of Chinese medicine by contemporary women in Taiwan. I want also to thank the East Asian Languages and Literature Department of Princeton University for its hospitality during the academic year 1986–87; the Needham Research Institute of Cambridge, England, where I visited in the summer of 1990; and the Sun Yat-sen Institute of Social

Sciences and Philosophy of the Academia Sinica in Nankang, Taipei, for its support during the fall of 1992. Especially I wish to thank the Institute for the History of Medicine and Medical Literature of the China Academy of Traditional Chinese Medicine in Beijing, its past and present directors Professors Li Jingwei and Zheng Jinsheng, and its faculty, students, and staff. Without their welcome and the resources made available to me over several trips to Beijing, my task would have been much more difficult.

At these institutions and elsewhere I found learned and helpful librarians, among whom I would like to thank especially Yang Kangwei of the rare book library of the Zhongyi Yanjiuyuan in Beijing, Diane Perushek and Martin Heidjra of the Gest Library at Princeton, Mi Chu Wiens of the Library of Congress, John Moffett of the Needham Research Institute, and James Cheng of the East Asian Library at UCLA. The Special Collections Division of the Louise M. Darling Biomedical Library at UCLA gave permission to reproduce the drawings of medicinal plants that ornament the chapter headings. These come from an 1896 edition of Li Shizhen's famous *Bencao gangmu*.

A grant from the National Library of Medicine of the National Institute of Health supported the initial stages of this research in 1986–87; and the Committee on Scholarly Communication with the People's Republic of China underwrote a travel grant covering research trips to Beijing in 1990 and 1992.

Many others have helped in a variety of ways. They brought their own diverse expertise to bear as critic and commentators, and called attention to many sources I would otherwise have missed. That long list includes Marjorie Becker, Carol Benedict, Bettine Birge, Beverly Bossler, Donald Brenneis, Cynthia Brokaw, Katherine Carlitz, Chang Chia-feng, Chang Chueh, Lucille Chia, Catherine Despeux, Barbara Duden, Patricia Ebrey, Fu Fang, Joanna Grant, Monica Green, Marta Hanson, T. J. Hinrichs, Hu Ming-hui, Huang Yi-long, Hsiung Ping-chen, Paul Katz, Kuriyama Shigehisa, Thomas Laqueur, Jen-der Lee, James Lee, Karen Leonard, Vivienne Lo, Susan Mann, Kenneth Pomerantz, Reiko Shinno, Paul Unschuld, Ann Waltner, Yi-li Wu, Zhang Jingli, and Zhao Pushan. My graduate students David Bello, James Liebold, Liu Xun, and Meng Zhang gracefully combined research assistance with comments and suggestions of substance. Above all, these and other colleagues and students at California State University at Long Beach and the University of Southern California, and at seminars and conferences at the University of Chicago, UC Davis, UC San Diego, UCLA,

Harvard, the University of Pittsburgh, and elsewhere have by their critical interest sustained my pursuit of knowledge in the intersections of Sinology, gender studies and medical history.

At the University of California Press, editors Sheila Levine and Dore Brown were unfailingly supportive and efficient, while my copyeditor Evan Camfield never allowed me to forget that the devil lies in the details. My neighbor and friend Lisa Johnson designed the original charts and figures. All of these people helped make a physical book a work of craft and its production a cooperative enterprise.

Los Angeles, California
October 1998

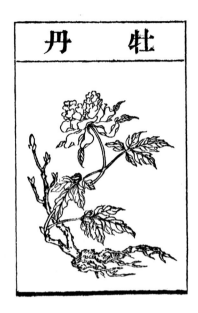

Medical History, Gender, and the Body

In the summer of 1982, while browsing in the library of Beijing University, I chanced upon a small volume anonymously published in 1715. Worn yet sturdily printed, bearing traces of some long-dead reader's inked-in punctuation marks, *On Successful Childbirth (Da sheng bian)*[1] turned out to be a popular guide to pregnancy and delivery, and it started me on the path that has led to writing this book. The excitement of reading it inspired me to search out an enormous late-imperial Chinese literature on health and medicine that circulated among the literate public as much as among professional healers. Even more, this text and others like it placed medicine in the context of elite domestic life and showed how the language of the body and body

1. Anon. ("Jizhai jushi"), 1715. See also Furth 1987.

processes constructed cultural identity. Much in *On Successful Childbirth* and many similar works seemed at first to tell a story familiar to feminist scholars of early modern Europe: a story of sex segregation and dense social rituals surrounding parturition, of tensions between male-dominated medical authority and a female sphere of health care associated with midwifery, of birth as a perilous and polluted life passage for mother and child. Above all, doctors repeated constantly that "in women Blood is the leader," and that "the disorders of women are ten times more deep-rooted and harder to cure" than those of males—tropes that inscribed gender difference on the female body, representing it as weak and hostage to reproductive necessity.

Fuke, or "the department of [medicine for] women," was the classificatory label Chinese physicians gave to that field of medical knowledge devoted to the disorders they deemed specific to women alone. My initial search to understand the body as a site of gender ideology in Chinese history drew me deeper into the literature of *fuke* as an integral part of China's ancient medical traditions and as a lens for thinking about the culturally constructed body. This book is the outcome of that inquiry. Writing it has involved long explorations along three scholarly paths: the history of Chinese medicine, feminist interpretations of gender in China, and the cultural history and anthropology of the body.

Medical History

The history of medicine in China is where I begin. A two-thousand-year literary tradition lies behind it, and it remains a living practice. Important fundamentals of Chinese medical history have been introduced to Western scholars by eminent historians of science like Joseph Needham and Nathan Sivin in the English-speaking world and Manfred Porkert and Paul Unschuld on the European continent. All who work in the field have benefited from the vast energy and visionary humanism that Needham brought to his pioneering work on premodern scientific and technological contributions of Chinese civilization. Needham's prestige as a distinguished Cambridge biochemist added insight and authority to his claim that Chinese achievements in sciences from mathematics to astronomy and chemistry, and in technologies like engineering, shipbuilding, metallurgy, and agronomy, matched and even surpassed those of the European West before the seventeenth century. His massively researched project, still incomplete at his death in 1995, introduced the voluminous textual record of Chinese achievements and interpreted them as an honorable chapter in the history of a globally evolving universal science. Medicine was only one facet of Needham's protean explorations, and an incomplete one. Perhaps this was not only because of the sheer volume of Chinese records about medicine but because their theoretical foundations eluded the positivist framework of Needham's own "ecumenical" model of world-historical scientific truth.[2]

Scholars of China's medical history following Needham, like Nathan Sivin, have turned to an internalist strategy—explaining this ancient science in terms of its indigenous conceptual framework and the cultural assumptions of its makers, opening the way for relativist approaches involving alternative epistemologies.[3] By this route the field has recently attracted more attention from social and cultural historians and encouraged my feminist perspective. Much of this book reconstructs the rich but neglected learned tradition of *fuke* over the long span of the Song, Yuan and Ming dynasties (960–1644), a tradition that today is identified with obstetrics and gynecology. My later chapters focus more narrowly on the sixteenth and seventeenth centuries and on the social relations of healing as seen through medical case histories and literary sources. Here I can more easily show how theoretical orientations translated into clinical strategies. Medicine also reveals itself as a social practice not dominated by the role of the elite doctor, where the management of illness might also appear as a domestic skill, as amateur literati learning, as a humble craft or as a religious practice based in ritual. Here sick people and their families negotiated with various kinds of healers—both male and female—who were valued as service providers but who did not command an unquestionably authoritative "science." In the historically specific context of late Ming elite culture, Chinese medicine was em-

---

2. Joseph Needham's monumental series is *Science and Civilization in China* (abbreviated as SCC), 1954– . Originally projected at seven volumes, it eventually ballooned into many more. However, Needham never completed a volume on basic medicine, and his various shorter essays on medical topics are being edited by Nathan Sivin for posthumous publication in the series. Among the completed volumes, his *Celestial Lancets* (with Lu Gwei-djen, 1980) explored acupuncture and moxibustion, while the topic of bodily self-cultivation for longevity was the theme of a volume originally projected as part of the series on chemistry, which was published separately (with Lu Gwei-djen, 1983) under the title *Spagyrical Discovery and Invention: Physiological Alchemy*. It was characteristic of Needham to analyze this complex of yogic meditation exercises known to Chinese immortality seekers as *nei dan*, or "internal alchemy," under the rubric of macrobiotic chemistry. I discuss the practice of *nei dan* in the Ming dynasty in chapter six.

3. See Sivin 1987, 1995a, 1995b, 1995c.

bedded in both cosmology and daily life, shaped by social relations that diffused power, and used in a world where the inner functioning of a human body was publicly knowable primarily through signs and speech.

The historical specificity of such a medical culture is illuminated by both similarities and dissimilarities with Renaissance and early modern Europe. In much of what follows it will be clear how much I have benefited from the insights and interpretive approaches of such recent social historians of that period in European medicine as Roy Porter, Barbara Duden, and Thomas Laqueur. Porter's work has popularized medical history from below, showing how a patient-centered approach to the early modern clinical encounter in England changes our historical understanding of medical authority and makes a truly social history of medicine possible. Duden has read eighteenth-century German medical case histories as revealing a phenomenological language of experience through which the historicity of a pre-Enlightenment body itself may be known. Laqueur, in considering the history of anatomy from the Renaissance through the nineteenth century, has shown how medical knowledge of the gendered body, once understood as a human manifestation of a metaphysically grounded hierarchy of Being, became essentialized in a biology of two basically incommensurable sexes.[4] My debt to these scholars will be apparent to every reader who knows their work.

Unlike the European humoral medicine these historians analyze so imaginatively, Chinese medicine has been seen as outside of history, both timeless and contemporary. It remains a living therapeutic system for millions of people today—a fact that is both an aid and an obstacle in reconstructing its past. The ethnographic present can, if carefully used, illuminate possible meanings of historical evidence. Among many fine anthropological studies, I have learned particularly from Arthur Kleinman's analysis of the clinical encounter in the pluralistic medical culture of Taiwan in the 1970s and from Judith Farquhar's subtle reading of the epistemology of medical knowledge as taught and practiced in a contemporary college of traditional Chinese medicine (TCM) medical college in Guangzhou.[5] Still, it is dangerous to accept the evidence of today's living tradition uncritically. In the PRC particularly, Chinese medicine is a well-established branch of the state health-care system.

4. Porter 1985; Duden 1991; Laqueur 1990.

5. Kleinman 1980; Farquhar 1994. TCM is conventional shorthand for Chinese medicine today, distinguishing present practice from the tradition in its original historical settings.

Maoist ideology has elevated it to the status of a national cultural treasure, producing researchers committed to their own version of a Whig history of Chinese medicine as a proto-science both "empirical" and "dialectical." To people outside Asia, on the other hand, Chinese medicine remains romantically traditional — an indigenous folk system, the domain of the anthropologist, easily mystified as a countercultural holistic art of Oriental healing, in opposition to hegemonic cosmopolitan biomedicine. Neither of these oppositions — tradition versus modernity, or science versus folk superstition — point to fruitful analytic categories for my subject. Rather, they encourage the discredited binary oppositions of Orientalism, the mutually reinforcing and totalizing stereotypes of East-West difference in the global discourse of colonialism. Such binaries are just as problematic when they valorize Eastern wisdom and spirituality as when they condemn or rationalize Asiatic scientific backwardness. The contemporary practice of TCM in both mainland China and Taiwan has taught me much about the medical world of my sixteenth- and seventeenth-century texts: about the doctor-patient relationship, about the art of diagnosis and prescription, about popular health habits and medical pluralism. But TCM today operates in a world vastly changed from the late Ming dynasty, whether the issue is patterns of fertility and mortality, technologies of knowledge, or the Chinese social system. Understanding the specificity of such changes is itself a useful antidote to Orientalist reasoning.

Gender

A feminist history of medicine in China is imaginable today partly because it builds upon the work of social historians who since the 1980s have been excavating the premodern Chinese woman as a historical subject. Among Euro-Americans, pre-twentieth-century Chinese society has been popularly defined by Confucianism, an ethos whose patriarchal foundations appear to be confirmed by anthropological accounts of China's patrilineal, patrilocal joint family system and lineage organization. Institutions like arranged marriage, son preference, footbinding, concubinage, and sex segregation extending to the exclusion of women from public office have fleshed out a feminist stereotype of Chinese women as profoundly subordinated. Moreover, such Western constructions of Asian women's victimization have been subtly

complemented by the judgments of China's own nationalist moderniz-
ers, who in their zeal for revolutionary change have identified traditional
womanhood with feudal backwardness. Looking beyond such politicized representations, feminist historians like Patricia Ebrey, Dorothy
Ko, and Susan Mann have sought to compare prescriptive norms with
evidence about women's social practice and their self-perceptions in specific historical contexts.[6] Without being apologists for the Confucian
gender system, they have tried to understand both its internal diversity
and its overall durability. Without seeing women's lives through the
politicized prisms of resistance or accommodation, they have tried to
show the roles that were possible and the sorts of subjectivities these
roles fostered. Among many topics they have illuminated, several are
particularly relevant to my study.

Both the place of the family in society and the norms of gender difference were constructed by Confucian moralists around a bifurcation
of spheres into inner (*nei*) and outer (*wai*) — terms that demarcated separate spaces but also claimed a complementarity between them. Since
the family as "inner" was understood as a microcosm of the state as
"outer," responsible for its own sphere of social order, functions that
today are thought of as public were aspects of family life. Most economic
production and much education, worship and ritual life took place at
home or on family farms. In this context the imperial state not only
recognized the family as a foundation of social order but also left substantial legal as well as social powers vested in it. Here as elsewhere, the
doctrine of separate spheres did not separate women from their male
kin within the household, while circumstances drew many women beyond the walls of domestic compounds as workers, travellers and so-
journers. As Dorothy Ko and Francesca Bray have argued, inner and
outer are best imagined as nested and overlapping spheres whose boundaries shifted with circumstance, while the family model of the state gave
the conduct of domestic life more than private significance. Identifying
a wife as an "inner person" (*nei ren*) constructed her femininity via bodily location rather than biology, a spatial habitus that taught female
gender in the idiom of a socially complex domain of family life. All of
these factors were at work in the management of sickness, which took
place largely at home.

The idiom of inner and outer points to the fact that ideas about
gender difference were not easily separated from those about the social

6. See especially Ebrey 1993, 1995; Ko 1994; Mann 1997.

roles of men and women. Patricia Ebrey and others have shown the importance of kinship in defining a woman's powers and in differentiating among different groups of women. Identities as daughter, wife or mother were among the most significant social markers for women in Confucian society. Emphasizing this, some scholars accordingly bifurcate the bodily and the social to locate traditional Chinese gender in kinship and other social hierarchies, minimizing the significance of the body as a site of the Chinese feminine.[7]

In this interpretation, popular among postcolonial scholars, body-based systems of gender construction look like a unique invention of the West's modern scientific revolution, transported to China complete with the baggage of science, social Darwinism, and the ideology of political revolution and economic modernization—baggage that included a project of female emancipation. There is some truth to the view that gender relations changed significantly in the twentieth century as Chinese learned the modernist axiom that only science can decipher the body's nature and represent it in truthful relationship to social norms.[8] However, the very ideological power of scientism to define Chinese modernity suggests what its secularizing teachings undermined: the old imperium's conviction of unity between Heaven, Earth, and Humanity—a natural philosophy without sharp boundaries between sacred and secular or between nature and culture. To seek to locate gender exclusively in either social roles or natural (bodily) attributes is to lose sight of other possible worlds encompassing both.

In this context inner and outer, which led away from the body in the foregoing discussion, are also categories that can lead back to it. Demarcating relationships of gender and social space, inner and outer were also a yin yang pair, linking patterns of social organization with larger overarching patterns in Chinese cosmology. Most broadly, the Chinese concepts of yin and yang constructed an interlocking network of signs binding a wide range of phenomena to a common system of signification that was metaphysically grounded. As part of this system, the categories of male and female were understood as both natural and social, and their bodily powers were given spiritual significance as fitting microcosmic participants in a universal order. Inner and outer, then, were not purely about gender boundaries demarcating domestic and public space; they were relationships in the natural world as well, including the human

7. Barlow 1994.
8. See Dikötter 1995.

body. This can also be a starting point for exploring how gender difference was naturalized in medicine.

While focusing on family and kinship as central, feminist historians of gender in China have also been concerned with exploring spheres of female activity beyond the functions of wife and mother. They have shown that women's work as economic producers was significant; they have analyzed female religious expression and looked into the stigmatized yet glamorous demimonde of prostitutes and courtesan entertainers. Literary historians in particular have brought to light a voluminous body of poetry and other writings by women of the Ming and Qing, demonstrating the high level of classical education attained by some elite women and the opportunities it afforded them as teachers and, to a limited extent, as participants in literati discourse.[9] Medicine can contribute to filling out this picture of female activity. Certainly literacy for women, as for men, provided one avenue to medical knowledge, and some women were economically productive health workers within and without the domestic setting.

However, the Chinese medical culture of *fuke* was perennially concerned with the gestational functions of women, defined as menstruation, pregnancy and postpartum recovery from childbirth. This emphasis brings us back to women as wives and mothers. The importance of reproductive medicine is reinforced by demographic estimates that marriage at a relatively early age (18–20 years) was a near-universal destiny for Chinese women throughout history, while infant mortality was high (estimated around three hundred per thousand on average). While seeking evidence for reproductive failure in macroeconomic conditions producing poor nutrition and disease, James Lee and his collaborators have recently argued that cultural factors, including conscious reproductive strategies, gender norms and sexual practices, also may help explain demographic patterns. Their figures suggest that completed marital fertility was on average low to moderate—four to six children, as against seven to eleven for comparable groups in early modern northwestern Europe.[10] These Chinese demographic patterns, then, hint of the basic

9. See Hu Wenkai 1985; Widmer 1989; *Late Imperial China* special issue on "Poetry and Women's Culture in Late Imperial China," 13.1 (June 1992); Widmer and Chang 1997.

10. Lee and Campbell 1997: 83–102; Lee and Saito, forthcoming. For the social historian, demographic estimates like these raise as many questions as they answer. Stevan Harrell (1985, 1995), Liu Ts'ui-jung (1995a, 1995b) and others work with Ming-Qing lineage genealogies that were originally composed to trace patrilines. These records underreported births in general and vital facts concerning daughters in par-

social contexts in which *fuke* was practiced, but also of medical norms surrounding reproductive processes. They evoke a social history of patriarchal kinship structures — the joint family system that allowed young couples to marry without responsibility for maintaining an independent household but required them to live under the authority of elders, and sex-selective child mortality that led to recurrent shortages of brides. By contrast, however, the history of medicine and the body in China seems at first to take a different direction, toward a natural world imagined in terms of transmutation, process, and change that relativizes all static hierarchies.

The Body

If the history of medicine is one path this book follows and feminist history is a second, the two meet in a consideration of the body. Histories of the human body are a recent and still experimental product of American and European scholarship. Intellectual roots for such a project extend back to the insights of the cultural anthropologists — their ethnographies of the diverse explanatory and symbolic systems that have shaped understandings of bodily experience in different human communities — and to the philosophical relativism of Nietzsche and the phenomenologists. Michel Foucault dramatized the possibilities for historicizing the body with his cumulative work on disease, madness, criminality and sexuality in eighteenth- and nineteenth-century Europe. Instead of Enlightenment rationality consolidating the findings of modern science, Foucault saw an epistemic rupture producing "games of truth" by which human nature came to be redefined. Instead of knowledge systems producing liberal emancipation and progress, Foucault saw nineteenth-century biology, psychology, medicine and the social sciences as imposing new forms of social discipline embedded in law,

---

ticular. Better sets of data come from the eighteenth- and nineteenth-century records of Manchu banners, explored by Lee and Campbell, and from colonial Taiwan. The broad constants I have summarized here conceal wide variability in figures on both marital fertility and child mortality, linked to region, economic conditions and social class ("the rich get children," in the words of Stevan Harrell 1985). Nonetheless Lee and Campbell's work breaks new ground for feminist analysis by reconstituting family records in an effort to reveal reproductive behavior. They point to long intervals between marriage and the birth of the first child and to "early stopping"—a last pregnancy in a woman's mid-thirties — as evidence of low coital frequency. They point to skewed sex ratios correlated with sibling birth order as evidence for sex-selective infanticide.

education and politics — disciplines powerful enough not only to police society but to shape the psyche's own subjectivity. If Foucault's notion that "discourses of power" are diffused in the personal relationships of daily life was a riposte to Marxist class analysis, his idea that "discursive formations" of language construct culture turned inquiry into the epistemological foundations of knowledge of the human body away from a materialist base. The most intimate dimensions of embodiment — our health and normality, our disease and suffering, our sexuality, the very boundaries of flesh and spirit that shape the self — all these could be related to a phenomenological body of experience that is felt and lived in, and is conditioned by culture.

While not necessarily embracing all the radical epistemology of a Foucauldian project, subsequent scholars have fleshed out the contours of a post-Enlightenment bourgeois body shaped by the impact of technology and science, by regimens of sanitation and hygiene, clothing and adornment, sexuality and sports. Not surprisingly, some of the most interesting work has historicized bodily gender. Using the representations of Galenic and Renaissance anatomy as evidence, Thomas Laqueur has argued for the relative novelty of the modern belief in a profound bodily difference between males and females that is demonstrated by the facts of biology. When Barbara Duden turned to accounts of illness in eighteenth-century German medical case histories, she exposed a female humoral body of fluxes and plethoras, of warm and cold wombs, of reproductive seeds and fruits, profoundly unlike the body of modern pregnancy. From another direction, Duden's account of the startling new reproductive technologies of DNA mapping, of sonograms, amniocentesis and fetal monitors constructs a biotechnical fetus that even our mid-twentieth-century grandmothers would have found alien. All of these authors have offered a common critique of modernist assumptions that the language of bioscience constructs an epistemologically privileged, truthful account of an ahistorical natural body.[11]

By and large, this postmodernist wave is just beginning to wash up on the shores of Chinese studies. Although there have been a few exploratory exceptions, notably the essay collection *Body, Subject and Power in China,* edited by Angela Zito and Tani Barlow,[12] the most familiar

---

11. See Laqueur 1990; Duden 1991; Duden 1993. A further sampling of a huge literature, in addition to Foucault's major works (*The Birth of the Clinic,* 1973; *Discipline and Punish,* 1979; and *A History of Sexuality,* 1978–1985), might include Corbin 1986 on odor and hygiene, Hollander 1978 on clothing, Stafford 1991 on visual perception.

12. Zito and Barlow 1994.

Euro-American scholarship on the subject has shown us a Chinese body that has been not so much historicized as Orientalized: imagined as an embodiment of the life forms of the East as opposed to the West. When R. H. Van Gulik wrote his classic work *Sexual Life in Ancient China,* it was as a Freudian admirer of what he saw as a healthy and pleasure-affirming Chinese ars erotica free of the repressions and perversions that were the unfortunate legacy of Christian sexual morality in the West.[13] In his important work on religious Daoism, Kristofer Schipper imagines a body of transmutation and generativity containing the seeds of its own rebirth; honoring the feminine, neither ascetic nor licentious, the Daoist self-cultivator strives for a sacred form of corporeality embodying pacifism, equalitarianism and nonstriving.[14] As I have already suggested, in any number of works the Chinese medical body has been praised as holistic, embodying ideals of psycho-physical integration and human harmony with the natural world, ready to teach alienated Western man and woman the secrets of self-healing and inner peace. All of these accounts are haunted by their opposite: a Western body bifurcated between body and soul, objectified as a material object shaped by regimens of modern science, and associated with a range of Darwinian attributes—competition, individualism, human domination of nature and the European domination of Asia.

All of these idealizations of an Oriental body have been based on the self-fulfilling oppositions of colonialist cultural discourse. They have found common ground with Asian self-interpretations because the Chinese have thought about the human body in terms of their own grand binary of nature, yin and yang. Classificatory, yin and yang align all phenomena as complementary opposites based on qualities of light and dark, day and night, male and female, hot and cold, and myriad extrapolations from these. Dialectical, yin and yang explain process and change as the product of the movement of such opposites in ceaseless alternation. There is no doubt that the concepts of yin and yang are fundamental to Chinese cosmology, and therefore to indigenous Chinese understandings of the workings of the human body, but the romance of yin and yang as Oriental philosophy is based on a one-dimensional and idealized reading of a polysemic field of meanings. One of my goals in writing about the Chinese medical body is to show this protean conceptual tool kit at work in different specific contexts and to historicize it adequately, including exposure of its metaphorical contradictions. It

13. Van Gulik 1974; Furth 1994.
14. Schipper 1993.

is to dissolve the discourse of symmetrical opposition between East and West by situating Chinese bodies in their own complex history.

Any critical analysis of culture and the human body leads easily to a consideration of gender. The old Chinese binary of yin and yang no less than the teachings of modern biology has provided prime examples of the way cultural agendas shape human notions of what is natural. While the first wave of feminist scholars of the 1970s took for granted that the body is an obvious foundation for the perceived differences between the sexes, the Foucauldian and later feminist critiques of bioscience successfully demolished this belief. Subsequent efforts to distinguish between sex and gender, between a physical substratum of biological difference and the cultural attributes of masculinity or femininity with all their baggage of values and social practices, also came increasingly under attack. Foucault argued that erotic desire itself is not so much a natural biological drive as a set of plastic impulses today understood through the prism of a distinctly modern discourse of incitement.[15] Jeffrey Weeks argued that coupling not only is surrounded by social rituals and moral judgments but is even performed according to culturally distinct erotic scripts.[16] Judith Butler proposed that gender is in fact a performance of the body, a cultural aesthetics of self-fashioning that constructs modern sexual identities.[17] All of these perspectives have worked to undermine the solidity of the idea of biologically based sex, suggesting that the categories of male and female are literally invented in the course of discursive cultural practices.

As a cultural historian I have found this a powerful, even seductive, tool of analysis, and much that follows will show its influence. My history of classical Chinese medical thought and practice is a history of texts that can be read on many levels, texts that were and are unstable over time, and through which we can see competing and conflicting models of embodied gender. I find symbolic bodies that tell stories about the social world, bodies of power that are shaped and disciplined

15. The phrase is from *The History of Sexuality* vol. 1 (1978: 17–18). As sex became the subject of scientific study, its importance in social life was enhanced by the discussions of biologists, doctors, psychologists, and educators, even before reactions against Victorian decorum opened the path to our twentieth-century "incitements" to pleasure via the discourses of popular entertainment and consumerism.

16. Weeks 1986. In arguing for an anti-essentialist approach to sexual meanings, Weeks has adopted the notion of a "sexual script" from interactionist sociologists. It calls attention to codes of sexual behavior that not only prescribe what is normal or abnormal but shape the production of desire itself.

17. Butler 1990, 1993.

by social rituals, fashion, morality, or law, cosmic bodies that metonym-ically replicate the universe as a whole and figure ontological meaning, as well as subterranean bodies expressing human fears and desires. By shifting their readings over time and speaking something other than an author's intentions, texts do their work as concrete bearers of a socially conditioned cultural meaning which shapes individual consciousness. Gender systems are built of such things.

But while gender may usefully be defined as a kind of cultural per-formance of bodily roles, bringing that perspective to a study of health and disease raises questions about the limits of the cultural construc-tionism that has been such a powerful stimulus to body history. As the historicity of the body is affirmed, problems of interpretation become epistemological. Essentialist categories constructing identity out of the presumably natural bodily characteristics of race, gender, or demo-graphic population disappear, but along with them I find also disap-pearing any body knowable in its materiality to be part of a stable epis-temological order. This debate has produced an impasse between those who maintain a positivist commitment to nature as bioscience defines it and radical relativists whose skepticism is bolstered by Marxist or phenomenological epistemologies.

I could speculate about why such a deconstructionist strategy has been especially attractive to recent feminist theorists and others strug-gling with the contradictions of today's identity politics. While this po-sition is a tempting one for some, many social historians and anthro-pologists of medicine try to relativize post-Enlightenment scientific understandings of the body without rejecting the knowability of a nat-ural world, including a corporeal body, to which the language of health and disease refers. Thus Charles Rosenberg prefers to say that culture "frames" disease rather than "constructs" it, while Margaret Lock, speak-ing of "cultures of biomedicine," argues that though there may be no "real biology out there entirely separate from the way in which we ap-prehend it," it is also mistaken to speak of biology as purely represen-tational, knowable only through culturally plastic discourse.[18]

On the one hand, the body cannot be considered an object. The word itself is shorthand, a product of limitations of English that do not hobble the Chinese *shen* (or the German *Leib,* for that matter). Just as *shen* is sometimes translated "body/person," and just as *Leib* refers to the sen-tient living organism rather than the physical object that is the German

18. Rosenberg and Golden 1992; Lock 1993.

Korper, so the real subject here is an embodied and functioning human being bounded more profoundly by time than by space, shaped more deeply by the processes leading from birth to death than by the structures of size, shape or volume encasing her.[19] But on the other hand, basic bodily functions—menstruation, conception, childbirth, lactation—cannot be treated just as the products of the languages through which they become culturally known. As functions that human beings in some sense share with animals, they stand across cultures as stable, materially grounded forms of human embodiment. There is a limit to the ways in which Chinese bodies are different from our own—or from each other. Boundaries of gender, too, appear more stable when the subject is a gestational body as opposed to a body of generation or the body erotic.

Textuality, Language, and Experience

Finally, in returning to discourse, I am made to recognize how my themes—history and medicine on the one hand, and gender and the body on the other—both require consideration of problems of textuality, language and experience. First, whatever the body may be, it enters culture as soon as we begin to speak of it. Here the theoretical problems of the knowability of an "objective" body intersect in an interesting way with the historiographical problems of the knowability of the past. I think historians have to believe that the texts they analyze are necessarily incomplete traces of past lives. The medical writings I discuss here were produced for use as memory aids, as household manuals or other guidebooks, as pedagogical tools, or as reportage of a clinical encounter. To complicate matters further, beginning in the tenth century C.E., print technology became available in China, and the medical system, like other domains of learning, gradually adapted to the shifts in relationship between knowledge and power fostered by print culture, encouraging both the codification of medical classics and the discursive polyphony of mechanical reproduction. Many surviving texts were not originally meant to be public. Printing them often appears to have been something of an afterthought. Some were esoteric writings passed down as part of rituals linking masters and disciples in medical lineages; others were householders' or clinicians' notes. I find anonymous and multiple

19. For *shen* see Elvin 1989: 267–349; for *Leib* see Ots 1994: 116–36.

authorship, texts cobbled together out of a shifting bricolage of component antecedents and commentary, many-branched variant manuscript traditions, and everywhere traces of oral transmission via family lineages and personal master-disciple relations. All of these call attention to medicine as a practice carried on outside the text, and to the centrality of the clinical encounters and personal relationships that constructed medical culture not in formal literary discourse but in knowledge-producing practices.

Yet these fragmentary texts also use language in complex ways to evoke the body. Their language about nature, cosmology and events — that is, the language claiming to describe the world beyond the self — is intermixed with a language of symptoms and sensations, words that point to a culturally dense phenomenology of experience. In confronting the language of illness we cannot refer simply to a world "out there"; we must also "read" our own bodies' realms of sensation, and imagine bodily experience framed in other words than our own. To the extent that the medical language of my texts takes this irreducible form, it constitutes, and does not merely represent, the culturally animated body. Moreover, this phenomenological aspect of language is an invaluable historian's tool, allowing me to hear the voices of the sick speaking through the doctors' narratives.

While I privilege language as the vehicle by which the mute presocial body enters the cultural domain, medical language is only partially phenomenological. In thinking about discourse as it shapes bodily experience — the relationship between language and embodied self-fashioning — I read medical language as communicating on three planes: the structural, the phenomenological, and the metaphorical. The first is a language of logical relationships and abstract qualities — claims about "nature" and "science," if you will. The second is a language of sensation, whereby hidden bodily events are named as symptoms and made a shared social property. This is how sick people and healers arrive at a common understanding of malady and of the processes by which suffering might be relieved. The third dimension, the metaphorical, is important because of the plastic, open-ended way in which words can shift meanings and associations, giving play to a diversity of connotations and associations. Metaphor is a particularly rich shaper of gendered and other social meanings of experience, while also potentially a domain of freedom enabling the new. As metaphor, language often seems to speak the social in ways that reinforce cultural hegemony, but it also may allow subversion, transgression or invention.

The Road Ahead

The three themes I have outlined—medical history, gender studies and the culturally constructed body—are analytically distinguishable here. However, just as medicine as a technology of knowledge produces a discourse on gender, and the discourse on gender leads to questions about the body itself as a subject of historical and social inquiry, so I can't keep these three strands separate, but instead interweave them in my narrative. Keeping them in mind as a ground, I have organized my figure, or story, to carry the reader forward in a sequence.

I begin by presenting *fuke* as part of the internal history of a premodern science, understood in terms of the ways it produced knowledge, the clinical issues that engaged practitioners, and the institutions that supported or constrained them. This largely unfamiliar medical system must be described globally as an imagined whole before it can be deconstructed and its inner historical tensions exposed. Here I have to explore a Chinese historiographical tradition that has so idealized its classical origins and the continuity of its transmitted medical wisdom that it successfully conceals much of the strangeness of its own past. I argue that patterns of change in this premodern scientific system were shaped by decentralized authority; by forgetting as well as by learning; and by the eclectic use of past knowledge as bricolage, preserved or adapted or reassembled at will. Here gender is not only a topic in itself but a new perspective illuminating medical pluralism and eclecticism and the subtle interconnections between medicine and ritual and religious beliefs. Gender also focuses us on the domestic domain as the site where most medical knowledge was produced, and on the dialogical nature of that production.

In chapter one, "The Yellow Emperor's Body," I start with a schematic and largely ahistorical introductory overview of classical medical thought. In chapters two through five I take up the history of *fuke* over the seven hundred years from the tenth to the seventeenth centuries. These chapters explore the historiography of a learned tradition and its shifting institutional contexts, and through these the multiple ways in which medical discourse constructed female gender. Chapter five, on the medical culture of the late Ming dynasty, also begins to focus in on the sixteenth and seventeenth centuries and on the regional centers of Jiangnan in the Yangzi delta. Chapter six, "Nourishing Life," complements my discussion of female gender by looking at male gender through the rich repertory of late Ming Jiangnan medical writings on sexuality, fertility and longevity.

Chapters seven and eight shift focus from prescriptive texts to narratives of the clinical encounter, where disease is experienced as personal history and embedded in the social relations of healing at the bedside. In these chapters I look at the relationships of male and female healers and their clients in the domestic context. I also discuss how gender, class and kinship shaped the pluralistic world of practice for both male and female medical specialists in Ming society. I explore patient voices and argue for the complex agency of women whom readers know mainly as subordinates in one of history's most successful patriarchies. Case narratives use every dimension of medical language—formal, experiential and metaphorical—in the context of stories. These stories show the socially embedded nature of illness as a fragment of biography. Here the categories of the culturally imagined body and the social relations of gender can come together as part of a single history.

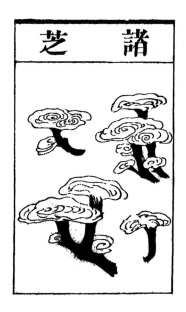

CHAPTER I

The Yellow Emperor's Body

The phrase "the Yellow Emperor's body" cannot be found in any of the classical texts that comprise the canon of Chinese medicine. I devised this phrase and use it here not as a scholarly summary of references contained in the medical classics but as an interpretive model. Two issues need to be kept in mind in thinking about it, one conceptual and the other historiographical. The conceptual issue is embedded in the problem of translation. From early on, the term *shen* (the closest classical approximation to our English word "body") sometimes referred to the physical form of the human being, that which could be weighed, measured, or covered with clothing, and sometimes to the "self" as a sentient person with a lived history and subjective consciousness.[1] Medical classics did not take *shen* as their object of study but spoke instead

---

1. In the classical language *shen* often carried both connotations, suggesting meanings like "body/person" (Elvin 1989). *Shenti,* the biological body, is a modern neologism.

of an ensemble of functions. Such a body encompasses psyche and emotions, blurring the mind-body dualism that makes our English-language "body" the object of our own gaze; it also privileges process over structures, effacing the anatomical foundations of the biomedical body we think of as the norm today. Nonetheless, this unfamiliar body is not a dematerialized abstraction but, like the biomedical one, is based on point of view—a selection from the overwhelming multiplicity of phenomena available. Biomedical bodies also can be thought of in terms of functions—reproductive, metabolic, endocrine, or psychological, for example. From another perspective, anatomical structures considered independent of function are no more than inert attributes of a corpse; disembodied, the mind ceases to exist. The phrase "the Yellow Emperor's body" is a metaphor calling attention to the conceptual point of view needed for us to connect classical medical theory to the human organism it was meant to explain.

The second interpretive problem is how to understand "the Yellow Emperor's body" in relation to the historiographical record of classical Chinese medicine. The Yellow Emperor, one of the mythical sage founders of civilization in China, was revered as the inventor of the medical art of acupuncture. The most famous of medical classics represents him as a mighty ruler who acquired the secrets of health and longevity by humbly seeking the wisdom of Qibo, a commoner physician. Any search through the classical tradition for a normative medical body begins with their imagined dialogue. It was first written about between the first century B.C.E. and the seventh century C.E. in manuscript traditions that took as their title *The Yellow Emperor's Inner Canon* (*Huangdi neijing;* hereafter *Inner Canon*).[2] In the context of its own era the *Inner Canon* was "a collection of interrelated short writings from distinct medical lineages at different times."[3] In fact, beginning with the second-century (C.E.) *Canon of Problems* (*Nanjing*), medical scholars have repeatedly devoted themselves to resolving discrepancies to expose some synthetic truth assumed to inhere in the classic. So in constructing a normative body with reference to the *Inner Canon* I have ample prec-

2. There are three surviving texts of the *Huangdi neijing*. Of these the *Su wen* (Basic Questions) and *Ling shu* (Divine Pivot) have been known since the Tang dynasty based on editions by Wang Bing (fl. 762). The third, *Tai su* (Grand Basis), is attributed to Yang Shangshan (fl. seventh century C.E.). Since it disappeared from circulation in the Song era, it was less important in shaping later canonical understandings. For a history of the textual tradition, see Sivin 1993.

3. Sivin 1993: 198.

edent for my rhetorical strategy. Generations of interpreters have assumed that China's early medical canons agreed on essentials that form a harmonic whole. By imagining the norm as embodied in the Yellow Emperor himself, I call attention to its metaphorical links to a body politic of kingly power. By evoking the myths surrounding the Yellow Emperor I ask readers to see this body first of all as cosmological rather than biological.

During the centuries when the textual tradition of the *Inner Canon* was being formed, philosophers of the Han dynasty (221 B.C.E.–C.E. 220) were coming to imagine the world in terms of a universal system by which all phenomena of Heaven, Earth and Humanity could be categorized and their transformations known. From these basic building blocks, philosophers elaborated various superstructures of symbolic correlations that patterned the relationship of a vast range of phenomena. In the version adopted as an official cosmology authorized by the Han court, the system became one of the theoretical foundations of imperial rule, accepted as expressing the truths of natural and social philosophy. One reason the *Inner Canon* became a germinal text was because it drew upon basic features of this cosmology — *qi*, yin yang and Five Phase theory — to explain health and disease, firmly establishing correlative relationships between the cosmos and the microcosm of the body.[4] (See figure 1 for a chart of symbolic correlations and the body.)

In the cosmos, *qi* named the fundamental energy at life's source, the unitary One prior to all differentiations. A tiny bit of this Heavenly *qi*, bestowed at conception and embodied as human "primordial *qi*" (*yuan qi*), maintains life and growth, supports generative vitality and declines with age. Its exhaustion means death.

Yin and yang as forces of change governed the differentiation of this primal *qi* into the myriad phenomena of the world and their subsequent transmutations. The cyclical mutations of nature were propelled by yin and yang as an overarching binary principle of growth and decline governing the tempo and pattern of change in phenomenal things. Archaic Chinese may have first understood them as the changing aspect of things in the play of light and shadow, shifting with the movements of the sun. As the world in the aspect of shadows, yin evoked darkness, cold, moisture; that which is hidden, latent or passive; the moon, night and the feminine. Yang symbolized brightness, the sun, fire, warmth, activity and the masculine principle. By analogy yin and yang regulated the

4. Sivin 1995a: 5–37.

Zang Organ System 臟	Yin/Yang Configuration 陰陽	Five Phases 五行	Channel 經絡	Cardinal Direction 方	Seasons 時	Color 色	Planet 星	Government 部	Taste 味	Smell 臭	Emotion 志	Sense Organ 官	Secretion 液
Liver 肝	yang within yin (lesser yang)	wood 木	zujueyin 足厥陰	east 東	spring 春	green 青	Jupiter 太歲	General 將軍	sour 酸	sour/sweaty 臊	anger 怒	eyes 目	tears 淚
Heart 心	yang within yang (greater yang)	fire 火	shoushaoyin 手少陰	south 南	summer 夏	red 紅	Mars 熒惑	Lord 君主	bitter 苦	scorched/burnt 焦	joy 喜	tongue 舌	sweat 汗
Spleen 脾	"arriving at yin," or equilibrium	earth 土	zutaiyin 足太陰	center 中		yellow 黄	Saturn 鎮星		sweet 甘	aromatic 香	worry 思	lips 唇	ordinary saliva 涎
Lung 肺	yin within yang (lesser yin)	metal 銀	shoutaiyin 手太陰	west 西	autumn 秋	white 白	Venus 太白星	Prime Minister 相傅	pungent 辛	rank 腥	sorrow 憂	nose 鼻	nasal mucus 涕
Kidney 腎	yin within yang (greater yin)	water 水	zushaoyin 足少陰	north 北	winter 冬	black 黑	Mercury 辰		salty 鹹	rotten 腐	fear 恐	ears 耳	saliva produced at base of tongue 唾

Figure 1. Symbolic correlations and the Yellow Emperor's body. Adapted from Needham 1962: 262–63, and Porkert 1974: 117–46.

movement of bodily *qi*, and thus the path, momentum and direction of both normal and pathological change in the body. They also ordered the qualitative oppositions of the body into masculine and feminine aspects, and into its spatial divisions of upper and lower, inner and outer regions, extending to its somatic attributes of heat or cold, moisture or dryness.

In Han cosmology other patterns of change in the natural world were grouped according to Five Phases (*wu xing*) identified with Wood, Fire, Earth, Metal, and Water. These Five Phases, here named in cosmogonic order, or sequence of production, also could be imagined as adversaries overcoming one another in different sequences of change. These phases were associated with fundamental material phenomena, somewhat like the four elements of ancient Greek thought, but always understood dynamically rather than as material substance alone. Applied to the human body, Five Phase theory explained the dynamic relationships and bodily affinities of five basic systems of visceral function (*zang*), loosely associated with Liver, Heart, Spleen, Lung and Kidney. Stressing function over anatomical structure, however, the *Inner Canon* imagined these systems in a political metaphor as a working bureaucracy in which "somatic posts" are charged like officials with certain duties, each responsible for a sphere of activity.[5] By adopting cosmological theory, the makers of the *Inner Canon* helped naturalize it as a fundamental belief system, not only incorporated into the cosmos at large and into the imperial body politic but also explaining a natural human body that experienced health and disease according to time and circumstances that the larger patterns rendered intelligible.[6]

5. The phrase is from Sivin 1995a: 12. Although the same Chinese terms are used today for biomedical organs, writers in English use capital letters to remind readers that in TCM they designate functional systems only vaguely connected to anatomical structures. Thus Liver has the function of Blood storage; Heart regulates the movement of Blood and governs consciousness; Spleen stores and regulates energy from food; Lung regulates the *qi* of breath and also keeps internal and external energy in proper channels, guiding the pathways along which inner circulation streams flow (*ying*), and the energy field defending the body's surface boundaries (*wei*); Kidney governs reproductive function and the stores of primordial *qi* (*yuan qi*), the original source of life. General introduction to the medical body may be found in Sivin 1987 and Porkert 1974.

6. See Sivin 1995a. For correlative cosmology itself, see Needham 1962: 232–91. Needham's is still the most eloquent appreciation of this cosmology as an organicist philosophy of Nature wherein, by contrast with Greek notions of linear causality, the universe of things is systematized into "a pattern of structure by which all the mutual influences of its parts were conditioned," taking up their place in a "field of

A second important repository of cosmological thinking in early imperial China was the *Book of Changes* (*Yijing*) — one of the Confucian "five classics" of antiquity, especially as it was explicated by Han dynasty philosophers in a series of appendices collectively known as the *Ten Wings* (*Shi yi*). Cryptic and haunting as befits its archaic origins in divination and omen, the *Book of Changes* weaves its web of enchantment out of the formal aesthetic of numbers: its symbols were based on a binary code of broken and unbroken lines grouped into eight trigrams (three lines each) and expanded into sixty-four hexagrams (all possible combinations of six lines each). But this abstract mathematical code was read as images (*xiang*): metonymic emblems of change in a world of action and movement, capable of evoking the abstractions of formal time — diurnal and lunar cycles, calendars of earthly or heavenly events — and also of figuring human situations in all their circumstance and contingency. The *Book of Changes'* deepest meanings pointed beyond phenomena to a hidden, even numinous revelation, and it generated its own particularly untrammelled form of correlative cosmology. However, interpreters of the *Changes* also understood yin and yang as basic organizing categories — known through the relationship of unbroken lines (yang and odd numbers) to broken ones (yin and even numbers). Further correlations related the eight trigrams to the Five Phases as well. Moreover, the *Changes* related macrocosm to microcosm through bodily images of sexual generation as cosmogenesis and of the universe as a family. The first eight basic hexagrams, constituting the universe as a whole, were given the roles of father, mother, sons and daughters (three of each), mapping biological kinship onto cosmography. Although the trigrams and hexagrams of the *Book of Changes* played no part in the texts of the *Inner Canon* itself, their symbolic repertory was used to talk about the body by medieval alchemists and Song dynasty metaphysicians alike, and so passed into medical language. Song (960–1279) and later medical authorities turned to its symbols for correlations of yin yang and temporal relationships, including figurations of the generative body of fertility and longevity.[7]

---

force alongside other particles similarly responsive" (285). Needham called this a "Whiteheadian" universe of patterned resonances, "reticular and hierarchically fluctuating, not particulate and singly catenarian" (289). He suggests that such a viewpoint might have more affinity with what he calls the decentralized "endocrine orchestra" of mammalian functioning than does the Newtonian mechanical model of causation. Schwartz 1985 provides a revisionist account of correlative cosmology, correcting Needham's neglect of religious and socio-political aspects. See 350–82.

7. For the *Book of Changes* and the body, see Fung Yu-lan 1952.1: 382–95; and Needham 1962: 304–40 passim. For medicine and the *Changes*, see Wang Dapeng

The Yellow Emperor's body must be looked at first as derived from this ancient cosmological system. This is not to contrast it with the seemingly more reliable modern body of bioscience. I have already talked about how all bodies, ancient and modern, are haunted by the languages of culture through which they are known, and must in a sense be prisoners of discourse. My point is rather like the one Thomas Laqueur made in contrasting the "two-sex world" of modern biology and the "one-sex world" of medieval and early modern European natural philosophy.[8] The latter's Galenic body of humors and fluxes was understood in the context of a "metaphysics of hierarchy" that ordained a Great Chain of Being ordering nature and society. If the Galenic body fitted into a system of neo-Platonic forms, its epistemological status was not radically unlike that of the Yellow Emperor's body, which was known in the patterns of correlative cosmology relating Heaven, Earth and Humanity in harmonious hierarchy. Both were truthful as a system of signs among others that allowed people to order the universe as meaningful. These signs were neither relevant to the body alone nor were they excluded from it.

Furthermore, such ancient bodies were not merely metaphysical or speculative. If systems of correlative correspondences are always overdetermined, providing an excess of possibilities for interpretation, people all the more easily could relate the universe of signs to what was seen, heard, felt or practiced in their daily lives. Chinese and Galenic philosophers of nature were both practitioners of Levi-Strauss's "science of the concrete," while their cosmologies, like today's sciences, were valued because they appeared as guides to how things work. That is, the gender relations I am going to talk about next were naturalized in the body because people experienced them in their social lives and saw them in the patterns ordering the cosmos at large. The body in turn spoke truths that then were mirrored in the world.

Gender Difference
and the Yellow Emperor's Body

Modern bioscience lies on our side of an epistemological gulf which today marks the naked body as a natural organism as the

---

1981 and Miu Junchuan 1981. Farquhar 1996 describes how a contemporary TCM doctor uses *Changes* symbolism in clinical reasoning.

8. Laqueur 1990: 26–62.

primary source of authority about its own human nature. The biological essentialism that results from this view has profoundly shaped the conceptual basis for sex as we now understand it. In this process scientists are vested with the authority that used to belong to philosophers, priests and kings. Thomas Laqueur is the most influential interpreter of the early modern shifts in the European imagination of the body whereby "an anatomy and physiology of incommensurability replaced a metaphysics of hierarchy in the representation of woman in relation to man."[9] Laqueur uses Renaissance anatomy to argue that before the Enlightenment and scientific revolutions gender ideology was embedded in a "one-sex" body. Here the male body was taken as the ideal human norm and the female was explained as a variant, either a less perfect version, following Aristotle, or an anatomically homologous variant, as Galenic science taught. Based on his account, three typologies of bodily gender can be found. The first is identity: that is, male and female are variants of a single human body. The second, homology, is closely related to the first: the two sexes have structurally or functionally equivalent or matching bodies. The third model is the modern biological one of difference: male and female bodies are qualitatively dissimilar. Feminist readings of the modern "two-sex" model discussed by Laqueur stress the subtextual imputation of female inferiority wherever bodily gender difference is found. I start my search for gender difference in the Yellow Emperor's body by asking whether it fits any of these alternatives or is illuminated by contrast with them.

At first glance, generalizations about the maladies of women in all historical periods appear to tell a familiar story about "difference." "The disorders of women are ten times more difficult to cure than those of males," went the proverb attributed to the "sage of medicine," Sun Simiao (581–682), who compiled an encyclopedia of pharmacy that set the clinical standard in the literate tradition between the Tang and Song dynasties.[10] In the Song period physicians said—using their favored medical idiom, political action—"In women, Blood is the leader" (*Furen yi xue wei zhu*). Such aphorisms, repeated endlessly through the centuries, suggest at first a stereotype of women as "the sickly sex" reminiscent of the "sick woman of the upper classes" of North Atlantic societies in the Victorian era.[11] But an examination of what the Chinese medical

---

9. Laqueur 1990: 6.
10. Sun Simiao, *Beiji qianjin yaofang,* juan 2, 14.
11. English and English 1978.

classics had to say about bodies in sickness and in health requires us to consider the Chinese model of bodily gender difference in another light. The search for gender in classical Chinese medicine must first follow the multiple significances that are given to yin and yang as organizing principles of the heuristic Yellow Emperor's body.

Ordinary Chinese language has always had terms for male (*nan*) and female (*nü*) that name a category presumed to be natural, independent of gendered kinship roles or cultural baggage of the sort implicit in the common word for "woman" (*fu*, literally a married woman). However, following the *Book of Changes*, doctors liked to pair these with the first two foundational hexagrams, *qian* and *kun*. *Qian* and *kun* spoke of cosmogenesis through the metaphor of the coital couple and evoked yin and yang as male and female generative principals; *qian* and *kun* also spoke of the father and mother as microcosmic embodiments of the truth—in the words of the neo-Confucian philosopher—that Heaven and Earth are one family. Here is homologous gender in the body, not as similar anatomical structures mapped on one another but as matching and interdependent functional processes, patterned like the synchronized movements of dancers in a duet.

However, this is only the beginning of the story of yin and yang in the Yellow Emperor's body. It was through yin and yang that gender could be seen as an attribute of nature itself within the body and without, and by association the qualities of myriad natural phenomena could be linked to gendered meanings. Yet yin and yang were highly multivalent concepts, logical and relational as well as qualitative and metaphorical. When referring to the momentum and direction of change and transmutation, yin and yang explained the workings of time; when structuring a binary of complementarity or of hierarchy, they established relations of equality or inequality. When doctors spoke about formal relationships at work in dynamic body processes, this logical and relational language had any number of points of reference.

Body functions were ordered in yin yang pairs at greater or lesser levels of generality. Some yin yang binaries established relationships as complementary opposites organizing temporal process where change is defined as the movement from one pole to another. In the movement from night to day or from summer to winter, for example, yin and yang forces are matched evenly over the long run, and the rise of one is balanced by the decline of the other. Since the moment of apogee, say high noon, is also the turning point which leads to the reversal of direction (here toward night), latent aspects of a phase were considered as "yin within yang" or "yang within yin." As Judith Farquhar has shown in her study of contemporary TCM, in this sense yin and yang operate to identify the path, momentum and direction of both normal and pathological change in the body.[12]

The second type of relationship orders yin and yang in a hierarchy, and here change is a matter of encompassment or generation—the embrace of the lower into the higher, or the generation of the second from the first. In the microcosm of the body, as in the universe, *qi* named the original, primordial sources of life energy, but *qi* also was differentiated as the yang aspect of discrete functional vitalities. Paired with Blood or with Essence, *qi* was the yang aspect of such a hierarchical yin yang binary. Both models of the relationship of yin and yang—the hierarchical and encompassing, and the complementary and equivalent—had a place in medical discourse.

A pattern of yin and yang as complementary opposites, transforming from one pole to another, underlies the standard account of the basic systems of visceral function (the *zang* and *fu* organ systems) and the flow of *qi* sustaining the living organism. If *qi* circulated as primary vitality through the whole, its energy came to be imagined as flowing along six yin and six yang circulation channels (*jing*) connecting extremities to vital centers. The pulses (*mai*) that are a sensible throbbing near the skin surface were understood as signs of energy flowing at deeper levels. (A seventeenth-century depiction of these channels is illustrated in figures 2a–2n.)[13] Yin and yang identified inner-outer pairs (traceable along the inner and outer surfaces of arms and legs), and also the connections between these channels and the inner organ systems that were also grouped into yin and yang sets. These visceral systems of function are nameable as anatomical organs but understood primarily as functional ensembles. *Zang* functions (involving the five organ systems linked to the Five Phases: Liver, Heart, Spleen, Lung and Kidney) were yin because they were associated with the interior, deeper layers of vital function and with the preservation and nourishment of primary vitalities of *qi* and Blood or *qi* and Essence (see figures 2a–2e). The yang category of *fu* functions—usually identified with stomach, large and small bowels, bladder, and gallbladder—were more eclectic and super-

12. Farquhar 1994.
13. The seventeenth-century illustrations show that by the Ming dynasty, two additional channels, the Superintendent and the Conception, had expanded the total to fourteen.

ficial by comparison. The common explanation for the grouping is that they perform functions of transport and exchange with the outside (see figures 2g–2l).[14] Seen as a whole, the twelve channels and their associated visceral systems organized yin and yang around the symmetries of inner and outer, and the organization of bodies was identical in males and females.

In this body, generative functions of reproduction were the domain of the *zang* functional ensemble of Kidney, identified with Water, the most yin of the Five Phases. Another way of talking about generative vitalities rooted them in a Vital Gate (*ming men*) and Cinnabar Field (*dan tian*) located somewhere beneath the navel in all human beings. The Vital Gate also had an indistinct morphological association with Kidney. Here concentrated primordial aspects of reproductive vitality deeper than visible male or female genitals or functions, and associated with primordial *qi* and life itself. In sum, in the body ordered around the cardinal channel system, the sexual domain was yin for males and females alike. In keeping with this, yin place (*yin chu*) or yin instrument (*yin qi*) were commonplace classical terms for the genitals in both sexes.[15] Medical authorities also sometimes used *yin zhong* for the generative center behind the navel, further affirming the affinities between yin, Kidney, human reproduction and primordial vitality.

In the Yellow Emperor's body, however, vitalities associated with its generative powers circulated along other paths as well. The medical body also possessed a number of "singular channels" (*qi jing*) — singular in that they did not form yin yang pairs. Ancient accounts of the singular channels are contradictory, suggesting eclectic origins; one standard view was that they regulated interior energy flow rather than exchange with the outside. Three of these channels were connected with generative functions. The Superintendent channel (*du mai*) and the Conception channel (*ren mai*) that pass along the dorsal and ventral axes of the

14. In the language of the *Huangdi neijing*, the yin *zang* were "full" but never "replete," suggesting the importance of storing primary vitalities and protecting them against dissipation and loss, while the *fu* systems were "replete" but never "full," suggesting their excretory function (*Su wen* 11.1:37). The standard enumeration of *fu* is of six, not five, organ systems, including the mysterious "triple burners" (*san jiao*) (figure 2j), relic of a little-understood eclectic strand in early medical thought. Further, at some point, a sixth yin channel identified with the "Heart envelope" (figure 2f) was added. By this process, the major organ systems gradually came to be identified with six yin and six yang paired cardinal channels. For details see Sivin 1987: 124–33; and Porkert 1974: 110–11.

15. See *Zhongwen da cidian* 35:386–87,393; *Su wen* 6.1:24, 31.2:92; *Ling shu* 13.6: 316.

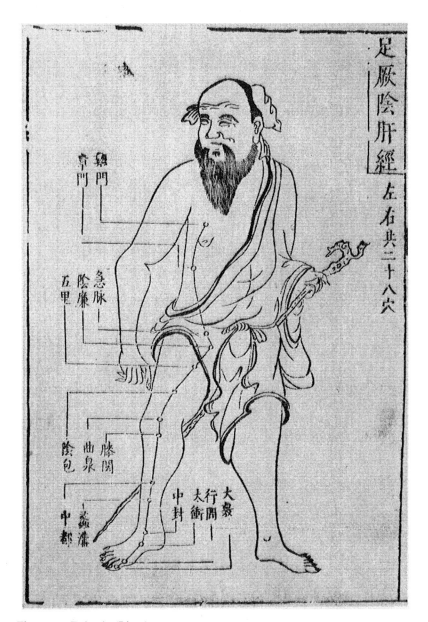

足厥陰肝經

左右共二十八穴

魚門
章門

急脈
陰廉
五里

陰包

膝關
曲泉

中都

中封
行間
太衝
大敦

Figure 2a. *Zujueyin* (Liver)

Figures 2a–2n. The fourteen cardinal channels of circulation. From *Shanbu yisheng wei lun* (Subtle Discourse on Nurturing Life) by Li Zhongzi, an early seventeenth-century doctor and medical scholar who lived in Shanghai. The originals are from the woodblock edition held in the Gest Library, Princeton University.

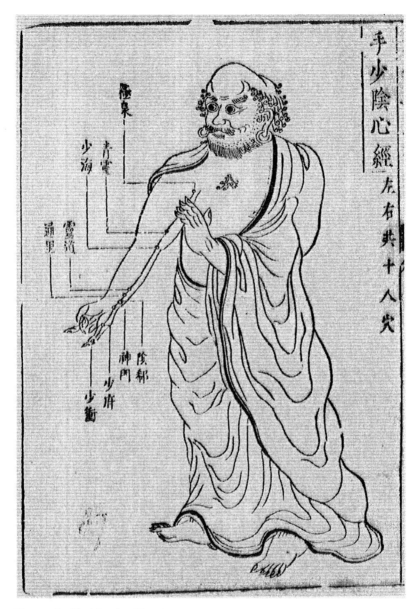

Figure 2b. *Shoushaoyin* (Heart)

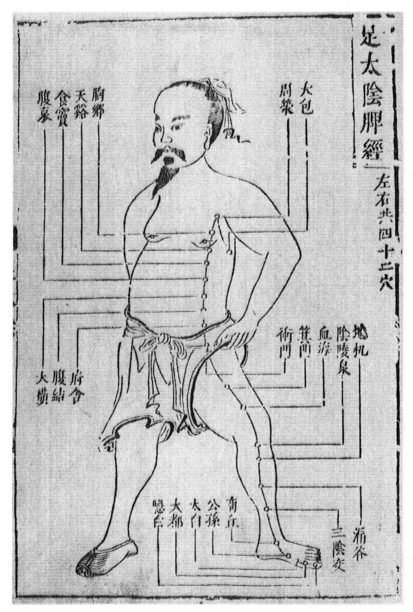

Figure 2c. *Zutaiyin* (Spleen)

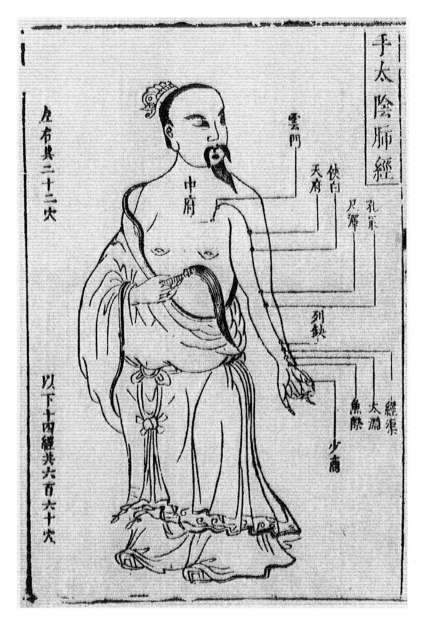

Figure 2d. *Shoutaiyin* (Lung)

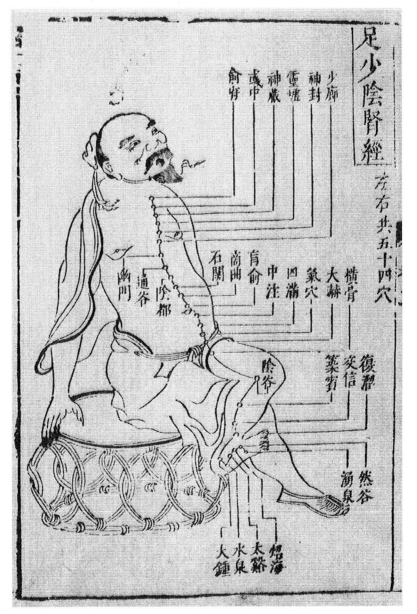

Figure 2e. *Zushaoyin* (Kidney)

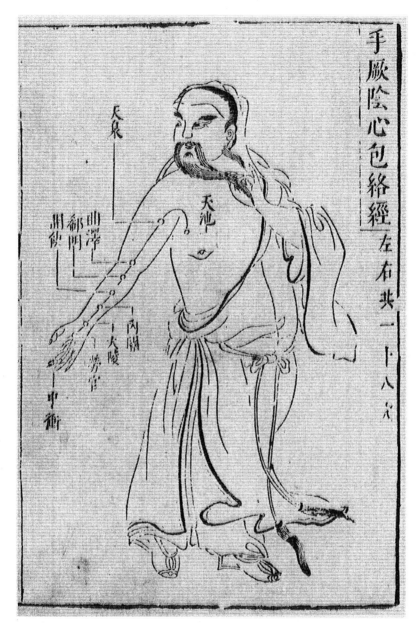

Figure 2f. *Shoujueyin* (Heart Envelope)

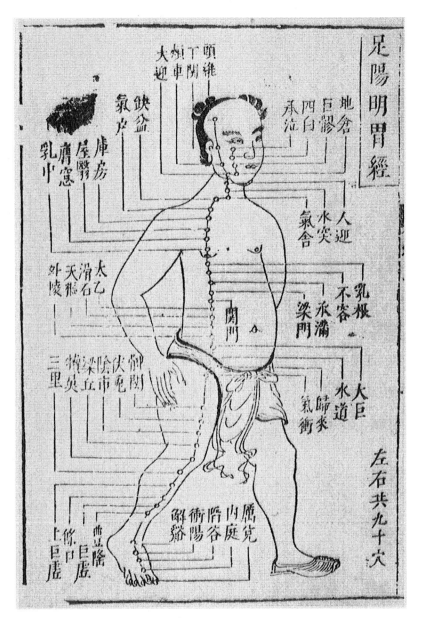

Figure 2g. *Zuyangming* (Stomach)

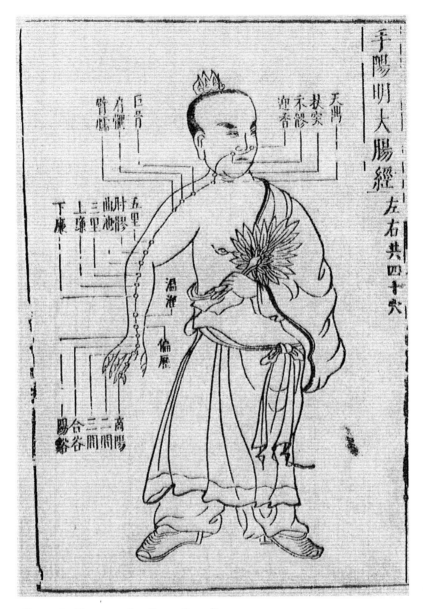

Figure 2h. *Shouyangming* (Large Bowel)

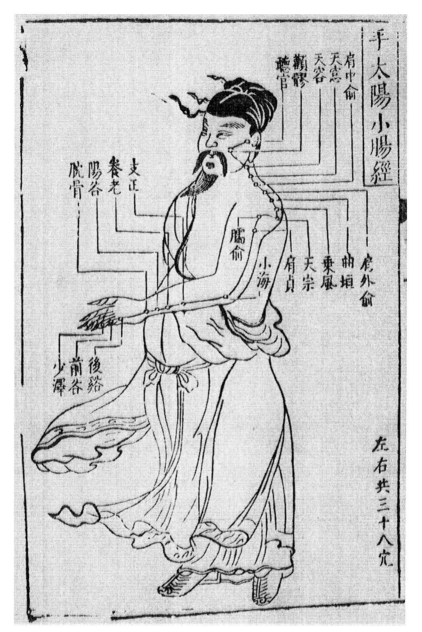

Figure 2i. *Shoutaiyang* (Small Bowel)

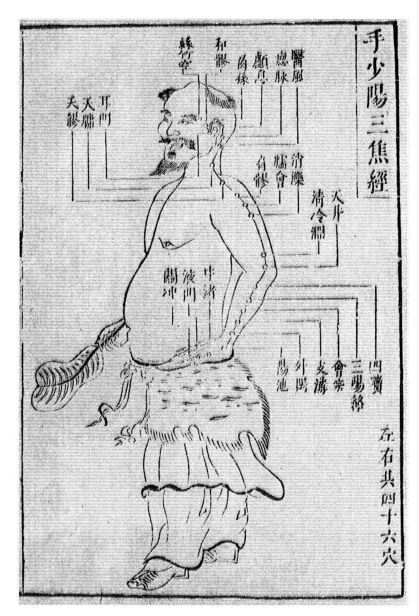

Figure 2j. *Shoushaoyang* (Triple Burners)

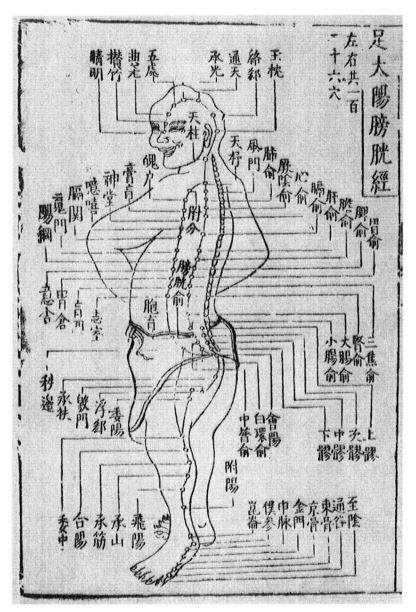

Figure 2k. *Zutaiyang* (Bladder)

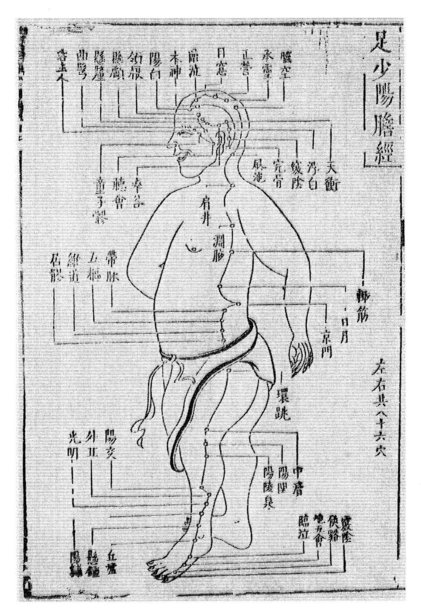

Figure 21. *Zushaoyang* (Gallbladder)

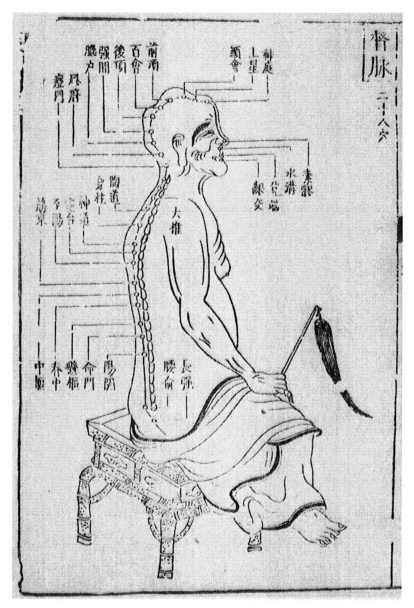

Figure 2m. Superintendent (*du mai*)

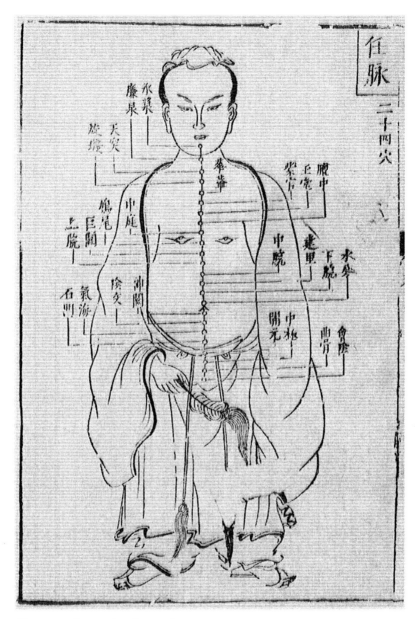

Figure 2n. Conception (*ren mai*)

body respectively, moving from the genital region to the brain and back, were associated with the management of male sexual function and the cultivation of longevity by "returning [seminal] Essence to nourish the brain." On the other hand, when the Conception channel was linked up with the singular Highway channel (*chong mai*) — imagined as an internal central body crossroads — the association was with the functions of reproduction in women, with fertility and fecundity.[16] (See figures 2m and 2n.)

In medical language "Conception" (*ren*) was often understood as a homophone for "pregnant" (*ren*). Nonetheless, the womb (*bao*) itself played no significant role in the system of body organization.[17] Functionally passive and insignificant in comparison with the *zang* or *fu* functional ensembles linked to cardinal circulation channels, "womb" as organ was not associated with the Kidney system and not central to the medical representation of reproduction. Rather than synecdochally signifying "woman," the womb was one of a number of supplementary leftover parts fitted into a scheme of bodily organization whose main thrust is in describing vital process, not visible form or anatomical structure.

Here female difference based on the womb as anatomy was reduced to an irrelevancy. The Conception channel connected the generative centers around the navel in all bodies, and pathologies associated with the Highway channel — tumors, internal growths, hernias, and swellings of the genitals and lower abdominal cavity — afflicted both males and females. Still, some singular channel functions hinted at sexual dimorphism in the energy pathways used in generative function by males and females respectively. In later medical thought the Conception and Superintendent channels were added to the twelve cardinal tracts as a pair, for a total of fourteen (see figures 2m and 2n). They were understood as playing a central role in the bodily cultivation of longevity, a predominantly masculine enterprise. The Highway channel remained singular, coupled with the Conception channel when the subject was female gestational functions.

16. The *Ling shu* said, "The Highway channel and the Conception channel both arise in the womb, ascending within the back to make the sea of *jingluo* [crossroads of yin energies somewhere in the center of the trunk]." *Ling shu* 65.2.1:435. The history of interpretation of the "singular tracts" is convoluted. The *Canon of Problems* said they function to channel energy overflows (Unschuld 1986: 322), but later commentators preferred to think of them as integrative interior circuits.

17. Beyond noting its affinity with the *qi* of Earth, the *Inner Canon* had little to say about the womb. See *Su wen* 11.1:37.

With this as background we can turn to the *Inner Canon*'s classic account of the sexual growth and development of boys and girls. They are portrayed as the work of a single human body of dynamically inter-penetrating yin yang vitalities. At the same time male and female are homologous partners in generative function; their complementarity as a yin yang pair is evoked through the convention of correlative cos-mology that odd numbers are yang in resonance and even numbers are yin. In this way the two sexes develop parallel and equivalent bodies and capacities:

> At seven years of age [*sui*][18] a girl's Kidney *qi* is flourishing; her adult teeth come in and her hair grows long. At fourteen she comes into her reproductive capacities [*tiangui zhi*]; her Conception pulse moves and her Highway pulse is abundant; her menses flow regularly and she can bear young. At twenty-one her Kidney *qi* is stabilized, and so her wisdom teeth come in and her growth has reached its apogee. . . . At eight [*sui*] a boy's Kidney *qi* is replete; his adult teeth come in and his hair grows long. At sixteen his Kidney *qi* is abundant, and he comes into his repro-ductive capacities [*tiangui zhi*]; his seminal essence overflows and drains; he can unite yin and yang and so beget young. At twenty-four his Kidney *qi* is stabilized and so his bones and sinews are strong, his wisdom teeth come in and his growth has reached an apogee.[19]

The text of the *Inner Canon* here integrates channel energy flows and functional organ systems. The combined Highway and Conception channels are seen in their governance of female fertility and fecundity, but the master system remains the Kidney, seat of primary life vitalities shaping the generative powers of both sexes. Accordingly, in the human body of medical imagination, changes in teeth and hair mark the devel-opmental curve of sexual life, and so they also are governed by the Kid-ney system. With age "Kidney *qi* weakens, hair falls out and teeth wither." Here the most important secondary sexual characteristics are not (like beard and breast) gendered anatomical features, evoking erotic dimorphisms of the flesh. Rather they locate both male and female bod-ies in time, marking off the years of reproductive capabilities from im-maturity on the one hand or old age on the other. What moderns would understand as menopause is identified in the same way as menarche, simply as an event in the life passage, similar in character if not in timing

18. Age in *sui* was computed from the time of conception and normally recorded with each new year, making a person's numerical age in *sui* one year older on average than a modern calendar would calculate it.

19. *Su wen* 1.3:8–9.

for males and females alike. Just as females cease to menstruate, males' semen becomes scanty, and the ills associated with this are not particular to a pathology of the climacteric but are part and parcel of the ungendered feebleness of old age.[20]

The *Inner Canon*'s classic account of the sexual body followed a rhetorical strategy that was repeated through the ages: the formal relationship of yin and yang itself (here expressed in symbolic numbers) was assumed to explain the relationship of the sexes in a satisfactory way. Gender homology evoked the ideal complementarity of male and female as a potentially fertile pair. Throughout, the most important signifiers of bodily gender remained yin and yang. These interpenetrate in all bodies, and all bodies are microcosmic, resonating with the yin yang rhythms of Heaven and Earth manifest in the cycles of nature.

We have left the categories introduced by Thomas Laqueur behind. Unlike the Galenic human "one sex" patterned on a male norm, the Yellow Emperor's human body is more truly androgynous, balancing yin and yang functions in everyone. Moreover, the very term "sex," which in Laqueur's analysis names a physical difference between males and females interpreted through the lens of gender ideology, appears a misnomer. Except possibly for the hint of sexual dimorphism in the functioning of the singular channels discussed above, the Yellow Emperor's body has no morphological sex, but only gender. Yin and yang do not get their meaning because they are attributes of something else, in bodies or in nature. Rather than labelling a gender which is defined on other grounds, yin and yang are the foundations on which the language of gender rests. In the language of literary theory, yin and yang are the signified, not the signifiers.

What happens within the androgynous body when we find yin and yang in relationships that are hierarchical and encompassing? Such a

---

20. The modern construction of "menopause" (*gengnian qi*) that is read back into TCM by today's practitioners is in fact a product of nineteenth-century bioscience transported to Asia. The term came into use as a medical syndrome specific to women with the modern spread of scientific medicine. See Lock 1993: "The Making of Menopause," 303–30. Earlier humoral practitioners in Europe imagined the "climacteric" as a moment of critical transition in the life cycle of men and women alike, often associated with numerical and other versions of "the [seven] ages of man." These earlier views were much closer to the spirit of the Chinese *tiangui*. Though *tiangui* today is translated as "puberty," the classical Chinese term, based on an allusion in the *Huainanzi*, called attention to the Heavenly North, source of the Water of creation in cosmography. These generative waters of the body were conventionally believed to be exhausted in women at age forty-nine (seven times seven) and in men at sixty-four (eight times eight).

pattern emerges when we look at yin and yang manifest in the paired primary body vitalities like Blood (*xue*) and *qi*.[21] As one of the most important of these pairs, Blood and *qi* referred to underlying bodily vitality and not to any particular function. In this sense Blood is the yin aspect of *qi*. The *Inner Canon* linked gender with yin and yang, Blood and *qi*, in this way: "Heaven and Earth establish the pattern of above and below for all things. Yin and yang pattern [the functions of] Blood and *qi* in males and females. Left and right form the path that yin and yang follow [i.e., the sun's path from east to west];[22] Water and Fire are yin and yang's visible manifestations; by yin and yang all things can come into being."[23]

As a yin yang pair flowing along the circulation channels, Blood and *qi* have a special relationship to generation, and hierarchies of gender are a part of this. In terms of the basic cosmology outlined in the *Book of Changes*, Blood is receptive (*kun*). In thinking of body functions, the medical men put it that "Blood follows *qi*." Unlike *qi*, Blood is always paired and cannot operate independently. By contrast, "unitary *qi*" (*yi qi*) transcends yin and yang, standing alone at the apex of the cosmic hierarchy and coming first in the temporal sequence of cosmogenesis.

Another hierarchical yin yang relationship is the pair Essence and Blood (*jing xue*). This is also an aspect of life energy in the functioning organism, but where the buried metaphor in Blood and *qi* could evoke the assimilation of food and the respiration of air as well as generative functions, the coupling of Essence and Blood suggests at the lower level the sexual powers of the body, and at the higher level these as an aspect of generative vitalities and primordial *qi*. At their most material, Essence and Blood name the male and female contributions to the creation of a child. Here Essence is semen, and Blood identifies the

---

21. *Xue* and *qi* was a very old binary referring to the animal powers of the body. Confucius had said, "In youth, before his Blood and *qi* are stable, the gentleman must guard against lust. . . . In old age, when Blood and *qi* are decayed, he must guard against greed" (*Analects* 16.7). In classical times, and in the *Huangdi neijing* accordingly, the preferred terminological order was to name Blood first, as befit a yin yang pair. Since Blood as a primary vitality in the Blood-*qi* pair is not reducible to blood as a body fluid, the word is capitalized in English.

22. I believe this directional logic derived from the placement of bodies of power in archaic ritual: the ruler, facing south, has the yang force of the rising sun on his left, and the yin setting sun on his right. Accordingly, the right (yin) side of the body had affinities for females, and vice versa for males.

23. *Su wen* 5.3:21.

woman's contribution to reproduction as a unity underlying all manifest forms of female reproductive fluid: menses or breast milk or the blood nourishing the gestating fetus.

At the next higher level, both seminal Essence and menstrual Blood are grouped together as "yin Blood" (*yin xue*), that is, common generative fluids paired with their *qi* aspect, Essence. In this sense, male seminal Essence (*jing*) is also yin, a specific form of a more general and primary yin, Blood. But at this higher level all sexual fluids and the specific vitalities underlying them are yin, encompassed by Essence as their yang aspect. At a third, even higher level, the pair Essence and Blood, which is yang in relation to sexual fluids, becomes yin when collectively named Essence in the dyad Essence and (*jing qi*). This latter, at the apex of the yin yang hierarchy, names the creative energy governing the critical moments of growth and coming-into-being when the transition takes place from yin poles to yang ones, and vice versa. (See figure 3.)

In sum, in the Yellow Emperor's body, the sexual functions of Blood and Essence are nested in a hierarchy of yin yang pairs where yin is encompassed by yang. In the medical body yin and yang alone might function as complementary opposites enabling the direction and momentum of bodily changes. But as generative vitalities, Blood, Essence and *qi* form hierarchical and encompassing yin yang relationships. Blood as yin and feminine may participate in a yang dyad of a higher order, but the principle of hierarchical ordering by encompassment always results in a genderized code of symbolic relationships: Blood is encompassed by Essence and Essence-as-Blood is encompassed by Essence-as-*qi*. Just so is Earth encompassed by Heaven and woman by man. From one aspect male and female bodies are identical or homologous and gender difference is a relativistic and flexible aspect of the body. From another aspect the bodily powers associated with sexuality and generation participate in the gendered hierarchical ordering of the human microcosm and the macrocosm of Heaven and Earth.

Yin Yang and Gender in Clinical Reasoning

Yin yang relationships as a basis for the gendered body organized many aspects of therapeutic practice. The notion that the bodies of males and females are homologous along a shifting continuum of mixed and interpenetrating substances and energies means that there are

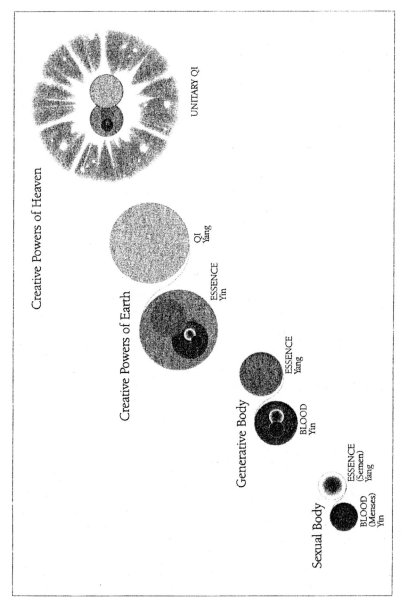

Creative Powers of Heaven

UNITARY QI

Creative Powers of Earth

QI
Yang

ESSENCE
Yin

Generative Body

ESSENCE
Yang

BLOOD
Yin

Sexual Body

ESSENCE
(Semen)
Yang

BLOOD
(Menses)
Yin

Figure 3. Yin yang hierarchy in the Yellow Emperor's body

multiple possible configurations of yin and yang within the body that might vary in individuals according to time and circumstance. Nonetheless, even as each individual body is ideally configured as balanced evenly between yin and yang forces, this balance is not stable, and the normal probability is that most males will tilt toward a preponderance of yang qualities, while in females an affinity for yin ones will prevail. Thus yin and yang come to name masculine or feminine aspects of bodily nature over a range of proportions that vary according to the individual. The proportion might be imagined quantitatively as a ratio, or imagined as a quality, like a color of varying intensities.

This logic is revealed in two canonical teachings on clinical practice: that of the *Canon of Problems* and the *Canon of the Pulse* (*Maijing*) on pulse differences in males and in females, and the teachings of the Tang medical master Sun Simiao on "separate prescriptions" for women. First, gender was presumed to influence the movement of energy along the cardinal channels as detected when a healer took his patient's pulse. A well-trained physician would be expected to read the pulse by pressing at varying depths on three separate locations on each arm and wrist, and to identify two dozen or even more distinct types of energy flow along the channels beneath the skin. Supporting theory linked different pulses to yin yang types, to the five *zang* organ systems, and to the major cardinal channel networks, and all this allowed for a sophisticated diagnostic repertory. In reading the pulse physicians were taught to consider sex (along with age, constitution and other bodily variations) in determining what kind of pulse variations might be considered normal.[24] The *Canon of Problems* went further, saying that patterns normal in one sex are pathological in the other.

> Pulse movements may be compliant or adverse [in direction]; in males and females they may be normal or abnormal. . . . Thus a male's pulse is stronger above the gate [on the upper wrist] and a female's pulse is stronger below the gate [on the lower wrist]. Thus in males the pulse is normally weaker in the foot section and in females it is normally fuller in the foot section. . . . When males display a female pulse it is a sign of deficiency disorder within; when females display a male pulse it is a sign of a disorder of excess in the extremities.[25]

24. *Maijing,* juan 1, in ZGYXDC 1:596: "The pulses of woman are normally inclined to be softer and weaker than those of males; in males a 'big' pulse on the left hand is as it should be; in females a 'big' pulse on the right hand is as it should be."

25. *Nanjing,* Unschuld text and translation, 259. I have altered his translation somewhat. See also Ma Dazheng 1991: 44.

Here the bodies of males and females had affinities for yin yang spatial relationships, and the pulse that did not match the sufferer's gender was deemed pathological.[26] Although not all yin pulses were gendered female, the specifically female pulse pattern was a yin one, and doctors normally were expected to know their patients' sex by pulse alone.

As with diagnosis, so with prescriptions and therapy. The subtlest of the physician's healing arts was the compounding of customized prescriptions built up out of a dozen or more individual materia medica. The goal here was the careful balancing of dominant and secondary ingredients and the matching of types of drug action and "flavors" (classified according to the Five Phases) with the sufferer's pathology. Rather than aiming at standard formulas for taxonomically distinct diseases, classically trained physicians prided themselves upon adjusting any prescription to the characteristics of the sick person as an individual and to illness as an ongoing process apprehended at a specific moment in time. In this light Sun Simiao's words "for women, there are separate prescriptions [from those appropriate for men]" might be read in alternate ways. The narrowest interpretation called attention to drug therapies for the gestational conditions unique to women in Sun's own medical thought — menstruation, pregnancy, delivery and postpartum illness. But broader readings justified the more extensive gynecological pharmacology found in actual works of medicine for women (*fuke*) of later periods of history. Eminent physicians could and did debate just when the rule for "separate prescriptions" should be invoked. The adjustment of a prescription to accommodate a female condition could apply to some but not all illnesses, or to some but not all individual females. It is easiest to see when medical texts identify an illness as gynecological; when other variables affect an individual case, it is more difficult to discern habits of adjusting the prescription to gender. In the prescription art, feminine yin qualities emerge as a variable along a continuum of persons, not as an absolute that divides medical bodies into two types.

How this might affect people's understanding of appropriate medication can be seen in an episode from a well-known classical novel, the eighteenth-century *Dream of the Red Chamber*. Everyone familiar with this novel knows the episode where the young hero, Baoyu, rejects a doctor's remedy for his maid, Shiwen; he says the doctor is prescribing as if she were male. By eighteenth-century standards, the doctor is using

26. See Ma Dazheng 1991: 44. For a Qing view see Lin Zhihan 1723: 98.

an old-fashioned approach to his client's commonplace Cold Damage fever (*shanghan* — designating a wide variety of acute infections). He includes "bitter orange" (*zhishi*) and "ephedra" (*mahuang*), which act powerfully on *qi* to purge and sweat. This will attack a delicate girl's yin fluids, and here the remedy is considered too strong for the adolescent female constitution. On the other hand, the anecdote shows that judgments about appropriate formulas are a matter of degree: Baoyu notes that bitter orange and ephedra are also too strong for himself — and this is one of the ways the author points up Baoyu's "feminine" qualities as an individual. In sum, the complementary logic of yin yang relationships will call for a balancing of these qualities in drug action adjusted to the corresponding configuration in each individual illness situation.

In sum, in everyday diagnostic and therapeutic situations, doctors considered the actual balance of yin and yang in a person's functioning, and health could be disturbed by excess or deficiency of either yin or yang. In any individual, whether male or female, the imbalances that so often tinged male bodies with disproportionate yang heat or female ones with intensified yin cold were in fact potential vulnerabilities, departures from the androgynous ideal of health. At the same time, at a more general level of medical reasoning, healthy males and females, when seen as a fertile couple, formed the matching yin yang opposites of homologous gender.

Gender Norms and Gender Boundaries

Unlike the "one-sex" model of classical European medicine, the body of classical Chinese medical imagination appears as genuinely androgynous. Yin and yang name the "feminine" and "masculine" as aspects of all bodies and of the cosmos at large. Such a logic would suggest room for variation and flexibility at the boundaries of gender. Sexual anomaly, though on the margins of discourse, revealingly constructs the normal, and medical writings on the subject show where the ideal of a naturally androgynous body of yin and yang was revealed to be in tension with the values of a strictly gendered social hierarchy. A particularly good example of this tension is found in a treatise attributed to a court physician of the fifth century C.E.: *Bequeathed Writings of Master Chu* (*Chu shi yi shu*). Beginning in the Song era Chu Cheng (fl. 423) was seen as a leading ancient authority on successful reproduction and what moderns might call eugenics.[27] This text is rich in pulse lore elaborating the homologous patterns of yin yang gender opposition: "The male's yang pulse movement follows an ascending path in compliance [with cosmic direction], so that the nadir [of the cycle of circulation in the body] and the Vital Gate [are felt] at the foot position of the right hand. . . . The female's yin pulse movement follows a descending path against the direction [of cosmic influences], so that the nadir and the Gate of Life [are felt] at the inch position of the left hand."

The pulse detected here at the Gate of Life reveals the condition of primordial *qi* and generative vitality; the reversal of movement, according to Master Chu, explains the protean eroticism of a hermaphrodite in whom yin and yang are "evenly balanced" and who is capable of male or female sexual roles: In the bodies (*shen*) of those who are "neither male nor female [*fei nan fei nü*], when influenced/stirred by a woman the male pulse beats in response; and when stimulated by a man, the female pulse is felt responding in compliance." Accounts of spontaneous changes of sex in humans and animals, cited as omens in historical annals of every dynasty, were seen by Chu and other medical authorities as remarkable but by no means outside the possible transformations of yin and yang. The transgressor of gender boundaries is a changeling, celebrated as uncanny evidence of the cosmos' creative powers of transformation.

However, the androgyny of the changeling, though subtly scripted around active or passive erotic roles,[28] was not a basis for any homosexual identity. The renowned Han dynasty physician Guo Yu could not be fooled when the emperor asked him to diagnose a homosexual "favorite" in disguise.

---

27. Chu Cheng was a court physician in the Southern Ji dynasty and was mentioned in its dynastic history. But his writings were unknown and not quoted by physicians before the Song dynasty, when they became popular as authoritative ancient wisdom on the nature of sex differences, conception, fertility, bodily inheritance, and the begetting of sons. The first known printed edition dates from 1201 C.E., with a preface claiming to be dated 936. An early reference to Chu Cheng in a Song medical work is found in the *Taiping sheng hui fang* (juan 63). (I am indebted to Professor Zhao Pushan for bringing this to my attention.) The cloudy history and sexual frankness of this text—it was said to have been carved on metal tablets and buried with its author—made the editors of the eighteenth-century encyclopedia *Siku quanshu* suggest that it might be a Song forgery. Whatever its original provenance, it found its audience in the Song and was treated as a somewhat controversial classic thereafter. For further discussion see Okanishi Tameto 1948: 507–9.

28. The notion of a sexual script follows Jeffrey Weeks 1986: 57–58.

> As an experiment the emperor ordered a male favorite [*bichen*] with lovely hands and wrists to lie down behind a curtain alongside a girl. He then had [Guo] Yu examine the pulse of one arm from each and asked him to identify the ailment. Yu said, "The left arm is yang and the right arm is yin. A pulse is distinctly male or female. But in this case it is as if there is a difference and your servant is puzzled as to why." The emperor sighed in admiration and praised his skill.[29]

In this tale the emperor appears to entertain the possibility of a third typology of body for some based on their sexual orientation, a possibility which the doctor rejects. Gender boundaries are affirmed without moralizing, and sexual roles alone are not presented as a bodily basis for gender identity.

Rather, it was sexual scripts implicating reproduction that produced the most value-laden accounts of gender boundaries in the body. In the teachings of Master Chu Cheng, classical medicine represented the sexual identity and sexual vigor of offspring as determined at conception by the result of a contest between the yin and yang energies of the mating couple locked in subtle competition for advantage. In coitus when yin is stronger, female offspring result. In considering the socially critical issue of how the sex of offspring is determined, medicine here acknowledged the powers of yin to match yang, but judged these powers negatively. Similarly, Master Chu taught that some kinds of yin yang (un)balance will produce undesirable configurations of bodily gender: "The daughters of a young father and an old mother will die young; a vigorous mother and a feeble father will produce feeble sons." In both these cases, the child is imprinted with the excess or deficiency of the generative vitality of the parent of the same sex rather than moved back toward the center by the opposite and complementary qualities of the parent of the opposite sex. Yin yang qualities emerge as adversarial, locked into a zero-sum game of success or failure, where imbalances of gender in one partner work to the disadvantage of the other.

In the late imperial reproductive context bodies "neither male nor female" were reinterpreted as defective, the products of "disorderly" configurations of yin and yang producing impotence and sterility.

> Normally *qian* and *kun* make fathers and mothers; but there are five kinds of "false males" [*fei nan*] who cannot become fathers and five kinds of "false females" [*fei nü*] who cannot become mothers. Can it indeed be

---

29. From the *Later Han History,* biography of Wang Fu, as excerpted in Chen Bangxian 1982: 61.

the case that defective males are deficient in yang *qi* and defective females have blocked yin *qi*? The false females are the corkscrew, the striped, the drum, the horned, and the pulse. The false males are the natural eunuch, the bullock [castrated], the leaky, the coward and the changeling.[30]

Here not only were some yin yang configurations understood negatively as unbalanced, but a line was drawn between normal and abnormal, not around erotic scripts but around reproductive capability. Thus even though human males were not pure yang and human females not pure yin, anomalies which impaired generative function were transgressive, distorted configurations of yin yang influences, establishing the boundaries of the ideal of normality. However, the catalogue of defects was subtly gendered: false females were sterile ("the pulse" is a woman with highly erratic menses) or physically configured in such a way that sexual penetration is impossible. By contrast, two of the five false males are functionally impotent, not physically marred, and the changeling's protean capabilities are allied with the powers of the male. In sum, when considering the socially critical issue of the reproduction of sons or daughters, classical medicine marked yin and yang as high and low on bodies labeled normal or abnormal and gendered either female or male, in more or less satisfactory replication of an ideal type evaluated according to reproductive capacity.

Deconstructing the Yellow Emperor's Body

The foregoing discussion of anomaly should alert readers to what is partial and incomplete in my narrative so far — to its gaps and fissures. What stands here is a reading of Chinese medicine that privileges the high tradition associated with the earliest texts of the Han to Tang dynasties. Any serious student of early China will know that the *Inner Canon* and associated medical classics are riddled with ambiguities and contradictions which have not been acknowledged here. Like generations of Chinese commentators throughout history, I have mined the

30. The quote here is from Li Shizhen, the great late-sixteenth-century pharmacologist (Li Shizhen 1596, 4:2971–72). Li and others attributed the teachings concerning *fei nan fei nü* to Chu Cheng, but the Ming-Qing editions of Chu I have seen refer only to those who "when moved by a male respond as a female, and when moved by a female respond as a male," that is, to the bisexual performance of the hermaphrodite. According to Ma Dazheng 1991: 208–9, the standard five-type classification began to circulate in printed medical works following the fifteenth-century physician Wan Quan.

historical archives to conjure up a holistic abstraction. Even as I select from those works and passages that were read as canon in late imperial society five hundred to one thousand years after they were written, I have filtered out the cacophonous voices that Ming-Qing Chinese had already forgotten so well that we twentieth-century outsiders can scarcely imagine them. The study of early medicine as it is being reconstructed by scholars today is exposing us to a strange landscape of magical surgeons and artful alchemists, of medical warriors gazing at the entrails of broken bodies on the battlefield, of shaman dancers and ritualists exorcising the demons of disease, and palace servants skilled in the arts of massage or breath control. This rich medical pluralism, with all its eclecticism and experiment, is lost here. I have provisionally assumed the dominance of a mainstream of medical thought, the coherence of a tradition and the possibility of positing a normative "body" handed down from antiquity in unbroken continuity with the past. Foucauldian theories of history as genealogy have made us skeptical of the claims of history to link us reliably to the past through any seamless narrative of continuity. However, I use the abstraction "Yellow Emperor's body" as an introduction here because one must start somewhere. It helps orient us, and it also reminds us that presumptions of continuity and coherence have been everywhere durable as organizing principles because they help order history as knowable. Such holistic patterns of imagining the Chinese medical body were commonplace in late imperial times, as they are today.

Overall, this account of the Yellow Emperor's body has focused upon yin and yang as logical and relational concepts without directly addressing their function as metaphor. When they name patterns of change, its momentum and direction, yin and yang operate as abstract, powerful illuminations of time. But time in human experience evokes characteristic forms of emotional pathos, reminding us that yin and yang are rich evidence for the way human language is saturated in metaphor. A dense matrix of qualities — sensuous and tangible as heat and light, aesthetic and moral as secrets of sexuality — is vital to an exploration of the world of meanings given historical Chinese bodies by the discourses of yin and yang in that culture. Metaphor is not just adornment or ornamentation but an essential aspect of linguistic meaning structures, and the flexibility of words as signs, their protean habit of shifting the ground of reference, derives powerfully from this metaphorical nature of thought. The Yellow Emperor's body can be called androgynous only because yin and yang in bodies have the potential to allude metaphorically to culturally coded gendered qualities bound up in a network of associations. As polysemic categories yin and yang both do and do not evoke any one metaphor to the exclusion of others, making the attributes of gender an ever-present if elusive aspect of their aura, resonances that are sometimes distinct, sometimes diffuse, sometimes hidden, but always potentially in play.

Beyond this, metaphors of generation were consciously and formally incorporated into representations of cosmogenesis in the macrocosm and of the genesis of the family in the microcosm. Gender then was potentially present whenever minds roamed these aspects of either cosmos or social world. From this perspective gender inhered in bodies not by virtue of biological fact but because human beings as embodied manifestations of the microcosm participated in the patterned relationships of Heaven, Earth and Humanity.

Moreover, metaphor also works within discourse beneath the surface to shift implications, to speak what is not said. Gender was potentially present whenever speakers' unacknowledged assumptions broke through the surface of language. The doctor's reflection quoted above on the "false male" and "false female" is just such an instance, where a syntactically ambiguous negative opens space for alternative understandings of gender boundaries. With this in mind, it is clear that I have barely touched the vast rhetorical substratum of gendered meanings that inhere in the medical classics by virtue of what they do not say, and by virtue of the social contexts in which they were produced, transmitted and constituted a cultural nexus. The *Inner Canon*, however subtle and abstract its construction of yin and yang as formal relationships in the microcosm of the body, spoke of people's social understanding of male superiority when its rhetoric imagined the body as a polity and health as kingly. The Yellow Emperor learns from the legendary physician Qibo that the prince becomes a sage as the body attains long life and the state attains good government. Man (*ren*) in the triad Heaven, Earth and Man, as elsewhere in ordinary language, was represented by the word that privileges the male as normative. Master Chu Cheng probably spoke to an audience of aristocratic males seeking heirs, if indeed his work was not the concoction of anonymous scholars several hundred years later who needed a cloak of ancient authority for a discussion of successful procreation and the body that, whatever its origin, addressed the same concerns among upper-class men of the Song.

Finally, the Yellow Emperor lives here in a body of generation, where gestational functions are virtually invisible. The next chapters will take up the history of "medicine for women" (*fuke*) as a recognized division of knowledge and practice, based on highlights of the textual record from the tenth to the seventeenth centuries (from the Song through the Ming dynasties). Cumulatively, this will take readers into deconstructions and reconfigurations of the heuristic Yellow Emperor's body that occurred as successive generations of healers considered the clinical problems of their female clients. In the Song era, medicine developed a holistic gynecology derived from the axiom that in women "Blood is the leader." Here the woman's generative body was seen as weakened by its gestational functions. In the Ming, a discourse on "nourishing life" taught that the male generative body must be guarded against sensual overuse while at the same time maintaining masculine sexual dominance. Throughout, medical men encountering the gestational body entered into a sphere where femaleness was essentialized as unclean. In the clinical setting there was a continual process of adjustment to shifting boundaries of gendered social relations. In sum, in the history of tensions between the spheres of generation and those of gestation, we can see how bodily androgyny was challenged by female difference. The history of *fuke*, then, takes as its point of departure the story of how the language of yin and yang, Blood, *qi* and Essence, imagined gestational bodies in relation to bodies of power and generation, and how metaphors of gender, a necessary part of the harmonic bodily whole, also continually disturbed it.

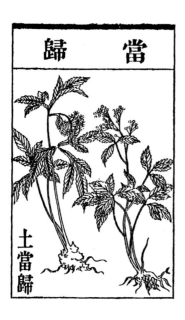

CHAPTER 2

The Development of *Fuke* in the Song Dynasty

Gynecology and Medical Innovation in the Song

All medical traditions have dealt with sick women as well as sick men, but not all have had a gynecology. At its base gynecology deals with medical disorders perceived and designated as gendered: that is, pathologies afflicting women alone, or taking different forms in males and females. For most of us today the concept of "gynecology" is fully laden with the understandings of biomedicine. We think of it in the structural language of anatomy as a specialty dealing with the pathologies of women's reproductive organs, or in the functional language of endocrinology as the science of regulating the female hormone system. The classical Chinese term *fuke*, today translated as "gynecology," has over the centuries designated a changing repertory of therapies for "wives" (a *fu* is a married woman), overlapping with those recommended for "birth" (*chan*, which might be thought of as an "obstetrics," or *chanke*). In the early imperial era this clinical tradition, invisible in the account of the Yellow Emperor's body discussed in the previous chapter, was an eclectic one, incorporating herbal drinks, medicinal pastes and washes, poultices and heat treatments, massage, moxibustion and acupuncture, ritual and diet,[1] transmitted in manuscript traditions independent of midwifery. It developed into a mature system of gynecology in the Song dynasty. Here I am not claiming that Chinese medicine was moving closer to modern gynecology or obstetrics. Rather, Song *fuke* was part of a broader movement of medical innovation that cannot be judged by the standards of bioscience. But the changes involved — in medical institutions and training, in the social position of healers, in the theoretical and clinical understandings of ailment and cure — make it possible for the first time to identify literate experts who were specialists in *fuke* and to identify a body of doctrine that related disorders deemed specific to women to the broader themes in medical discourse. All of medicine was reshaped over the three-hundred-year span of the Song, but the participation of *fuke* in a new learned synthesis, along with a similar incorporation of pediatrics (*erke*), brought hitherto marginal practices into the mainstream.

In the Song the *Inner Canon* and other works became codified as medical classics, and medical authorities aimed for a standard, orthodox model of the Yellow Emperor's body as a basis for clinical reasoning. Innovations in diagnostic method were designed to relate clinical decision-making to this body, and in a parallel process to explain the action of drugs on a level deeper than that of symptom relief. The aphorism "In women Blood is the leader" summarized learned doctors' efforts to apply new doctrines to find the roots of women's illnesses in holistic clinical patterns beneath the surface of ordinary symptoms. Following the Tang master's saying "For women there are separate prescriptions [*bie fang*]," they emphasized pharmacy over other therapies and expanded the repertory of *fuke* to include formulas for a wide variety of diffuse internal illnesses. They medicalized menstruation as a bodily signifier of ideal female normality identified with fertility. They deployed the language of the androgynous body to accentuate the gendered meanings of yin and yang, Blood and *qi*. In the Song dynasty medical thought appeared more concerned with female difference than either earlier or

1. Lee Jen-der 1996, 1997.

later in Chinese history. I contextualize this as reflecting learned doctors' commitment to the problems of maternal and child health under the prodding of a state anxious to make medicine an effective instrument of the imperium's benevolent rule, and under the aegis of a society that was revising its inherited models of kinship and family.

Innovation in medicine during the Song dynasty was not an isolated technological phenomenon. Over a three-hundred-year period, China's upper class was transformed from a small aristocratic elite to a broader one marked by scholarship and office holding, while the imperial monarchy strengthened both autocracy and civilian rule. During the first 150 years (the Northern Song, 960–1125), the institutional and doctrinal reform of medicine was part of an imperial agenda to spread good government by providing for the people's welfare and reforming unorthodox customs. Using the revolutionary technology of printing in medicine as in other domains of knowledge, the state sponsored a profound transformation in the nature of textuality and of literacy as a nexus of knowledge and power.[2] After ceding the north to the "barbarian" Jin invaders from the steppes in 1125, the truncated Southern Song state withdrew somewhat from its earlier imperial activism, but the economy burgeoned, producing unprecedented prosperity some have called China's first "commercial revolution." Buddhism ceased to dominate cultural and religious life, making way for a complex Confucian revival, which was aided institutionally by the growth of competitive examinations for office, and by a movement to reorganize kinship around agnatic lineages. This last particularly affected the lives of upper class women and children, as philosophical reformers turned their attention to the legal, social and ritual organization of domestic life. Both medicine and China's gender system were caught up in these manifold changes.

The official medicine of the preceding Tang dynasty had been based in the imperial capital, and served mainly to provide services to court, officialdom and the army. In the Northern Song, this bureaucracy was expanded and transformed to carry out an ambitious program of medical education, even extending to provincial government branches. State-appointed Song doctors gradually tied the production of medical knowledge more tightly to the learning in approved classical books, hoping to strengthen a literate medical elite and marginalize heterodox popular ritual healers (*wu*). To give practical support to reform, emperors and

2. See Cherniack 1994 and Chia 1996 for the emergence of print culture in the Song.

officials periodically ordered the distribution of free medicines against local epidemics and set up charity pharmacies. This strategy promoted a visible new stratum of learned physicians, distinguishable not only from the shamanistic *wu* but also from Daoist and Buddhist healers.[3]

The imperial state's policies, lubricated by the powerful new technology of printing, went hand in hand with a gradual shift in the social construction of medicine as a calling. From above, medical study and writing became fashionable among "gentleman admirers of medicine" (*shang yi shiren*) who promoted it as a humanitarian skill in the hands of scholars serving their families and society. From below, definitions of acceptable ritual practice shifted to stigmatize the southern *wu*, and even the title of Daoist Master (*Daoshi*) ceased to be a mark of the highest respect.[4] Instead, ambitious "medical craftsmen" from families of hereditary practitioners could benefit from the fact that the textual horizons of literate healers were no longer dominated by esoteric manuscripts transmitted from master to disciple, making it possible for them to train in the approved classics and textbooks. Popular stories about inspired healers told of the classic books in their knapsacks and medicine bags, and of itinerants who could recite portions of the *Inner*

3. From the time of the founding emperor Taizu, himself medically learned, a Northern Song imperial agenda was to raise the level of the empire's ordinary "medical craftsmen" (*yi gong*) through a program of standardized education disseminated from the capital. State-appointed physicians were charged with the ambitious program of compiling, editing and printing approved medical books. State bureaus developed standards for processing materia medica and codifying approved prescription formulas, and at times supervised distribution and sale as well. A separate medical school, the Grand Medical Office (*Taiyi ju*), founded in 1044, developed academic curricula, tested students, awarded ranks and degrees, and for a time was even charged with supervising prefectural medical officers. Although the history of the Grand Medical Office was uneven, and state medical ranks never competed in prestige with those assigned civil officials, medical orthodoxy was closely identified with state policies in both Northern and Southern Song dynasties. For the history of Song medicine, see Unschuld 1979, Hymes 1987, Li Jingwei 1990, Liang Jun 1995 and Chen Yuan-peng 1995, 1997.

4. The practices of many south Chinese *wu* conflicted with emerging neo-Confucian notions of ethical conduct, particularly in the crises of epidemics attributed to infestation (*zhu*) caused by malignant ghosts and spread through contact with the sick. *Wu* encouraged families to abandon afflicted relatives, and called for ritual burning of sufferers' clothing, possessions and sometimes even dwellings. I want to thank T. J. Hinrichs for allowing me to see the discussion of these issues in her dissertation chapter "Medicine, Shaman Suppression and the Transformation of Southern Customs in the Song." The gradual decline in the prestige of medical practitioners identified as Daoists is documented for one Jiangnan prefecture in Hymes 1987, but it is generally still not well understood.

THE DEVELOPMENT OF *FUKE*   63

Canon by heart.[5] In sum, as it became more common for a gentleman to be learned in medicine, so a medical man could seek to be known as a gentleman.[6]

In this way the emerging Song identity of "literati physician" (*ru yi*) came to signify a cultural ideal of good medical practice, and, more ambiguously, an improved social position for the most learned group of doctors. If few actually combined healing arts with a Confucian philosophical education—as the emperor Huizong, who first promoted the concept, envisioned—a good many more could claim the title as an informal honorific.[7] Such men liked to quote the aphorism of the eminent Northern Song scholar-official Fan Zhongyan: "If you cannot become a good prime minister, you can become a good doctor." Slowly, mostly in the Southern Song, as literacy expanded (measured both as an absolute number and as a percentage of the population), more doctors wrote books and more learned amateurs joined the ranks of published medical authors. The textual development of Song gynecology was part of this larger movement.

Consolidating *Fuke:*
Ordering Illness and Organizing Healers

Using newer approaches to nosology, *fuke* became an academic subject taught in a state-approved curriculum, and gradually practitioners, visible first in the imperial palace and then beyond, gained prestige from being associated with it.

One of the signs of the systematic gynecology of the Song era was the application to women's disorders of a paradigm of diagnosis that made it easier to relate diverse symptoms to holistic body functions.

5. Stories about doctors from Song informal essays (*biji*) are collected in Tao Yuanfeng 1988.

6. Chen Yuan-peng (1995, 1997) has studied a wide range of Song-era literati writings, including biographies, *biji* and prefaces, to construct the complex social negotiations of the roles of gentleman and doctor in a rank-conscious society. He argues that the promotion of medicine by elite scholars was just as important as state sponsorship in reshaping medical culture. His conclusion is that although the social gap between a genteel amateur of medicine and a person who practiced for a livelihood was generally clear, over time more men from hereditary medical families were recognized as literati physicians, while the vocation of doctor was taken up by some men from established scholar families.

7. For the emperor Huizong's edict calling on scholars (*ru*) to study medicine, see Liang Jun 1995: 100, and Chen Yuan-peng 1997: 182–86.

When medical experts began to group the signs and symptoms of distress into deep patterns, they left earlier, more rudimentary systems of disease classification behind. Song learned medicine had inherited from Zhang Ji of the Eastern Han (25–220 C.E.) traditions associated with his short treatise on "the thirty-six disorders of women."[8] In the early Tang Sun Simiao (581–682) was the first medical master to stress the importance of the female contribution to successful reproduction, opening his encyclopedic work on pharmacy with three chapters of "separate prescriptions" for female fertility, pregnancy and postpartum.[9] Here as on other topics, Chao Yuanfang (fl. 605–616) was the classic source of understandings of the etiology of disease based on the system of cardinal channels and circulating vitalities developed from the *Inner Canon*.[10] However, the limitations of early *fuke* show themselves in the construction of the "miscellaneous disorders" (*za bing*) of women around the rubric of *daixia* — "below the waistband."

In the Qin-Han era, *daixia* had named women's reproductive malfunctions in terms of an energy field holding the womb in place and regulating the flow of fluid discharges from the vagina. The *Inner Canon* understood *daixia* as a region of the female body where *jia* — abdominal swellings and tumors — might appear.[11] Catalogues of *daixia* ailments in medical classics, like Zhang Ji's thirty-six disorders of women and Chao Yuanfang's "thirty-six *daixia* ailments" or his "eight *jia*" referred to aberrant bloody and other discharges by color, flow and odor, or identified abdominal masses by shape and feel.[12] But such symptoms were not

8. The *Jin gui yaolüe* (Essentials of the Golden Casket) of Zhang Ji (Zhang Zhongying) contains three chapters that Ma Dazheng 1991: 40–43 calls the earliest *fuke* text. Zhang was most famous later as the author of the *Shanghan lun*.

9. Sun Simiao, *Beiji qianjin yaofang*, juan 1–3. See Lee Jen-der 1997.

10. Chao Yuanfang (fl. 605–616), *Zhubing yuanhou lun* (On the Origins and Symptoms of Disease). Chao's work was a major point of departure for Song nosology. He did not discuss pharmacy. Juan 37–44 discuss the disorders of women.

11. See *Su wen* 60.1.3:161: "Disorders of the Conception channel: in males the seven internal *shan* [herniated swellings]; in females *jia* [tumorous swellings] and *ji* [accumulations] of the *daixia* region." However, when Ma Dazheng 1991: 27 looks for canonical origins of the modern reading of *daixia* as leukorrhea, he finds it in a passage of the *Ling shu* that links light-colored discharge from the genitals to a pathological draining of brain marrow due to poor digestion of grains. The original did not use the term *daixia*, and it is not even clear the disorder was associated with female genital discharge as well as male. However, the *Ling shu* passage may help us understand contemporary folk interpretations of *daixia* in Taiwan, where I have found that women associate the disorder with consumption of indigestible "cold and raw" foods.

12. See Zhang Ji, juan 1, in SKQS, vol. 734, 12. The summary in juan 22, 185, identifies them with the *daixia* region. For Chao Yuanfang, see juan 38, in ZGYXDC

explained according to any consistent model of disease process. Over the course of the early imperial era, the concept of *daixia* was given new meanings. Integrated into the system of energy pathways, an older eclectic "belt channel"(*dai mai*) became another ungendered "singular" channel, encircling the waist like a belt, but in this process the term lost its privileged association with the womb as an organ.[13] In thinking about the energies underlying reproductive function and malfunction in women, Chao Yuanfang led later classical theorists to imagine them flowing along the Highway and Conception pair of channels. On the other hand, early imperial doctors like Sun Simiao continued to use *daixia* as an umbrella nosological term for reproductive disorders marked by genital discharges and lesions, aberrant flows of menstrual blood, abdominal pain and infertility.[14] In Song *fuke* these rudimentary umbrella classifications, whether thirty-six disorders, eight *jia*, or *daixia*, became obsolete.[15]

Of course the changes of the Song era can be read as an incremental process drawing upon rich if scattered accounts like these from earlier medical history. But I think we should not take the claims for continuity presented by Chinese medical authorities, either Song or subsequently, at face value. Song doctors' appeals to tradition were highly selective, and their classical revivalism was a mode of innovation, as so often happens. Basic among these innovations was what I call "pattern diagnosis" (*bian zheng*), which spread gradually in the twelfth and thirteenth centuries. This was less a method of diagnosis in the modern sense than a strategy for grouping the multiplicity of individual symptoms into a smaller number of broad categories that in turn could be related to each other dynamically.[16] Eventually the

---

2:790–92, 794–95. Chao also uses the term to refer specifically to abnormal vaginal discharges, associating these with sterility and menstrual irregularity as well. From Chao on the eight *jia* (794), we can see that early authorities did not always distinguish between tumorous swellings, abnormal vaginal discharges and aberrant forms of menstrual bleeding. See also Ma Dazheng 1991: 41–43, 93–94.

13. For *dai mai*, see *Su wen* 44.3:125.

14. Sun Simiao, *Beiji qianjin yaofang*, juan 4, 63–65. Sun speaks of the "thirty-six ailments" and of the "one hundred disorders of the *daixia* [region]."

15. For a seventeenth-century survey by a scholar of the medical classics, see Xiao Xun 1684, juan 7, in ZGYXDC 5:717–20.

16. As a modern term, *bian zheng* is sometimes translated as "manifestation type determination" (Sivin 1987: 109) or "syndrome differentiation" (Farquhar 1994: 56). I prefer "pattern diagnosis" for the older version. A Northern Song exposition may be found in the writings of Kou Zongshi, considered one of the founders of the new movement. See juan 1 of his *Bencao yanyi*, in ZGYXDC 2:53.

patterns came to be standardized as the "eight rubrics" (*ba gang*), which clustered specific symptoms as signs of a root (*ben*) pattern identified with some combination of yin/yang, cold/hot, inner/outer or depletion/repletion factors. Correctly naming the underlying pattern at work structured a healer's understanding of his clients' problems in a way that pointed directly to clinical strategies, that is, to appropriate prescriptions. The skilled diagnostician had to discern these root patterns linking immediately experienced signs and symptoms to holistic functions. Like other divisions of medical practice, *fuke* was affected by the new sophistication of theory, and medical experts developed new "separate prescriptions" for a wide variety of systemic, internal "miscellaneous disorders," now seen as gendered forms of illness. The term *fuke* itself, hitherto a marker for chapters or sections of ungendered master narratives, came to designate a subdiscipline within medical learning. *Chanke*—the traditional term for obstetrics and the major one identifying gendered texts in earlier writing—gradually became subsumed within the larger category. Menstruation, as a visible manifestation of the underlying functioning of the reproductive female body, gained weight in medical diagnosis, resulting in an elaboration of menstrual nosology and a corresponding simplification of *daixia* to a more limited range of vaginal discharges. Men of learning began to consider alternative theories concerning the mechanisms underlying conception, and in particular those affecting the sex of offspring. Finally, literate medicine began to pay more attention to issues surrounding parturition. Cumulatively, then, in the Song dynasty medicine was more concerned with female difference than it ever had been before, and perhaps more than it was to be later in imperial history.

Fuke as a distinct department of medical knowledge first became visible in the organizational structure of the Imperial Medical Bureau, which specialized in medical education. Where Tang dynasty state medicine had been organized around only four divisions—pharmacy, acupuncture, massage and ritual—the Song system privileged internal medicine (*neike*) and introduced *fuke* and pediatrics (*erke*) as two of nine separate sections.[17] Traces of academic curricula include twelfth-century records of examination questions on menarche, pregnancy and postpartum disorders. Among leading Song medical authors on *fuke*, Qi Zhongfu,

17. For a while there were thirteen. See Ma Dazheng 1991: 146–47, and Liang Jun 1995: 99–100. Hsiung Ping-chen 1995: 6–10, shows the parallel development of Song pediatrics.

Guo Jizhong and Chen Ziming all held appointments as professors.[18]

Song learned discourse on *fuke* was primarily the work of experts attached to the state medical bureaus who, among other duties, served the imperial palace. As elite innovators at court, they intruded onto an existing domain of medical practice we know very little about. The textual traces of pre-Song healers serving palace women certainly include ritualists and shamans as well as herbalists, acupuncturists and masseuses, and among these female healers occasionally appear. The Qin-Han palace had its *daixia* doctors (*daixia yi*), while in the early imperial era practitioners called female doctors (*nü yi*) or childbirth doctors (*ru yi*) attended palace women. Ritual and other unspecified female healers were also part of the scene. While there were stories of famous male healers who saved women in childbirth with acupuncture, these were medical emergencies, not ordinary deliveries. So if childbirth was the sphere of female healers, pharmacy and acupuncture were represented as male preserves. Whatever the popular source of the eclectic cornucopia of remedies for gestational problems that crop up in surviving pre-Song texts, "separate prescriptions" for women, after all, were taught to males.[19] It is hard, then, to disentangle the effect that Song learned *fuke* had on female practitioners from its impact on a variety of popular and ritual healers and their techniques.

Medical stories from the women's quarters of the imperial palace, sparse as they are, may offer the best clues that in fact gender boundaries of medical practice shifted in the Song. In the Northern Song, as earlier, the palace had its own separate household bureaucracy, which included low- and middle-ranking female functionaries in charge of materia medica and other health services for the several thousand women who lived and worked in the inner court. A tale of a royal illness shows an informal network of women with healing skills at work: when the empress Meng (1086–1101) suffered dizzy spells from "Wind," her attendants performed incantations and prepared *fu* charms[20] to cure her. When her daughter

18. Ma Dazheng 1991: 147–49. Sources disagree as to whether the Nanjing *shu-yuan* where Chen Ziming taught in the twelfth century was an official or a private academy. See Hymes 1987: 31.

19. For Han-Tang medicine, see Lee Jen-der 1996. See also Ma Dazheng 1991: 145–46; Chen Bangxian 1982: 33–35, 72, 87, 98, 182; Tao Yuanfeng 1988: 111–18. Lee itemizes surviving pre-Song formulas for pregnancy, labor and postpartum. From early on there were warnings about the risks of acupuncture for gestational problems.

20. *Fu* charms were pieces of paper on which esoteric ideographs were written. As medicine they were burnt and the ashes drunk with liquid. Although associated with Daoism and often prescribed by itinerant Daoist healers, *fu* charms did not

sickened, the empress's sister "who knew medicine" was summoned, in spite of palace rules against visits from outside.[21] I read these sorts of stories as showing elite women's everyday use of females expert in both ritual and pharmacy.

But beginning in the Northern Song, side by side with this kind of story are reports of palace service by literate males with expertise in *fuke*. These physicians did not so much displace earlier female healing networks as represent the expertise of males claiming a more comprehensive and deeper knowledge of the female body than their own predecessors. Interestingly, two lineages of *fuke* practitioners told stories in later centuries of a famous woman ancestor who had served in the Northern Song palace and established their family's medical traditions, suggesting that some male physicians gained both expertise and access through women members of their own families. According to one account Mistress Wang (*Wang furen*), who treated the empress, was heaped with honors and was able to see that her "sons and grandsons" succeeded her, establishing the Guo line of famous hereditary *fuke* experts. In another version of this story, the Guo family first became famous for a set of thirteen "peony prescriptions" for women's disorders, said to have been given to the founder, Guo Zhaoqian, by a mysterious Daoist; his grandson, Guo Jingzhong, gained access to the palace when his mother, a Mistress Feng, went there to attend the empress. Over time other males, some apparently from commercial pharmacies in the capital, joined them.[22] In the middle of the twelfth century a hereditary physician, Chen Yi, gained fame when he prescribed successfully for the empress, and the emperor rewarded him with permission to practice in the inner court on a regular basis. The ceremonial fan that Chen was given to carry as a passport on entering the women's quarters became the signature of his family's hereditary *fuke* practice thereafter.[23]

---

necessarily require a religious specialist to prepare them. Examples from the text of Chen Ziming are shown in figure 6, p. 118.

21. Chen Bangxian 1982: 277, 281, quoting the Song dynastic history biography of Empress Meng.

22. The Guo family established long-lived medical lineages in Zhejiang, and these narratives were transmitted in Ming editions of the *Zhejiang tongzhi*. My interpretation here comes from Professor Zheng Jinsheng, who believes that two branches of the Guo lineage, long separated from one another, had slightly different recollections of their founding ancestors. "Wang" and "Feng" could sound alike in Zhejiang dialect. Some Ming family practitioners even invented mythical female ancestors as founders of their medical traditions. See Zheng Jinsheng 1996.

23. For Chen Yi, see He Shixi 1991, 2:412–13; and Ma Dazheng 1991: 183–84. The Chen family practice flourished in Zhejiang for centuries, and in the late Ming dy-

Under the last Northern Song emperor, Huizong (reigned 1101–1126), *fuke* had a patron who featured advice on pregnancy and pediatrics prominently in the *Canon of Sagely Benefaction (Sheng ji jing)*, a work of medical philosophy written over his own signature and made a required textbook for the state medical examinations. Huizong also established a special Office for Health and Long Life (*Baoshou cuihe guan*) for the palace inner court.[24] In sum, under Huizong and other Northern Song emperors, medical ranks for specialists in *fuke* were acquired both through the state examination system and as a recognition of doctors from town or country who performed successfully when summoned to court to deal with emergencies in the imperial household. These doctors in turn could use their fame to establish hereditary family practices.

And so the increased prestige accorded *fuke* as medical curriculum, and the reputations gained for male healers tending palace women, gradually lent dignity to what had been an area marginal to learned medicine. In 1220, in the closing years of the Southern Song dynasty, a professor of the Grand Medical Office, Qi Zhongfu, sat down to compose a work titled *One Hundred Questions on Medicine for Females (Nüke baiwen)*, seeing himself as a pioneer in an enlightened age:

> Our august emperors of the present dynasty, following the precedents of the sages before them and pitying the people's suffering, have established medical education and codified the "thirteen departments of knowledge [*ke*]," each with its special practices. In keeping with the [ideals of] the Zhou dynasty, today not only does medicine have its own officials but also its own learning, and within that learning there are departments. For the first time there is specialized knowledge concerning the women's chambers. Surely it should not fail to be written in books? I have made a study of this specialization in medicine. Not daring to be lazy and disregarding my own ignorance, I have gathered many prescriptions and compiled them into a volume called *One Hundred Questions on Medicine for Females*.[25]

---

nasty two *fuke* texts attributed to Chen were published by his descendants. Ma relies heavily upon these rare texts for his reconstruction of Song *fuke*.

24. The *Sheng ji jing* was promulgated under the emperor' name in 1118 C.E. Reflecting Huizong's personal metaphysics, this text interpreted the *Huangdi neijing* in light of the Daoist classics and the *Yijing,* and claimed the Yellow Emperor as philosophical sage. It was an important source for Song *fuke* master Chen Ziming. However, after the fall of the Southern Song it was criticized as heterodox, and no printed edition is known before 1887, when Chen Xinyuan produced one based on manuscripts incorporating the Song-era commentaries of Wu Ti. For the Baoshou Cuihe Guan see Chen Bangxian 1982: 242. I cannot find any details about this organization beyond the date of its founding, 1114.

25. Qi Zhongfu, preface, 1220. Although this preface makes clear Qi's hope for imperial sponsorship in publication, the first known printed text of this work was

Although Qi Zhongfu thought of his work as a bedside manual for family use, it may well have been the first book to address gynecology on a equal basis with the gestational issues of pregnancy and postpartum: the first fifty of his one hundred questions dealt with menstruation and "miscellaneous disorders." A few years later Chen Ziming (1190–1270), member of a successful Zhejiang medical lineage and professor at a Nanjing academy (*shuyuan*), produced a more comprehensive medical treatise on *fuke* directed largely at a learned readership of experts. Compared with Qi Zhongfu, Chen's evaluation of contemporary clinical standards was critical. Commonplace writings, he said, were neither thorough nor systematic: "Doctors [of *fuke*] are limited to the simple and easy, and can't search deeply for an all-round view. Some only try a single prescription, and if it doesn't work they wring their hands helplessly." The *All-Inclusive Good Prescriptions for Women (Furen ta quan liang fang)*[26] was an encyclopedic gynecology as well as an obstetrics, summarizing the historical achievements of literate medicine as Chen evaluated them. Of the eighty titles and fifty doctors Chen cited by name, the majority were authorities of his own dynasty.[27] Far more than Qi Zhongfu's, Chen's summation of Song theory and practice was the basis for later learned understandings of the inherited tradition. It underscored the difficulty of healing women with the prefatory words, "Medicine is difficult, *fuke* is especially difficult, and all the stages of birth [*chanke*] are both dangerous and difficult."

Song *Fuke*'s Body of Blood and *Qi*

A good place to see the emerging discourse that culminated in Chen's work is to start 250 years earlier with the tenth-century pharmacopoeia the *Imperial Grace Formulary (Taiping sheng hui fang)*, compiled by Wang Huaiyin and a team of court-appointed doctors be-

published in Nanjing in the Ming dynasty. Following Ma Jixing, I assume that the Wanli edition of 1571 (with a preface by Xu Gu telling of the discovery of the text in the library of a local scholar) may be accepted as a Song work. For Yuan and Ming variant texts see Ma Jixing 1990: 226.

26. Chen Ziming, *Furen ta quan liang fang*, 24 juan. First compiled in 1237 and revised for publication in 1284. The quotations are from Chen's original preface, the main source of knowledge about his life. The 1985 edition edited by Yu Ying'ao et al. seeks to be faithful to the thirteenth-century original. Yu's preface discusses extensive alterations found in subsequent widely circulated Ming versions.

27. Ma Dazheng 1991: 181–82.

tween 978 and 992.²⁸ One of the first of the state's ambitious publication projects of medical synthesis and standardization, it took fifteen years to complete and represented a summary of medical knowledge of the prescription art in the early decades of the Northern Song. The *Imperial Grace Formulary* devoted twelve of its one hundred chapters to *fuke*, and the later Southern Song masters Qi Zhongfu and Chen Ziming were indebted to many of its nosological and pharmaceutical strategies.

The point of departure for Song medical practitioners was the early Tang picture introduced in the three chapters on women's disorders in *Prescriptions Worth a Thousand (Beiji qianjin yaofang)* by the renowned Sun Simiao. Although specific therapies from these chapters played only a limited role as guides to later practice, in the Song dynasty and afterward almost every important writer on the subject quoted some or all of Sun's compelling account of the female medical body:

> It is said that the reason there are separate prescriptions for women is because they get pregnant, give birth and suffer from uterine damage. This is why women's disorders are ten times more difficult to cure than those of males. The Classic says: women are a gathering place for yin influences, dwelling in dampness. From the age of fourteen [*sui*] on, their yin *qi* wells up and a hundred thoughts run through their minds, damaging their organ systems within and ruining their beauty without. Their monthly courses flow out or are retained within, now early, now late, stagnating and congesting Blood and interrupting the functions of central pathways. The injuries from this cannot be enumerated in words. Internal organs are now cold, now hot, now replete, now depleted. Bad Blood within leaks out, and energy channels are used up and drained empty. Sometimes immoderate diet causes damage, sometimes they have sexual intercourse before their [vaginal] itching sores have healed. Sometimes as they relieve themselves at the privy above, Wind from below enters, causing the twelve chronic illnesses. All of this is why women have separate prescriptions. If an illness is due to the *qi* of the four seasons, or to the divisions [of day and night] and to imbalance of cold and heat or of repletion and depletion, it is no different from that of men; only potent [*du*] medicines are to be avoided if they fall ill [of these] when pregnant. For miscellaneous disorders [*za bing*] that are the same in women and men, one should consult the main chapters of this work. Nonetheless, females' longings and desires are more intense than those

28. *Fuke* is discussed in juan 69–81 of the *Taiping sheng hui fang*. For a history of the text, see Ma Jixing 1990: 173. For the value of its *fuke*, see Ma Dazheng 1991: 158–60. Although it was reprinted twice in the Song, this work disappeared from circulation afterward.

of their husbands, and they are more frequently stimulated to become ill. Add to this that in women envy and dislike, compassion and love, grief and sorrow, attachments and aversions are all especially stubborn and deep-seated. They cannot themselves control these emotions [*qing*], and from this the roots of their illnesses are deep, and their cure is difficult.[29]

Alone among early medical masters canonized in the Song, Sun Simiao had emphasized the social importance of therapy for women and children. Doctors, he had said, who are called to preserve life, should remember that life begins with birth. So he placed the disorders of women and children in the first chapters of his encyclopedic pharmacopoeia. But his actual text on *fuke* emphasized illnesses during pregnancy and postpartum. It was left to the authorities of the Song era to grapple with the contradictory implications for gynecology of his famous passage. On the one hand, Sun's claim that disorders of external origins and "miscellaneous disorders" were no different in the two sexes would appear to minimize the importance of the female body as a site of gender difference. On the other hand, Sun's holistic "gathering place of yin influences" represented the embodied female with a cluster of resonant popular images saturating the yin yang dyad with metaphors of the feminine. As the single most famous passage of *fuke* from earlier medical classics, Sun's words show how easily the abstract yin yang of the androgynous body could be rhetorically overwhelmed. This is a female body marked by instability of boundaries: open to invasion, now penetrated sexually or chilled by invading winds, now leaking and draining what cannot be contained. Blood is the visible sign of this instability, now overflowing without, now subject to hidden blockages and stagnation. In Sun Simiao's imagery this Blood as yin was a holistic figuration of woman's bodily nature.

Song *fuke* linked these resonant figurations with the developing language of diagnostic theory based on pattern analysis. Ma Dazheng argues that the relationship of yin and yang on the one hand, and of Blood and *qi* on the other, formed the scaffolding of the new therapeutic reasoning, used by a wide variety of Song authorities to name patterns in female illness.[30] While some experts, like the authors of the *Imperial Grace Formulary*, stressed women's natural affinity for yin, such a ten-

29. Sun Simiao, *Beiji qianjin yaofang*, juan 2, 16. Quoted in the *Taiping sheng hui fang*, 2183; Chen Ziming, juan 9, 288; Qi Zhongfu, juan 1, 2b; and many others.
30. Ma Dazheng 1991: 149–52.

dency, in keeping with Sun Simiao's views, was a mark of vulnerability. The physician's goal was to restore an equal balance between the two, in keeping with the *Inner Canon*'s cryptic aphoristic definition of health: "tranquil yin and hidden yang." Accordingly one standard therapy, adapted from the *Imperial Grace Formulary*, was to assist Blood by prescribing medicines to repress *qi*. On the other hand, the dyad Blood and *qi* could be deployed in the formal reasoning of pattern analysis to claim a natural and healthy hierarchy within the body. "In women Blood is leader," doctors said, claiming to interpret the *Inner Canon*.[31] However, where the relevant passage in the ancient text both treated Blood as a fluid and suggested that repressing *qi* should be the therapeutic strategy appropriate to sick females, Chen Ziming reasoned as follows: "In males one regulates *qi*, in females one regulates Blood. *Qi* and Blood are the [foundation] of living consciousness [*shen*], and one must handle them with great care. In women Blood [function] is the root [*ben*]; when the function of *qi* and Blood are both manifest, the psyche [*shen*] is naturally clear. If the so-called 'Blood Chamber' is not blocked up, *qi* is harmonious; if Blood congeals, then Fire and Water contend [causing illness]."[32] Yang Shiying, a Southern Song authority, put it this way: "Males and females both have Blood and *qi*, yet people say that in women Blood is fundamental. Why? Because their Blood is in ascendancy over *qi;* it is stored in the Liver system, flows through the womb and is ruled by the Heart system; it ascends to become breast milk, descends to become menses, unites with semen to make the embryo." He then reminded his audience that such action was not by Blood alone; Blood, after all, follows *qi*.[33]

These statements suggest the broad strategies followed by Song *fuke* in its depiction of Blood. The first, based on the assumptions of

---

31. Here the classical point of departure was *Ling shu* 65.2.1:435–36: "The Yellow Emperor said, 'Women do not grow a beard. Is this because of a lack of Blood and *qi*?' Qibo said, 'The Highway and Conception pulses both arise in the womb and ascend along the interior of the back to form the sea of cardinal pathways [*jingluo*]. They move to the body's surface along the right side of the bowels, ascend to the throat, separate to connect to the lips and mouth. When Blood and *qi* are abundant they fill the skin and warm the flesh. When Blood alone is abundant it moistens the skin and grows hair. Now women have a surplus of *qi* and a deficiency of Blood because they repeatedly lose Blood [menstruate]. The Conception and Highway pulses do not invigorate their mouth and lips and so they don't grow beards.'"

32. Chen Ziming, juan 1, 12, quoting the preface to an unidentified work, *Chan bao fang* (Prescriptions from the Birth Treasury).

33. I have taken this quote from Ma Dazheng 1991: 151–52. Yang was a well-known Southern Song physician from Fujian, not particularly identified with *fuke*.

homologous gender, produced a view of Blood and *qi* as a yin yang pair dominant in female and male respectively. The second strategy, as it reasserted the primacy of *qi* in female bodies as well as male, called attention to the buried metaphor of yin and yang as hierarchical and encompassing: Blood was feminized as secondary and dependent in the hierarchy of bodily energies, unable to stand alone as a primal body vitality as *qi* did. Both strategies, however, allowed the Blood-*qi* dyad to be used like other dyads in pattern analysis—as defining the root pattern that determined therapy in a given case. Finally, as yin and Water, identified with sexual functions and body fluids that were transformations of one another, Blood was what underlay both generative and gestational body functioning in females. Although in their material manifestations they flowed from the body as waste, menses and the blood of childbirth partook of the vital function of underlying yin Blood.

Menstruation

According to the Yellow Emperor's model of the body, the generative body was at deepest level the same in both sexes, but the gestational body was woman's alone. Menstruation, which manifested both the generative and gestational aspects of Blood, accordingly became a major focus of Song gynecological theorizing. The older medical literature contained some hints that menstrual blood was understood as tainted by "the power of pollution"—sexual intercourse during the menses was early on criticized as unhealthy for both partners, for example.[34] But the generative virtues of menstrual blood were not much emphasized either. By the end of the Song dynasty, however, menstruation had assumed a place as the first, and often the longest, section of a work of *fuke*. Here primary aspects of Blood in the Blood-*qi* dyad were linked to all manifestations of reproductive blood, while menstrual disorder in turn was explained holistically as implicating other illnesses. Song doctors learned to classify menstrual symptoms according to the categories of pattern analysis into combinations of yin/yang, Cold/Hot, depletion/repletion types of syndromes. Finally, time's cycle in the microcosm of the body made the menses a model of natural rhythms akin to the tides and moon, a metaphorically rich sign of female health and fertility.

34. See for example Chao Yuanfang, juan 39, in ZGYXDC 2:829.

"Heavenly true *qi* flows with it; peaceful and harmonious, it doesn't miss its proper time, and we call it 'monthly [*yue* = moon] Water.'"[35]

As Chen Ziming put it in his opening chapter, "In treating illness in women, one must first regulate the menses, so I place this first."[36] He summed up the reasoning by which menstruation was linked to the deepest levels of body function by invoking yin yang poles, the cardinal channel system and the cosmology of Five Phases. Classical channel theory had been silent or inconsistent in its references to the menses. Four different channel groupings were variously offered as functional regulators of the menses: the Conception and Superintendent pair, Conception and Highway pair, Heart and Small Bowel pair, or the singular *daixia* channel encircling the waist.[37] Following the *Imperial Grace Formulary*, Chen Ziming offered the following standard Song view of the matter: "The Highway and Conception pulses arise from within the womb [*bao*] at the sea of *jingluo* pathways connecting the *shoutaiyang* [Small Bowel] and *shoushaoyin* [Heart] channels. These channels form an outer/inner pair linking functional centers of Bowel and Heart, and regulating the descent as menses and the ascent [after birth] as breast milk."[38]

In this account Chen Ziming supported the tradition that went back to Chao Yuanfang and the *Inner Canon*, linking female functioning to the Conception and Highway channels while subordinating the womb as organ to their system of circulating energies. Here as elsewhere the network of channels played a primary role in Chen Ziming's clinical reasoning, but therapeutic reasoning based on links between channels and organ systems received attention as well. "The Heart system produces Blood" and "the Liver system stores Blood," while both of these systems depend upon the metabolic function of digestion centered in the Spleen-stomach system. Thus any menstrual disorder might be sign of a root in serious dysfunction of the circulation of Blood and *qi* in the channels, or in central *zang* organ systems, affecting Blood as a primary vitality in the Blood-*qi* pair. Similarly, damage to any one of these underlying functions might destabilize menses.

Menstruation permitted a deep reading of surface signs. It provided

35. Qi Zhongfu, question 5.

36. Chen Ziming, juan 1, 10.

37. See Xiao Xun, juan 1, in ZGYXDC 5:651.

38. *Taiping sheng hui fang*, 2271; Chen Ziming, juan 1, 13, almost identical wording. See also Qi Zhongfu, question 7.

a variety of symptoms: early or late, heavy or light, pale or dark, clotted or watery, in all possible combinations. These were fertile ground for "eight rubrics" diagnostics. Blood as menses was a mutation not only of semen or breast milk, but of multiple manifestations of bodily fluid. In its aspect of "monthly water" (*yue shui*) it might be a harmless residue voided like urine, but within menses could dry up and reappear as oedema—water-swollen tissues—or drain out as diarrhea, or under the impact of cold congeal into tumorous swellings, or reverse course upward as bloody sputum or bleeding gums.

Beyond such material transformations of menstrual fluid, menses showed its underlying significance above all in its periodicity (*yuejing*), its healthy predictability (*xin*) as sign of a fertile reproductive body. Medicines that addressed menstrual anomaly aimed first to "regulate." "Menstrual regulating" (*tiao jing*) formulas proliferated, fostered by learned medicine's growing infatuation with complex, individually crafted prescriptions. They functioned both as points of departure to treat illness and as preventive medicine aimed at ensuring fertility and general female health.

While the "eight rubrics" style of pattern diagnostics was used to elaborate the nosology of menstrual dysfunction, this mode of reasoning supplied a critical standard simplifying the nosology of *daixia*. In the Han, Zhang Ji's "thirty-six disorders of women" had made vaginal discharge, bloody or otherwise, almost a master code for all female illness, and Chao Yuanfang had written of "twelve kinds of *daixia*." Although Chen Ziming and Qi Zhongfu continued to treat *daixia* as potentially serious, threatening barrenness and chronic depletion syndromes, they criticized "the confused itemization [of thirty-six] and the many separate prescriptions for each." They prescribed for only two kinds of discharge: red and white, signs of yang heat and yin cold. Here Song authorities drew firmer boundaries between abnormal kinds of menstrual flow and what today's experts would call leukorrhea.[39]

Such shifts are keys to a subtle alteration of the codes by which the female body was read. Abnormal vaginal discharges took a back seat to

39. See Qi Zhongfu, questions 49 and 50; Chen Ziming, juan 8, 258; and Ma Dazheng 1991: 166–67. There seems to have been no consensus on what underlying patterns were at work in *daixia*. Chen Ziming spoke of external pathogens of Heat and Cold in interaction with Spleen-stomach system malfunctions, while Qi spoke of corruption and thinning of Blood from Cold Damage. Chen Ziming still classified *daixia* by the five colors associated with the Five Phases (following the *Canon of the Pulse*), but his prescriptions were for red and white types only.

irregular menses, shifting the pathological sign from the foul to the unpredictable, from the physically repugnant to the measurably unreliable. The ideal of menstrual regularity, functioning harmoniously under the hierarchical and encompassing governance of Blood and *qi,* could even be seen as Song gynecology's answer to the disorderly, unbounded yin body of Sun Simiao's medical imagination. In terms of gender ideology, menstrual regularity as an inner process identified with ideal normality was coming to serve as a primary bodily signifier of female difference.[40] Femaleness came to be constructed around this manifestation of the interior body that is unseen but revealed in the menstrual flow — its periodicity attesting to free and ample circulating vitalities within. As a generative fluid, menstrual Blood was comparable to male seminal Essence, also understood as a yin distillation of primal Blood. Thus the closest masculine counterpart to the menstrual cycle was the generative rhythm of timeliness in sexual potency — imagined as "daily" — but medicine suggested no masculine version of menstruation itself.[41]

"Miscellaneous Disorders" of Women

The *Imperial Grace Formulary* was a vast encyclopedia of more than one thousand disorders listed by name. In any medical system, naming illness is a critical step whereby the body's experience enters culture and is rendered intelligible to the sufferer. Naming here did not identify discrete diseases so much as list myriad signs and symptoms that it was the physician's duty to combine into meaningful functional patterns. The *Imperial Grace Formulary,* like Chinese nosology generally, classified disorders under the headings of signs (which could be observed by outsiders), symptoms (that is, indications of inner bodily distress which had to be reported by the sufferer) or syndromes, the physicians' grouping of these. Any medical text presented all three in bewildering profusion and combinations. Many illnesses were identified by signs that anyone would recognize: a cough, a nosebleed, skin eruptions, diarrhea or vomiting. Symptoms, however, named inner distress in humoral lan-

---

40. This is persuasively argued for late imperial China by Bray 1997.

41. In European humoral medicine, by contrast, periodic bloody rectal discharge in males was sometimes seen as analogous to menstruation in women. Arguing that such discharges in both sexes were nature's way of releasing a plethora of humors, seventeenth-century physicians sometimes called a hemorrhoidal swelling in a man a "golden vein." See Pomata 1984.

guage of bodily heat and cold that cannot simply be translated into the temperature measurements of biomedicine: one afflicted with a "Cold womb" (*bao leng*) or "depletion Heat" (*xu re*), for example, experienced infertility or weakness in a thermal idiom. Many vital indicators of illness were named in words that to an outsider's eye are anything but transparent: stasis (*yu*), fright (*jing*), congestion (*yu*), blockage (*pi*) or reversal (*jue*) linked sensations of inner distress to vagaries of *qi* flow. Aggregate terms like Wind stroke (*zhongfeng*), Cold Damage (*shanghan*) and Blood Wind (*xuefeng*) constituted a doctor's expert shorthand for loosely grouped syndromes that encompassed variable signs and symptoms.

Both symptoms and syndromes were often simply called *zheng*, blurring the boundaries between them. But what biomedically acculturated readers see as classificatory laxness gains richness and meaning when interpreted instead as the verbalization of the experiences of illnesses, giving names to their plenitude of sensation. As elsewhere in the preindustrial world, there was no physical examination to speak of, and many signs as well as symptoms were reported rather than observed by the attending physician. The doctor was respectful of bodily boundaries which by custom were impossible to breach very far. Since the sufferings hidden inside the body were known chiefly through the sufferers' own speech, the language of diagnosis began with everyday idiom, where the vocabulary of healer and patient was shared.[42] Nosological categories — those naming disorders — had to rely upon this level of the experience of illness, and patient report supplied the knowledge of the body, not just the material for a diagnosis. If pulse readings were a doctor's privileged knowledge, outside the clinical dialogue even the technical yin yang binaries of his pattern analysis remained connected to the phenomena of illness experienced as heat or cold, or bodily emptiness or fullness, or the movement of breath and blood. Thus the nosology of the syndromes clustered under the rubric "miscellaneous disorders" in women is only one example of how at bottom Chinese medicine depended upon

42. My discussion here is indebted to Barbara Duden's superb interpretation of the relationship of learned doctrine to popular cosmology in *The Woman Beneath the Skin: A Doctor's Patients in Eighteenth-Century Germany* (Harvard, 1991). See chapter one, "Toward a History of the Body," 1–49. Historians of Chinese medicine like Porkert and Needham, in attempting to dignify Chinese medical concepts by Latinizing terminology, have, in my view, exaggerated the conceptual gulf between learned and lay understandings in traditional China. Duden's work shows how much our interpretation of premodern medicine is enriched by a phenomenological reading of the language of bodily maladies.

a phenomenological language of bodily experience arrived at in nego-tiation between speakers and listeners in the clinical encounter.

The vast majority of symptoms and syndromes discussed in the *Imperial Grace Formulary* were ungendered. No special prescriptions for women were indicated for any febrile disorders from Cold Damage (*shanghan*) or Warm epidemic (*wenyi*) — the largest, most important syndrome clusters thought to arise from pathogenic *qi* in the environ-ment. This was in keeping with Sun Simiao's classic statement that dis-orders due to external agency were no different in males and females. Diarrheas, dysenteries, skin rashes, eczemas and oedemas remained un-gendered, as did all of the many disorders classified under parts of the body, whether external (such as eyes, nose or throat) or by reference to functional internal organ systems such as Heart, Liver and Spleen.

However, three broad internal syndrome clusters were given a place in the *fuke* chapters, indicating that in females doctors should look for signs of gender difference. First, Wind stroke (*zhongfeng*) was grouped under a master pattern functional disorders from Wind (*feng*). Wind was found both in the external world and within the body. It was iden-tified with the environmental *qi* of the four seasons of time and the five cardinal directions of space, which could assume destructive, unseason-able form, correspondingly manifest in pathological internal changes — rapidly moving symptoms and sudden loss of function. As Shigehisa Kuriyama has so eloquently put it, Wind evoked random and irregular changes in the body's internal weather system, identified with cosmic forces of change and time gone awry.[43] The paradigmatic Wind attack was a stroke, apoplexy, paralysis, coma, or perhaps a fit marked by rav-ings or convulsions. Working more slowly, pathogenic Wind might lodge in the limb that withered, the extremity that was numb, the rheu-matic joint, the palsied tongue.

The second broad cluster, depletion fatigue (*xusun, xulao*), assembled afflictions marked by slow, chronic wasting, where the sufferer grew emaciated and debilitated, accumulating a host of secondary symptoms from pallor, indigestion and shortness of breath to hair loss, hot sen-sations on palms of hands and soles of feet, and palpitations, while also experiencing a destabilized psyche marked by disturbed dreams or in-somnia, fits of melancholy or anger. Coughing with bloody sputum was an important but not definitive symptom in this syndrome. The third

43. Kuriyama 1994. He is looking at the early classical medicine of Han and Six dynasties.

cluster, "swellings and accumulations" (*jiju*), produced as "swellings," masses, tumors, lumps or circulation blockages where the movement of *qi* up and down was impeded. Sometimes palpable and sometimes not, "accumulations" might be seen or felt as moving or fixed, or be known through the impairment of digestion, urination or defecation. As illness labels, this kind of symptomatic nosology represented only the beginning of diagnosis, which ideally proceeded to distinguish patterns according to the eight rubrics, pointing to the circulation channels and functional organ systems believed affected and to the quality and momentum of the pathology. In this situation a gynecological version of a disorder usually implicated a root pathology affecting functioning of the primal energy associated with Blood, or the Blood-*qi* pair.

In keeping with this, *fuke* emphasized disorders from Wind presumed to agitate and destabilize Blood and *qi*. The *Imperial Grace Formulary* named Blood Wind (*xuefeng*) as a syndrome cluster in its *fuke* but not in its ungendered chapters. Blood Wind could be implicated in attacks of Heart fright (*xin jing*), in which Wind affects Heart and disorders psyche, producing fright and palpitations, mental confusion and melancholy; of "fidgets" (*fenmen*) (feverish sensations, restlessness, pains in limbs, dry mouth); of "roving flux" (*zou zhu*), in which Wind *qi* pursues Blood moving about the body, causing roving pains; or of "bone ache" (*gu tong*), in which hurtful Wind lodges in flesh and skin next to bone. Since Blood and *qi* suffusing healthy skin could be destabilized by Wind, Wind-generated itching and irritation of skin, or hives (*yinzhen*), also were included in *fuke*, as were prescriptions for attacks of madness, since both agitated (*kuang*) and apathetic (*dian*) forms were associated with Wind as well.[44]

If Wind could provoke disordered Blood in women, the second internal syndrome category, depletion fatigue, was gendered through the agency of sexual function and emotion. Among various types of depletion fatigue the "seven damages" usually described male problems: Kidney weakness, impotence, wet dreams and "dreams of intercourse with ghosts," spontaneous seminal emissions, genital sores and discharges. Depletion fatigue, then, was a broad syndrome of internal disorders impairing sexual function as part of an overall pathogenic process, as well as those where sexual excess was adduced as part of an etiological pattern. In addition, depletion fatigue in its various manifestations had an especially close association with affective disorder. Of the "five fa-

44. *Taiping sheng hui fang*, 2155, 2167, 2170, 2173, 2177.

tigues," three are strongly emotional: fatigue from grief, fatigue from worry, and fatigue from striving. The syndrome's affinity for women could be based on the propensity to emotionality that Sun Simiao had articulated.

As disorders of uncontrolled emotions and of sexual function, depletion fatigue in women might manifest itself in sterility or menstrual irregularity, often if not always linking specific symptom clusters with erratic movements of yin Blood. "Infertility in a woman, if it is due to illness rather than bad fate or a horoscope incompatible with her husband's, will always involve Blood fatigue."[45] It may be suspected, moreover, when Blood strays from orderly function, randomly moving about: divided Blood (*xue fen:* menses cease and Blood is transformed into water, swelling tissues with oedema), or Blood Wind fatigue (*qi* and Blood are depleted and menses are irregular, perhaps as an aftermath of childbirth), or "Blood flowing from nose" (an adverse movement upward of what should flow down). Thus separate prescriptions, constructed with an eye to preserving female fertility, were recommended for Cold fatigue, Hot fatigue, fatigue with cough, with vomiting, with vomiting of Blood, and so on.

Finally, the most dangerous, life-threatening forms of depletion fatigue—"bone steaming" (*gu zheng*)—required "separate prescriptions." To today's readers, such advanced fatigue, eventually penetrating to bones, sounds like the tubercular "consumption" of early modern European medicine in its patterning of physical decline, respiratory distress, emotional volatility and sexual excitability. The sufferer experiences shortness of breath, loss of appetite, fierce sweats, cold extremities, dreams of intercourse with ghosts, irrational likes and dislikes, hot and cold spells, coughing and pain in the side, and bloody sputum until the disorder has afflicted all five *zang* organ systems and the slide toward death is irreversible. There was no suggestion that bone steaming was particularly common in women or in the young; indeed, the text is clear that all can suffer, but it suggests that in males and females the root may be different. "In males the root of the disorder is swellings or obstructions of lower abdomen; in females it is Blood and *qi*."[46]

The third broad category to be considered is swellings and accumulations, which appear due to blockage of the movement of yin and yang *qi* up and down the body's central pathways. Some show at the surface,

45. *Taiping sheng hui fang*, 2191.
46. *Taiping sheng hui fang*, 2203.

some present as intestinal blockage; some are visible when a person has just eaten, some when the body is empty; some itch, others hurt, and some can be fatal. Like all other major categories they can be classified according to yin and yang forms, and according to organ system. But in males they were associated with malfunctions of digestion and elimination (today we often read them as hernias), while women's *ji* or *ju* swellings were identified with reproductive disorder and digestive symptoms were treated as secondary. Particularly important were the eight *jia*, after the account by Chao Yuanfang. "The eight *jia* in women occur when due to pregnancy, childbirth and menstrual function, the Blood pulse's creative function (*jing qi*) is not regulated."[47] One of the eight is "turtle *jia*":

> When menses has just come she engages in physical activity that causes her to sweat, and she does not change damp clothes promptly. She may get her feet wet, sleep in a draft, and waken suddenly in confusion; and before she is steady on her feet and before her color is normal, she may become excited by some pleasurable sight; her *hun* and *po* souls are moved and her five internal organ systems experience a sudden sense of vacancy. If she bathes and doesn't leave the water promptly and her spirit is not collected, water *qi* and pathogenic *qi* both enter into her "triple burners" and move about in hiding there. They may obstruct the movement of fluids, preventing their egress. So she grows turtle *jia*, accumulations as big as a small plate causing sharp belly pains and movement up and down of bad *qi*. . . . if the swellings grow to the size and shape of a hand or foot, it is incurable.[48]

With *jia*, then, the gynecological syndromes will remind moderns of uterine fibroids or other tumors, or ovarian cancers. The Song woman's affliction, however, would be experienced as yin Cold and Damp, or related to menstruation as a vital whole-body function rather than to the womb as an organ. Since the genesis of an illness could lie in a fleeting moment of instability resembling soul loss, it would have a psychic dimension as well.

A final addition to this early Song gynecology was "foot *qi*" (*jiaoqi*). Here pathogenic *qi* gathers in the feet, producing swelling, numbness and pain; if the *qi* gradually ascends to strike the Heart, the sufferer may die. Twentieth-century doctors have read today's diagnosis of beriberi back into the earlier syndrome, some on the basis of the vivid description

47. *Taiping sheng hui fang*, 2243.
48. *Taiping sheng hui fang*, 2245.

of the symptoms found in the *Imperial Grace Formulary* itself. Tang
sources are more vague, but some physicians early on associated foot *qi*
with Kidney depletion, and thus with generative vitality.[49] The *Imperial
Grace Formulary* recorded its affinity with the warm, damp river valleys
of Jiangtong and Lingnan in the far south—and also reported it to be
more common in females than in males: "Women and maidens of the
capital district, and sometimes youthful scholars, are afflicted even when
they do not live in such places."[50] In the *fuke* section, it was classified as
a disorder of the "circulation channels of the womb."[51] Similarly, Chen
Ziming observed that "foot *qi* in women is different than in men. Males
suffer from weakness of the Kidney system, making them susceptible to
damp Wind; females, due to weakness in the channels [*luo*] of the womb
[*bao*], are struck by poisonous Winds. This is because the womb channels belong to the Kidney system."[52] Whatever observations may have
provoked the nosology of foot *qi* as a gender-linked disorder,[53] Song
fuke taught that it threatened generative vitality.

Chen Ziming's itemization of all of the "numerous ills" (*zhong ji*)
of women closely followed the nosology of the *Imperial Grace Formulary*.[54] Since Qi Zhongfu's simple question-and-answer format rhetorically addressed (presumably female) lay readers' queries about their
problems, he scattered his definitions in answers to fifty questions on
commonplace signs and symptoms. However, both authorities actually
added to the earlier work's gynecological repertory. Qi Zhongfu called
for "separate prescriptions" for thirst (*ke*) syndromes, which today are
identified with diabetes. Since, as Qi reasoned, in women this might be
linked to exhaustion of Blood, he attacked medical quacks for prescribing fiercely drying mineral infusions.[55] Chen Ziming added some cau-
tions concerning the important category of Cold Damage fevers. Like
the classic authority on these disorders, Zhang Ji (Zhang Zhongjing),

49. Wang Xi, *Wai tai mi yao*, juan 18, 491.

50. *Taiping sheng hui fang*, 1355.

51. *Taiping sheng hui fang*, 2178–79.

52. Chen Ziming, juan 4, 129, quoting the *Taiping sheng hui fang*, 2178–79.

53. Chen's modern editors hypothesize that Chen Ziming had noticed that
women with beriberi are infertile. See Chen Ziming, 129, editor's note. *The Cambridge World History of Human Disease* notes the special susceptibility of pregnant
women and nursing infants. See Kiple 1993: 607–8.

54. Chen Ziming, juan 2, 63–80. Chen's variant title—"numerous ills" instead of
"miscellaneous disorders" (*za bing*)—was based on the saying, "When the menstrual
pulse is irregular, numerous ills arise" (63).

55. Qi Zhongfu, question 38. He particularly objected to Five Minerals infusion.

Chen Ziming understood Cold Damage fevers in menstruating or postpartum women as apt to trigger "Heat entering the Blood chamber" (*re
ru xueshi*), destabilizing the flow of menstrual or postpartum Blood.[56]
His advice—to avoid the standard remedy of purgatives (*xia*) in favor
of medicines that induce sweating—was based on the assumption that
such serious fevers easily dry up fluids essential for the normal functioning of Blood. Nonetheless, even here we see the Chinese physician's
dislike of any invariable therapeutic rule, and his reluctance to contradict
classical canon.

> Although Cold Damage fevers differ in males and in women, so that in
> women one first regulates Blood and in males one first regulates *qi*, this
> is a general way of speaking. . . . If her center is drained empty, use White
> Tiger formula; if her stomach is replete, use Move *Qi* infusion [*Cheng qi
> tang*]. Why must one regulate Blood and only afterwards offer a laxative?
> Zhongjing's *Treatise on Cold Damage Disorders*, in refusing to consider
> women separately, has the virtue of teaching that one may follow the
> illness and decide on the basis of the syndrome to select medicine appro-
> priate to males.[57]

Chen's position may in fact have been a cautiously moderate one on a
controversial topic. Other anonymous Song authorities, whom he criticized, produced pharmaceutical manuals (now lost) exclusively devoted
to "separate" Cold Damage prescriptions for female use. These, Chen
said, claimed the authority of ancient authors for remedies that in fact
were new.

In discussing the "miscellaneous disorders" of women in this way,
Chen Ziming and other *fuke* authorities started by balancing the primacy
of Blood in females with that of *qi* in males; but they thought about
individual cases in terms of a normal range against which many people
would vary somewhat and some would be exceptions. In understanding
these as *fuke* syndromes, they were not claiming males were immune.
Rather, they were making claims about what we today might call a
statistical population, calling attention to a group with a range of likely
vulnerabilities that mandated adjustments in treatment.

56. Following Zhang Ji, "Blood chamber" was a commonplace classical term for
a woman's generative center, but exactly how it related to the womb, to Blood storage
or to reproductive pulses was debated by Song and later medical authorities.

57. Chen Ziming, juan 6, 175. These were among Zhang Ji's classic prescriptions
for Cold Damage fevers. White Tiger is for the early stages thought to be characterized by "repletion heat." Its leading ingredient is asphodel (*zhimu*) to drain Fire and
support fluids. Move *Qi* infusion, with rhubarb as a major ingredient, eases bowel
stagnation.

The Art of Pharmacy: Separate Prescriptions

As the discussion of female "miscellaneous disorders" shows, disorders were included in Song *fuke* texts when their authors wanted to alert doctors treating women to the need for "separate prescriptions." How different were such prescriptions likely to be in practice? The discussion of Cold Damage fevers above makes clear that doctors were thinking about a yin yang continuum of bodies—not forgetting that the individual case was also a unique event. In the *Imperial Grace Formulary*, model prescriptions in the *fuke* section indeed differ from those for similarly named disorders in the ungendered section of the work, but the differences are usually minor and difficult to interpret. In the treatment of most miscellaneous disorders, practice probably accommodated graduated variations of gender-based vulnerability in bodies that remained androgynous mixes of yin and yang, Blood and *qi*. However, separate prescriptions for any disorder in a woman were always understood as protecting reproductive vitality, while prescriptions for menstrual regulation and recovery from childbirth were also understood holistically, as panaceas.

A good place to look at the pharmaceutical results of this orientation is through the formulas and materia medica recommended by Chen Ziming under the heading of "all-purpose prescriptions" (*tong fang*) for women's problems—formulas that reflect the emerging standards of pattern diagnosis. The most famous of these, Four Ingredients infusion (*Siwu tang*), had been developed by the Northern Song Imperial Medical Bureau in the eleventh century. It privileges mild drugs that act on Blood and has remained a staple in the *fuke* repertory ever since. It is made of the following: angelica root (*danggui*), considered the premier drug for women for its Blood-nourishing properties;[58] white peony root (*baishao*), which also supports Blood; lovage rhizome (*chuanxiong*), a stronger substance in its action to move Blood and break up Blood stasis, therefore prescribed by some in smaller quantity than the others; and fresh Rehmannia root (*sheng dihuang*), a drug to move *qi* that balances the other three by cooling action to support the production of fluids. (In some Song versions, the dried, steamed form of Rehmannia root was deemed to be a more powerful agent reserved for serious cases,

---

58. On *danggui*, Kou Zongshi said, "It is useful above all for replenishing insufficiency in females." See juan 9 of *Bencao yanyi*, in ZGYXDC 2:67.

or to be used on those rare occasions when Four Ingredients was given to a male.)[59] Four Ingredients infusion balanced action on Blood in three instances with action on *qi* in the fourth; it stressed mild replenishing and nourishing over moving and draining. It was also easy to shift proportions or methods of preparation of individual drugs to accommodate different situations. Beyond this Chen Ziming offered several dozen variations based on additional ingredients targeting specific symptoms. Two or three of these four basic materia medica were included in almost all the other "all-purpose prescriptions" in Chen's book. At the level of symptoms, such prescriptions addressed problems of menstrual regularity and menstrual pain; at the level of pattern diagnosis for action on root pathologies, they "enlivened Blood" (*huo xue*), "replenished Blood" (*bu xue*), or "moved Blood" (*tong xue*). The Song reputation of Four Ingredients infusion as "a treasure for women" may be seen in the enthusiastic report of the late Song medical essayist Zhang Gao on how the formula worked holistically to cure chronic toothache in one woman and depletion-fatigue symptoms in another.[60]

Recovery from childbirth also required all-around strengthening of *qi* and Blood, for which all-purpose prescriptions were recommended. A standard formula was Buddha's Hand, which leads with "finger citron" to stimulate vital *qi*, supplemented with the strong Blood mover lovage rhizome and the all-purpose angelica.[61] This more potent formula balanced action on Blood and action on *qi* more evenly and was considered essential after birth. An even more complex combination was Chen's all-purpose "Pills Better than Gold" (*Sheng jin yuan*), where the leading ingredient is a concentrated form of white peony root (*baishao* [*yao*]), supplemented not only by angelica and lovage rhizome but also by tree peony bark and corydalis tuber (*yanhu* [*suo*]), all of which were for Blood, and by ginseng (instead of Rehmannia root) as the most powerful known stimulant of *qi*. This part of the formula maintains the balance found in Four Ingredients infusion of three parts action on Blood to one on *qi*, but with stronger ingredients on both sides of the equation. Further ingredients in Pills Better than Gold release at the

59. Chen Ziming, juan 2, 65–66; Ma Dazheng 1991: 155. Chen Ziming's commentary shows that some Song authorities believed that both males and females could take fresh root, but that the dry root should be reserved for males. In later centuries the dry form became the standard.

60. Zhang Gao, *Yi shuo*, juan 9, 35b/36a. Zhang (1149–1227) was a member of a medical lineage from Anhui province and author of a famous early collection of medical essays (*biji*).

61. Finger citron gets the name Buddha's Hand (*Foshou*) from its wrinkled appearance.

exterior (that is, induce sweating) and drive out Wind, acting on Heat: these are ligusticum root (*gaoben*), Dahurian angelica root (*baizhi*), and cinnamon. The final additions are white atractylodes (*baishu*) for Spleen-stomach function and white poria fungus (*fuling*) to support fluids and tranquilize. Such a broad-spectrum formula represented a more cumbersome and less elegant therapeutic strategy. Still, Chen claimed, Pills Better than Gold was deemed good for all depletions involving deficiency of vital energy, for internal pains, barrenness, Blood wind, numbness and pains in hands and feet, paralysis and stroke, red and white leukorrhea, vaginal bleeding, postpartum illness, depletion fatigues, urinary incontinence, thirst disease, possession by ghosts, bad Blood striking upward, Hot and Cold headaches, and emaciation. "It will cure all the myriad ills of women, old and young alike." Chen also recommended it for weak males "who are depleted and lack strength below."[62]

Chen's all-purpose prescriptions addressed patterns of disorder in the root function of Blood, while in serious cases they turned to *qi* to lead Blood back toward healthful functioning. They also show that this therapeutic strategy was not a fixed, inflexible one. Chen warned against ignoring individual symptoms: "Though we say these are all-purpose [*tong yong*], you should not mark your boat to find a knife [that has fallen in the water] or paint a stallion by copying a picture." These are aphorisms for action inappropriate to circumstance. All-purpose formulas were adjustable according to individual circumstances, and doctors implied that recipes for a typical woman could be suitable for weak males but not for robust males. The underlying logic was that in *fuke* the appropriate use of pattern diagnosis privileged the dyad Blood and *qi* over others available. This logic in turn ensured that formulas for reproductive disorder, including menstrual regulating formulas, were deemed a suitable foundation for treating a wide range of illnesses in women.[63]

Body, Emotion and Desire

Sun Simiao's famous eighth-century summation of illness in women had called attention to emotions in the etiology of gyneco-

---

62. Chen Ziming, juan 2, 72–73.

63. The standard eight rubrics (*ba gang*) in modern TCM are inner/outer, depletion/repletion, cold/hot and yin/yang. Blood/*qi* is not included. But in earlier centuries practice varied. For the use of Blood/*qi* in pattern diagnosis in Song, Yuan and Ming *fuke*, see Ma Dazheng 1991: 152–53, 204–5.

logical disorder. Song *fuke* took for granted that emotion played an important role in the "difficulty" of cure Sun had warned about. In classical medical thought, emotional and bodily pathology were not bifurcated around a body-spirit split; rather, madness was a symptom with roots in the whole organism. Nor did doctors think in terms of the psychosomatic, that is, a somatic displacement of fundamentally psychic problems. In the Chinese medical imagination consciousness (*shen* = psyche) was an aspect of the functioning of the Heart system, and emotion could destabilize Blood and cloud the psyche. But the path of influence also ran the other way: erratic motions of Blood might manifest themselves in the derangement of madness, the flare of Liver Fire in the surge of anger, the dispersal of *qi* in the withdrawal of melancholy. The "seven *qi*" of the *Inner Canon* tied emotion directly to movement of bodily *qi* without privileging psychological agency, and in keeping with this Qi Zhongfu explained that women are often frightened (*jing*) because the Heart rules Blood, directly affecting psyche. In all these classical readings there is no distinction between psyche and soma: fright as fear links directly to fright as descending *qi*, emptying out the bowels. Timorousness as timidity also evokes the flutter of palpitations.

Nonetheless, Sun Simiao had stressed psychic agency in his account of female susceptibility to "disorders of [emotional] influence" (*gan bing*), where affect-laden stimuli produce internal response, as when "fierce joy attacks yang; fierce anger damages yin."[64] As for women who "are sorrowful and weepy without reason, presenting the appearance of wraiths," their resulting Hot and Dry *zang* organ system syndrome may be because "their prayers to the ancestors have not been answered."[65] In the late Song, Zhang Gao understood such illness patterns as producing from the influence of the imagination alone a sensible alteration of bodily state, just as "thoughts of sour plums makes one's mouth water . . . or feelings of sympathy or hatred make one's eyes well with tears." Thus, although the standard clinical strategy was to treat psychic and physical symptoms alike through materia medica acting on the whole organism, Song medical reflections on female illness often stressed the specific agency of emotion in an overall process. "In treating the disorders of women, if you can both treat [*zhi* = cure] their longings and desires and ease their worries, not one will fail to be healed."[66]

64. Qi Zhongfu, question 21.
65. Qi Zhongfu, question 27.
66. Zhang Gao, juan 9, 33b/34a, "Women" (*furen*).

Although Song comments on female emotion often showed sensitivity to psychic agency as well as to social circumstances circumscribing female lives, discussion of female sexual desire was more evasive, eliding morally ambiguous emotions as aspects of bodily rhythms shaped by reproductive functions. Consider, for example, the discourse that Song authorities attributed to Chu Cheng about separate therapies for widows, nuns and maidens—differentiating them from married women.[67] Chen Ziming tied their medical problems directly to the thwarting of sexual desire and reproductive function at a stage of the life cycle characterized by "ample Blood" and readiness for conception.

> Dwelling in the inner quarters, their desires germinate but lead nowhere, until yin and yang contend; now Hot, now Cold, they have the symptoms of intermittent fevers which, prolonged, lead to fatigue disorders. Blocked menses, filthy white leukorrhea, phlegm buildup, headaches, heartburn, facial moles and warts, pains in joints—these are the illnesses of widows . . . the illnesses of those with ample Blood. The Classic says: when a male's Essence is ample, he thinks of a mate; when a girl's Blood is ample she becomes pregnant.[68]

In the case of widows and nuns, medicine portrayed desire as natural in mature women while tying it closely to reproductive function. Concerning maidens, desire itself was treated as problematic. The idea that youth was a phase of the life cycle marked by ascending yang forces competed with representations of adolescent girls as delicate. Doctors warned that it was dangerous to consider the Blood of maidens as naturally Hot. The blush was medicalized in both boys and girls as a sign of the delicate emotions of puberty disturbing Blood.[69] Further, in offering a medical mediation of the gulf between puberty and socially acceptable age of marriage, doctors followed the fashionable reasoning attributed to Chu Cheng. Adolescent girls should remain sexually unaware for ten years after puberty and be married promptly thereafter. For males the ritually recommended age of marriage was thirty,

67. See Chen Ziming, juan 4, 129, and juan 6, 167–68; Zhang Gao, juan 9, 36a/36b; and Qi Zhongfu, question 47. Neither the *Siku quanshu* nor *Shuo fu* texts of Chu Cheng contain any such passages, but the belief about him was an old one. "Chu Cheng treated widows and nuns according to different principles than wives and concubines," said Tao Hongjing in his famous fifth-century *bencao*. Tao praised this as an example of prescribing according to clients' specific circumstances. Quoted in Unschuld 1986: 38.

68. Chen Ziming, juan 6, 168.

69. Chen Ziming, juan 1, 22, quoting Kou Zongshi and an anonymous Master Zhang. See Qi Zhongfu, question 12, and Kou Zongshi, *Bencao yanyi*, juan 1, in ZGYXDC 2:53.

when a man's yang is "replete" (*shi*). Here gender homology of yin yang equivalence was overridden by assumptions tying a girl's marriage to bodily ripeness for birth, while the delay recommended for males encouraged them to gain experience in sexual continence and control. Socially, such medical advice criticized youthful dissipation in sons, while warning against families' readiness to marry off daughters too early in adolescence.[70]

Similar difficulties over the meaning of female desire surrounded discussion of female sexual fantasy. "Dreams of intercourse with ghosts" was an old medical syndrome understood as a form of possession afflicting women with weak bodily defense systems and depleted inner organs, inviting invasion.[71] In classical authors like Chao Yuanfang, such dreamers were victims of supernatural agency, weeping without reason and talking to the empty air—their affliction clearly kin to types of spirit possession found in popular religion. By placing the syndrome under the category of depletion fatigue, Chen Ziming emphasized its construction around weak bodily defenses inviting the incursion of "ghost pathogens" (*xie guimei*) from without, thus underscoring wayward emotions as a tragic aspect of affliction rather than morally improper fantasy. Qi Zhongfu thought that such dreams, which could produce *jia* swellings and cases of "ghost pregnancy," were especially prevalent among the many widows and nuns of the palace.[72] This construction of illness as spirit possession rendered a woman blameless while showing her as passive. When males, usually youthful, damaged their health from seminal emissions provoked by dreams of female ghosts, they were seen as succumbing to erotic temptation.[73] Respectful of the honor of their upper class clients, medicine showed a concern for female chastity.

---

70. See Chen Ziming, juan 9, 286–87; Chu Cheng, SKQS 734:547, "Wen zi" (Questions about descendants). These ideals of age at marriage derived from the *Book of Rites,* but upper class girls in the Song probably married soon after puberty. See Ma Dazheng 1991: 194–95, on the extreme youth of imperial consorts entering the palace. Patricia Ebrey found that in her gentry sample the mean age of marriage for girls was nineteen *sui* and for boys twenty-one *sui* but that the male range of deviation from the mean was much wider. See Ebrey 1993: 74–78.

71. See Chao Yuanfang, juan 40, in ZGYXDC 2:799; Sun Simiao, *Beiji qianjin yaofang,* juan 3:51.

72. Qi Zhongfu, question 47; Chen Ziming, juan 6, 173.

73. Judith Zeitlin comments that in literary texts ghosts are female seducers of men. The opposite—women possessed by male ghostly lovers—is recorded in ethnographic literature but not in fiction. (Personal communication.)

If for certain women, like widows or nuns, desire repressed was responsible for bodily imbalance and vulnerability, for others, like maidens, desire expressed led straight to the marriage bed. Although untimely (early) arousal was criticized in both sexes as dangerous to health, in maidens normal desire was linked to "ample Blood," that is, to procreative readiness. Interestingly, though in all these ways desire was understood as an aspect of female fertility, medical authorities did not talk about female orgasm as important to successful conception. In advising clients on how to beget heirs, Chen Ziming summarized the prevailing wisdom that emphasized timeliness in terms of yin and yang forces operating both within and without the body. Within, the man's cyclical rhythms are daily, the woman's monthly, establishing for her a monthly time for fruitful intercourse just after the end of the menstrual cycle and for him a procreative hour in harmony with the ascending yang energies of early morning — between midnight and dawn. To this might be added the yin and yang force field of day and month of the calendar year, as well as the astrological influences of lucky and unlucky days presided over by various star spirits. Thus, in thinking about fertility, Song *fuke* imagined the union of yin and yang according to sexual scripts that were more cosmic than erotic. The woman's sexual body was not separated from her generative and gestational body, and desire in both sexes was naturalized as a manifestation of the intentionality of Heaven and Earth rather than psychologized as erotic pleasure. Throughout, however, where the woman's fertility was an internal bodily readiness outside of her conscious awareness, the male was assumed to be in charge of timing and in control of the coital event.

From Homology to Difference

Song medical thinkers in developing *fuke* started out with the androgynous body of yin and yang and the model of gender homology in males and females. In theory, Blood was simply bodily *qi* in its yin aspect, the same in all bodies. However, when doctors theorized that "in women Blood is the leader," in fact they produced gender difference. Applying the emerging diagnostic theories of pattern analysis to locate Blood disorders at the root of a range of internal illnesses in females, they encouraged a holistic interpretation of the human body implicating reproductive vitalities in these cases. Diagnoses like these expanded on the well-established tradition of pharmacy for fertility and gestational disorders, to encourage "separate prescriptions" for a broad spectrum of diffuse ailments in female sufferers. Holistic reasoning also encouraged a medicalization of menstruation as a process with far-reaching significance for female health and as the preeminent bodily sign of female normality.

Although diagnosticians claimed that the primacy of Blood in women matched a complementary pattern of disorders rooted in malfunctions of *qi* in males, in practice Song medicine offered no parallel discourse of "medicine for males" (*nanke*). (*Nanke*, as an approach to male sexual dysfunction in Chinese medicine today, is a modern rearrangement of the historical tradition.)[74] As a yin yang pair, Blood and *qi* were not equivalent but always related through the encompassment of Blood by *qi*, reproducing gender hierarchy. Similarly, *qi* alone stood at the apex of the yin yang system, as the unitary representative of Heaven and of creation itself.

As a multivalent concept, Blood in Song gynecology could call attention to fluid, function or rhythm in turn, and to either superficial or primal levels of body function. Blood as a bodily vitality was not merely an abstract and formless yin *qi*. Blood's function was revealed in the movement of energy along circulation channels sensed through pulse diagnosis. It worked through breast milk as well as menstruum, and other yin fluids also, like semen, or the primal Water underlying saliva or sweat. Its function was manifested through the skin that reddened in a blush or erupted in an itching rash, but also through the disordered dreams of ghostly lovers, through the wasting of depletion syndromes or the congestions and stagnations of repletion syndromes, through fright attacks and pains in bones. In sum, although Blood as a bodily vitality was never reducible to blood as a material fluid, Blood remained tied to the world of phenomenal bodily experience.

Menstruation in particular presented Blood both as generalized bodily vitality on a higher level and as a specifically female function on a lower one. As an aspect of the yin yang dyad Blood and Essence, Blood functioned as a precious reservoir of generative power in both sexes, linked to inchoate energy centers like Vital Gate and Blood Sea. Menses as monthly discharge was an outward sign of these vitalities encapsulated as a "menstrual pulse," a predictable rhythm of movement, the micro-

74. Xue Qinglu 1991, the leading bibliography of surviving historical medical works, does not use *nanke* as a classification. I discuss the development of medical advice literature for males in the sixteenth and seventeenth centuries in chapter six.

cosmic replay of lunar cycle, the "monthly pattern" (*yuejing*) that was reliable (*chang*) and dependable (*xin*).[75] Spent successfully in generative function, Blood as Essence in females as in males was a precious resource to be husbanded, nourished and used to contribute to human and cosmic creation. But if menstruation was a marker of the woman's generativity, it was also an aspect of gestation, a process completing the work of generation that was both uniquely female and medically complex. To produce an adequate *fuke* Song physicians also had to think about birth. My discussion, accordingly, turns next to what medicine had to say about the Song woman's gestational body.

75. See Chen Ziming, juan 1, 10, 17. "It is seen every thirty days, as the moon waxes and wanes." See also Qi Zhongfu, question 9.

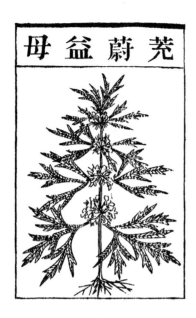

CHAPTER 3

Gestation and Birth
in Song Medicine

When Song experts in *fuke* applied pattern diagnosis to privilege Blood over *qi* in women, they produced a gynecology that modified the ideal of an androgynous body but did not intentionally break with it. Birth was another matter. Learned physicians attempted to incorporate the gestational body into their discourse by theorizing the transformations of pregnancy according to approved categories of yin yang and Five Phase reasoning. But at the same time doctors were drawn into a very different world of strategies for managing gestation and birth, where the fetus was imagined as a destabilizing intruder spirit and female blood was essentialized as unclean, requiring ritual procedures of purification and propitiation. In addition to tensions between these modes of interpreting body process, there were tensions between male and female spheres of social space in clinical relations. Thus, gestational processes did not easily fit into the holistic system of the Yellow

Emperor's ideal, and male medical authorities remained on the margins of the female sphere of birth. Birth, then, shows further how androgyny was challenged by difference. It also reveals more clearly how gender boundaries were negotiated as Song society both increasingly valorized motherhood, inviting elite healers to concern themselves with birth, and also gradually demanded a stricter sex segregation that constrained their clinical presence. Tracing the history of writing about birth also throws into sharp relief some important features of the medical system not limited to the practice of *fuke*. Here, I think, we can see more clearly how medicine was fundamentally a domestic activity carried on in the setting of the home, and how ritual was integrated into healing strategies. Moreover, texts on *chanke*—the obstetrical sphere of childbirth itself— were particularly fragmentary and changeable, showing with especial clarity how print as a mode of textuality claiming to produce public and standard forms of learning was destabilized by medicine's fluid, practice-based modes of producing knowledge.

Text and Context

"As childbirth approaches, the works of pharmacy have little to say."[1] This observation, which introduced a late Song handbook on parturition, encapsulates the ambiguous relation of literate medicine to the female sphere of childbirth. If pre-Song *fuke* was a minor aspect of medicine even in its learned form of prescriptions for pregnancy and postpartum, the management of labor and delivery appears to have lain outside the male medical mainstream altogether. It is true that from early imperial times popular stories told of obstructed labors cured by famous physicians, but typically the doctor was called by the woman's husband at the last minute in a life-threatening situation, and his emergency remedy involved acupuncture.[2] More often, classical medical

1. *Chanru beiyao* (Essentials for Childbirth Readiness), an anonymous handbook of the eleventh or twelfth century. For a history of the text, see Okanishi Tameto 1948: 504.

2. A famous early tale was of Hua Tuo, a semilegendary physician said to have lived in the third century C.E. He was called in by a General Li, whose wife had given birth to a stillborn baby. Reading her pulse, he declared that a second dead fetus was still inside and ordered acupuncture and a herbal infusion, which successfully delivered her of the twin. Some read this account from the dynastic history of the Three Kingdoms as implying he used manual or even surgical techniques, but others see this as an example of the magical arts of the *fang shi*. See Chen Bangxian 1982: 72.

masters alluded to esoteric ritual matters. In the sixth and seventh centuries, Sun Simiao and Chao Yuanfang advised parturient women to ensure safe delivery by observing unspecified techniques (*chan fa*) and procedures (*shu fa*). They were alluding to ritual precautions such as "the days of sojourning and the prohibitions concerning taboo days."[3] Their own chapters on *fuke* did not discuss these procedures or the birth process in detail.

A number of anonymous Sui and Tang works dealing exclusively with birth (*chan*), like the Sui *Birth Classic* (*Chanjing*) and the late Tang *Birth Book* (*Chan shu*), are partially known today from scattered excerpts preserved elsewhere. Those fragments that survive suggest that shortly before the dawn of print culture, handwritten manuscripts on birth circulated that combined elaborate ritual instructions with a repertory of herbal prescriptions and home remedies to assist labor and postpartum recovery.[4] Of this genre, only Zan Yin's *Birth Treasury* (*Chan bao*), an herbal from the ninth century whose contents were confined to pharmacy, made its way into print in the Song.[5] Other lost works known in surviving bibliographies simply by the generic title "Birth Chart" (*chan tu*) were classified under divination (*wu xing*), not medicine, and were probably purely ritual in nature. While this fragmentary record suggests to us today a rich lost world of folklore, religious belief and practical skills, most of it represents scattered debris that the Song architects of medical orthodoxy left behind.

It also points up how far printing, the new Song technology of transmission, gradually came to shape the contours of "tradition" as understood in late imperial China as well as in our own day. Throughout the Song dynasty, printed medical books, which were heavily state sponsored, represented only a small fraction of the knowledge and practice that continued as before to be transmitted orally or through handwritten

3. Chao Yuanfang, juan 43, 809–10; Sun Simiao, *Beiji qianjin yaofang*, juan 2, 30.

4. A comprehensive survey of surviving Han to Tang writings is in Lee Jen-der 1996. Most, like those preserved in the tenth-century Japanese encyclopedia *Ishinpo*, originally compiled by Tamba Yasuyori, dropped out of circulation in China even before the Song. The *Birth Classic* was already virtually unknown by the end of the Tang; the *Birth Book* circulated enough during the Song to be quoted by several authorities, then disappeared as an independent work. See also He Shixi 1984; and Ma Dazheng 1991: 101–5, 132–34.

5. A Sichuanese, Zan Yin was said to have attracted the patronage of the Provincial Viceroy, who consulted him about the high number of miscarriages among the women of his household. Zan offered his compilation to the official, who disseminated it. No editions of this work were published between the Song dynasty and the nineteenth century, and modern versions are based on a Northern Song handwritten text preserved in Japan. See Ma Jixing 1990: 134–35; and Okanishi Tameto 1948: 483–84.

manuscripts used by healers and householders. The few obstetrical books that survive — because someone printed them — lead me to consider the emergence of the public text itself as part of the story of how *fuke* became a tradition of learned medicine.[6] These works bear the marks of earlier (and perennial) modes of communication. Surviving printed texts vary in content and even in title; the genre is often that of "discourse" (*lun*), or oral instructions written down. Authorship is ambiguous. Stories about the works suggest they were preserved by happenstance. Yang Zijian's "Ten Topic Discourse on Birth" (*Shi chan lun*) (which may at times have been seven or fifteen topics) was said to have been written down when a practitioner visiting an aristocratic household was invited to stay and discuss his art with the local literati.[7] The twelfth-century *Childbirth Treasury Collection* (*Chanyu baoqing ji*) was printed after a practitioner persuaded a court physician to add prescriptions to make his "discourse" more valuable, that is, more learned. *Useful Prescriptions Ready-Made to Assist in Birth* (*Bei chan ji yong fang*) was published in 1140 when a literatus named Yu Chong decided to make the handbook written for (by?) the women in his family more widely available.[8]

Although all of these works were practical bedside manuals, none circulated in published forms after the fall of the Song dynasty. The last two works may have survived because the late Southern Song official who published an anthology of *fuke* and *erke* produced such a model of fine printing that copies were preserved in the libraries of several bibliophile collectors.[9] On the other hand, works by Chen Yi and Qi Zhongfu, now thought of as Song *fuke* classics, were probably passed down in handwritten copies by generations of family practitioners before they began to be circulated in printed form in the sixteenth century, not always under the presumed original author's name.[10] Only Chen

6. For the history of printing in the Song, see Chia 1996 and Cherniack 1994.

7. In *Yi yuan*, 1875; preface by Zhang Shengdao dated 1025. This anonymous compilation of rare medical works exists only in manuscript. I have examined the copy in the rare book library of the Zhongyi Yanjiuyuan in Beijing.

8. This date is estimated in Ma Jixing 1990: 223.

9. Zhu Duanzhang 1184, *Weishengjia bao chanke beiyao* (Essentials on Childbirth Preparedness from the Treasury of the House of Good Health). This anthology was compiled from works in Zhu's family library and published while he was an official in Nankang, Fujian. I consulted the reprint in the *Shiwanjuan lou congshu*, published in 1876 and held by the Zhongyi Yanjiuyuan in Beijing. For a history of the text see Okanishi Tameto 1948: 516–17.

10. A *fuke* attributed to Chen Yi was printed by a nineteenth-generation descendant in Ming Hangzhou. See Ma Dazheng 1991: 183–84; He Shixi 1991, 2:412–13. Another example is *Chan bao baiwen* (One Hundred Question Birth Treasury), 5

Ziming's *All-Inclusive Good Prescriptions for Women*, which incorporated material from many of the aforementioned compilations, preserved aspects of Song *chanke* as part of a continuous printed tradition. This fluid identity is well illustrated by the *Childbirth Treasury Collection* attributed to Guo Jizhong and Li Shisheng.[11] In later centuries, this was the best known Song obstetrical text and also the one that engaged most directly with medical theories of the time. But Li's preface, dated 1131, calls attention to the fact that in his day medical writings were still most likely to be private manuscripts kept for family use, more like household notebooks or collections of recipes than like public documents:

> I have collected a discourse of twenty-one topics on childbirth. Its views are subtle and sound, and nothing is left unexamined. In general, the doctors with national degrees print elegant books on pharmacy. Alas, [my work] has discourse [*lun*] but no prescriptions. The worthy Guo Jizhong, a famous doctor of the age, is especially expert in childbirth, so that his reading of the pulse and use of medicines have produced some remarkable results. He has expressed his willingness to use his family's collected prescriptions in an appendix to these discourses, making a more perfect whole. Truly the compilation will be an unusual book of benefit to all. Ancients tell us that the man who does not study medicine is not filial, and so there have been prescriptions and [medical] discourses that were not transmitted to the world. How can this be called humane?[12]

This work was known under several titles, identified sometimes with one and sometimes with both authors. Song sources suggest that some

---

juan. This is a variant of Qi Zhongfu's text attributed to more famous Yuan and Ming doctors, Zhu Zhenheng and Wang Kentang. Ma Jixing (226) believes that the late Ming publishers borrowed these famous names to make sales. I have also seen a three-juan version at the Library of Congress, with an undated preface claiming to be by Wang Kentang.

11. Guo Jizhong and Li Shisheng 1131, *Chanyu baoqing ji [fang]*, 2 juan. For the history of the many lost variants of this text see Ma Jixing 1990: 220, and prefaces collected in Okanishi Tameto 1948: 495–97. I have examined versions preserved in *ce* 6 of the medical anthology *Danggui caotang yixue congshu* and in Zhu Duanzhang's anthology, both of which include prescriptions in a second juan and modify the title accordingly. In his 1220 preface to *Nüke baiwen*, Qi Zhongfu referred to a work by Guo and Li consisting of twenty-one topics without the addition of prescriptions. This is suggestive concerning the form in which the earlier versions may have circulated.

12. See Okanishi Tameto 1948: 496. The same version of the preface is found in Zhu Duanzhang's anthology, thought to be the earliest surviving edition. This preface does not really distinguish between the manuscripts of hereditary family practitioners and those kept by private householders, but suggests the novelty of committing either sort of document to print. According to Chen Yuan-peng many surviving Song works on pharmacy were the work of "gentlemen admirers of medicine" who published family collections as a humanitarian enterprise. See Chen Yuan-peng 1997: 151–59.

now-lost early versions incorporated Zan Yin's *Birth Treasury* or Yang Zijian's "Ten Topics." Surviving versions include a second juan of miscellaneous prescriptions and advice for new mothers, added by some anonymous compiler. One surviving version, preserved in the early Ming Yongle imperial encyclopedia, also interpolates criticisms of many of the original "discourses" by a well-known later master of pharmacy, Chen Yan. Chen's criticisms appeared in his own work, *Prescriptions for the Three Types of Disorder* (*San yin fang*), compiled in 1174, and must have been added later to some Li-Guo text by someone else.[13]

The point here is not that the surviving texts are corrupt, as China's own eighteenth-century encyclopedists later put it in the *Siku quanshu*, but that Song knowledge about birth particularly resisted identification with an original "authentic" text or author. Rooted as it was in practice and passed on from person to person in clinical settings, the learning that shaped the management of birth remained fluid and its textualization malleable. Generations of later practitioners claimed Song origins for their expertise, but they did so on the basis of lineage affiliations, not by reading Song books. Of course, all kinds of Song medical publications drew upon the oral and written informal learning of practitioners. But in the case of *chanke*, no Song printed text ever came to represent a superior source of authority.

In sum, the predominantly female domain surrounding childbirth was particularly resistant to modes of knowing of the sort easily codified in print. When thinking about the gestational body in particular, I see literate medicine embedded in a cosmology and a culture of daily life that shaped its meaning, and in traditions of healing carried on within families. Traces of this show in the way Song writings on obstetrics concern themselves with ritual as well as pharmaceutical issues, with concrete symptoms and techniques of delivery as well as the repertory of cosmological speculation that the gestational body inspired in learned physicians. These writings are a flotsam surviving the wreckage of time, allowing long-standing practices to emerge into historical visibility. Still, Song concerns with textuality were not merely a matter of recordkeeping. As medicine was becoming a self-consciously literary discourse seeking to locate knowledge in authoritative, public, printed classics, it was also drawing closer to the problems of birth. Thus literate healers found themselves in enhanced positions of authority concerning gestation and delivery.

Classically trained doctors were learning to see themselves as masters

13. Ma Jixing 1990: 220; Okanishi Tameto 1948: 498.

of a learned technology with life-saving powers, superior not only to those of *wu* shamans but of uneducated "medical craftsmen" (*yi gong*) or Daoist healers (*Daoshi*) as well. But birth, like death, also made Song doctors think of fate — of things beyond the power of medicine to influence, and then of the fate of women, whom they saw as bound to reproductive necessity. A particularly famous statement came from Zhou Ting, early Northern Song editor of Zan Yin's herbal, whom Chen Ziming quoted in full to introduce his own advice on childbirth:

> "Male and female unite essences and *qi* is divided into yin and yang.[14] In reaching this goal the female is weakened, and her illnesses are quite frequent. Her natural endowment is frail because she has ordinary viscera within, yet in carrying a child through pregnancy she must be guided by constant norms. As for her food and drink, activity and rest, she is to observe many prohibitions and to restrain her emotions. When delivery approaches few can keep calm; this injures and wracks *zang* and *fu* organ systems; it shakes and damages bones and sinews. If any matter goes amiss, illness and calamity soon appear. Add to this ignorant doctors, who make her down many medicines until she is sorely afflicted, bringing her to the point of danger day by day until she is almost dead! Isn't this grievous! Of old the *Changes* said that the great virtue of Heaven and Earth is life, so we know that human birth is the foundation of natural order. So how can it be fated that birth puts human life at risk?"[15]

Here the Song doctor was asking existential questions about the place of suffering in a supposedly beneficent universe, while pointing to the doctor's mission of relief. In thinking of the "difficulty" of curing women, Zhou spoke specifically of the burden of repeated childbearing: "After two or three births, their Blood and *qi* are not yet weakened . . . but after four, five, or even as many as seven or eight times, the damage is grave." He counted nursing as a further drain in "commoner families" where mothers did this themselves.

The Song discourse on obstetrics took off from Zhou Ting's view of birth as both a natural process and a medical crisis mandating intervention. Doctors did not use a disease model, asking whether pregnancy and parturition were normally healthy processes or a kind of illness. When thinking of the natural they thought of a process like cosmo-

14. This refers to conception: unitary Heavenly *qi* is divided into yin and yang. This cosmogonic sequence is also the first in the creation of new human life.

15. Zhou Ting (fl. 982), preface to Zan Yin. See Chen Ziming, juan 16, 441–43. Though this edition of Zan Yin was lost, Zhou's preface was reprinted separately from the text in a number of places. See also Okanishi Tameto 1948: 485.

genesis, where over time Heaven and Earth achieve completion, extending life in the world. When thinking of this work as a human labor, they imagined a gradually accumulating deficit, the outcome of the necessary work of a mother's gestational body effecting the transfer of life from one concrete form to another. The female body in question was not weakened because it embodied any fixed biological essence, but in proportion to that labor as a function of time and use. Here medicine's limited offerings consisted both of remedies for specific dysfunctions and of technologies to protect and restore vitality and strengthen resistance. At the same time doctors allowed room for ritual practices from outside the sphere of classical healing that mediated birth's darker risks. In sum, birth had meaning in Song medicine as cosmogonic sign, as a bodily crisis needing symptom management, and as a ritual life transition. It justified medical paternalism, and made the goal of "good doctors" to help women cope with their allotted destiny, not change it.

Gestation and Birth: Time and Ritual

From the *Imperial Grace Formulary* to Chen Ziming, the surviving Song medical writings on *chanke* show a fascination with gestation and birth as a microcosmic enactment of the processes of creativity and change shaping all phenomena in the universe. Concern with birth as a clinical problem gained dignity when birth was considered as a replication of cosmogenesis according to the teachings of philosophical and religious classics. Song interpreters could turn to the Han philosopher Huainanzi's venerable account of the "ten months of pregnancy," which made the closely observed gestating woman's body into a sign linked to Daoist accounts of Creation—by which existence emerges from nonexistence as "One creates Two, Two creates Three, and Three creates the myriad things."[16] The emperor Huizong's eleventh-century *Canon of Sagely Benefaction* combined other accounts based on Daoist

16. *Huainanzi,* juan 7, "Jingshen," links creation and gestation this way: "The spirit [*jingshen*] is received from Heaven and physical form is the endowment of Earth. So it is said that One creates Two, Two creates Three, and Three creates the myriad things. All things are yin behind and yang in front. With the effusion of *qi* they unite. So it is said that in the first month there is a blob of fat, in the second a thread, and in the third a fetus [*tai*]. In the fourth month there are pulses, in the fifth sinews, in the sixth bone. In the seventh month [the fetus] is fully formed, in the eighth it is active, in the ninth it is boisterous, and in the tenth it is born."

traditions with Five Phase theory and a cosmological calendar that mapped the eight basic trigrams of the *Book of Changes* onto the sexagenary cycle of Heavenly Stems and Earthly Branches. Evoking the primal creativity of the Dao, gestation was figured as a potter's molding of clay or an alchemist's molding of metal. The ten months of prenatal development began with the Phase of Water, shaping the Kidney system first. Kidney was the primary embodied repository of primordial *qi*, identified with the Vital Gate, while the development of later fetal morphology proceeded in accordance with overlapping emblems of time and space: the abstract time figured in the order of the trigrams, the human calendar and directional coordinates of the Stems and Branches.[17]

If Huizong's version of gestation drew on the most exuberant cosmological numerology of Song metaphysics, a different set of deeply spiritualistic views left traces in the shamanistic pediatric manual the *Fontanelle Classic* (*Luxing jing*). Fetal life was successively animated by spirits (*shen*) and souls (*ling*) from an eclectic popular pantheon. There were the three *hun* souls in the third month and the seven *po* souls in the fourth month, followed by the spirits of the five *zang* organ systems in the fifth month, the navel anima (*qi ziling*) in the sixth, and the primal spirit (*yuan shen*) in the eighth. Here, flocking to take their places in the fetus, mingled the ancient Daoist spirit-denizens of the bodily microcosm, the anima (*ling*) of the reincarnated Buddhist soul, and the ethereal (*hun*) and material (*po*) aspects of the ancestral spirits worshipped in mortuary rituals.[18] Still other accounts, identified by Chen Ziming with the "sayings of venerable grannies," organized gestation around what midwives might have seen or felt—the morphology of aborted fetuses in the earlier months and fetal movement in the later ones.

In considering this lively repertory, Chen Ziming wrote as a reformer, rejecting the spiritualistic views of "Buddhist books" and "old shamans" on the one hand, and the "vulgarities" of "old woman" midwife practitioners on the other. At the same time he criticized the emperor Huizong for preferring Daoist philosophy to the orthodox Han dynasty cosmology of symbolic correlations. Chen preferred the model of the "ten months of pregnancy" offered by the medieval medical mas-

17. Huizong, *Sheng ji jing*, juan 2, 38–41. These pages were not quoted by Chen Ziming.

18. The *Fontanelle Classic* was excerpted in Liu Fang, comp., *You you xin shu* (New Book on Caring for the Young), a twelfth-century pediatric encyclopedia. See juan 2, 22. Chen Ziming, juan 10, 304, quotes a variant text. Huizong, *Sheng ji jing*, juan 2, 40, offers yet another version of the same genre.

ters Sun Simiao and Chao Yuanfang—a model that privileged the Yellow Emperor's symbolism of yin yang and the Five Phases working on the development of *zang* and *fu* organ systems through the action of the cardinal channels. Chen offered this model in *All-Inclusive Good Prescriptions for Women* as orthodox, "in accordance with the Classics."[19] (See figure 4.)

In this version each of the ten months is a cycle of change, moving from yin to yang poles and working through all the Five Phases. Fetal development occurs as primordial *qi* concentrates on each cardinal channel in turn, shaping *zang* and *fu* organ systems from inner to outer functions and body parts. A certain amount of empirical observation lay in the background of Chao and Sun's depiction of the gestational process: *pei* and *gao*—inchoate fatty blobs of the first two months—give way in the third month to *tai*, a human form with recognizable genitalia, preserving some of the English-language distinction between embryo and fetus. But in contrast to classical European accounts, Chen Ziming's ten months of pregnancy neither illustrated anatomy nor established a moment of "quickening" at which "descent of soul" occurs. In the occasional crude drawings added to popular texts, the developing fetus was carelessly rendered.[20] What mattered was the sequence of ten stages, calling attention to cycles of time, to the regularity and predictability of an ideal normal period of growth.

In this construction of gestation life in some basic sense begins at conception—so that at birth a person's age in Chinese count (*sui*) is already one year. Nonetheless, the yang moment of beginning is counterbalanced by the longer yin process of completion, and the embryo's value as life is a latent and potential one, to be actualized only gradually as gestation, birth and infancy lead to one's realization as a human descendant and ancestor-to-be. Although gestation takes place in a yin female body, the fetus is yang by virtue of its dynamic energy of growth, and the *qi* responsible for the developmental transitions of the ten months is Essence—the creative aspect of primary vitalities. In sum, the ten months of pregnancy taught about Nature and normality, giving

19. See Chen Ziming, juan 10, 303–5; Chao Yuanfang, juan 41, 803–4; Sun Simiao, *Beiji qianjin yaofang*, juan 2, 20–24.

20. I have no Song examples of pictorial representations. A Tang version found in the *Ishinpo* portrays the full figure of a naked woman, marking the governing cardinal channels month by month as well as a fetus in the belly. Late imperial drawings focus on the fetus independent of the body carrying it, but in no case is the fetus itself rendered with any care.

Month	Chen Ziming after Chao Yuantang			The Fontanelle Classic	"Venerable Grannies"
	Name	Phase	Organ/Channel Activated		
1	始胚 Embryonic Mud	yin and yang unite	Liver and Zujueyin channel	a pulse (mai)	a pearl of dew
2	始膏 Embryonic Fat	Essence matures	Gall and Zushaoyang channel	the fetus (tai) forms	a peach flower
3	始胎 Fetus Begins	the inner responds to the outer environment	Heart and Shoushaoyin channel	the yang spirit (shen) makes the three hun souls	male and female differentiate
4	始受水 Phase of Water	Essence acts to form blood	Triple Burners and Shoushaoyang channel	the yin anima (ling) makes the seven po souls	physical form is visible
5	始受火 Phase of Fire	Essence acts to form qi	Spleen and Zutaiyin channel	the Five phases differentiate and the five zang organ systems receive their guardian spirits (shen)	sinews and bones are formed
6	始受金 Phase of Metal	Essence acts to form sinews	Stomach and Zuyangming channel	the six musical notes are set and the navel receives its anima (ling)	hair grows
7	始受木 Phase of Wood	Essence acts to form bones	Lung and Shoutaiyin channel	Essence opens the apertures circulating light	the hun soul wanders and the child moves its left hand
8	始受土 Phase of Earth	Essence acts to form skin	Bowels and Shouyangming channel	the Primal Spirit (yuan shen) is ready; the true anima descends	the po soul wanders and the child moves its right hand
9	始受石 Phase of Stone	Essence acts to form hair	Kidney and Zushaoyin channel	the palace chamber is arranged for birth	thrice-turning-body moves about
10	All faculties ready	organ systems are complete and interconnected and the faculties of consciousness are ready		qi is sufficient; all form is manifest, and the Primal Principal within the head called the Mud Terrace gathers all the spirits together	qi is sufficient

Figure 4. The ten months of gestation: three Song views

gestation spiritual significance without recourse to the supernaturalism of popular religious views. Chen Ziming's imprimatur made this account a staple in the repertory of *fuke* and *chanke* thereafter.

However much the ten months of pregnancy might inspire or reassure as natural philosophy, clinical guidelines came from somewhere else. Qi Zhongfu's popular text—organized around questions and answers designed to help women interrogate their sensations and symptoms—constructed a pattern of change over the ten months based on a reading of female bodily experience. First of all, Qi's questions lumped the first two months together as a period of menstrual irregularity when she "hopes to be pregnant" but cannot be sure. Only in the third month have menses ceased (*ju jing*).[21] Then it is possible to understand why she feels "irritable and depressed [*xin zhong fenmen*], apathetic and listless, nauseated at the smell of food." Then also it is possible to speak of miscarriage. Subsequent questions suggest no monthly rhythms but speak of fetal movement, fetal fullness, fetal cold, fetal distress, fetal hiccups/belching, fetal incontinence and fetal fits—of the fetus as an inchoate internal presence experienced in terms of bodily derangements in the mother, progressively more vehement. These, as well as the unpredictable bouts of acute illness (fevers or dysenteries), may portend the random disaster of miscarriage. Qi's narrative took up the monthly passage of time again only when "in the eighth or ninth month both feet swell up."[22] Only after this point did Qi Zhongfu quote the classical account of gestation, unabridged, in the language of Chao Yuanfang and Sun Simiao. A user of the handbook, now on the verge of delivery, could turn to question seventy-eight ("What are the pregnant woman's ten months of gestation?") as way of summing up the process as a whole. To read about it here was to reflect on her body's contribution to the grand design of classical cosmology.

By contrast, the interrogation of symptoms suggested the unstable relationship of host and guest. Prescriptions were needed to tranquilize the fetus (*an tai*), stabilize the fetus (*gu tai*), or, as delivery approached, to shrink the fetus (*shou tai*) and make the fetus slippery (*hua tai*), while in the course of delivery itself labor-hastening (*cui sheng*) formulas

21. *Ju jing* is a technical term from the *Canon of the Pulse* for three months of interrupted menses. Sometimes the term was used to describe a type of amenorrhoea, but Qi here suggests that the three months' cessation of menstruation should be taken to signify pregnancy.

22. Qi Zhongfu, questions 54, 57–59, 77.

shared place with those that evacuated postpartum material. Here the body's spatial volume and physical structure were important, and drug action addressed physical mechanics more than holistic functions. Moreover, the gravest danger—miscarriage—meant that the many materia medica with a moving action on Blood or fluids were believed dangerous, as were bitterly cooling ingredients. Here "separate prescriptions" meant fewer medicines, not more, and the list of drugs prohibited in pregnancy was long. Chen Ziming offered a catalogue of fifty-nine in seven-character couplets, one of the many popularizations of this vital information.[23] Clinical strategies, then, addressed symptoms without relating processes to cosmology or time's rhythms and made only limited use of pattern diagnosis.

But there was yet another kind of time available for thinking about pregnancy and birth—ritual time based on days, months and years of the natural universe. This ritual time was calculated by astrological and divinatory calendars—constructions designed to bridge the chasm between the orderly sequence of heavenly bodies and the unpredictability of human event. Recorded in imperial calendars and farmers' almanacs, calculated by priests and diviners, time like this was not for contemplation only, but to pattern human activities in court and country—everything from the emperor's ritual schedule to the farmer's cropping season, the orientation of buildings or graves, and the calculation of marriage horoscopes. It was also deployed in a ritual obstetrics that profoundly shaped Song women's experience of childbirth.[24]

"Heaven is round and Earth is square," went the classical aphorism,[25] which also explained the design of the diviner's calendar and the geomancer's compass. The birthing woman—here representing Humanity and completing the triad—was enjoined to place herself according to the ritual "positions and directions" (*fang wei*) in proper relation to the cosmic influences of Heaven, Earth and Humanity bearing on the time and place of her delivery. All three were representationally linked through the names of ritual numbers: the Twelve Heavenly Stems (*tian*

23. Chen Ziming, juan 11, 325–26. Ma Dazheng notes that the number of materia medica deemed unsafe in pregnancy expanded steadily over the centuries between Song and Ming, beyond what he believes was reasonable. See 158.

24. In what follows I rely mostly on the accounts in medical texts, particularly Chen Ziming, the *Taiping sheng hui fang,* and Huizong's *Sheng ji jing,* supplemented by the very helpful discussion of traditional Chinese birth customs in Guo Licheng 1979. I thank Dorothy Ko for calling Guo's work to my attention.

25. This can be found in many sources, including the *Liji, Huainanzi* and the *Su wen.* It linked the round dome of Heaven with the human head, and the square Earth with human feet.

gan) and the Ten Earthly Branches (*di zhi*), which could indicate degrees of space as well as time. Stems and branches marked each of the points of the compass on square earth, the encircling degrees of the night sky and the cyclical periods of solar and lunar year, and also the months and years of an individual human life. This last was measured not by the public calendar of history and dynasties (which also used the same signs in the sexagenary sequence of dates) but by an individual calendar (*xing nian*) which ran from the sign of origin at *zi,* the hour of each person's conception, to the time of death.[26] Thus the fate and destiny of an individual life were imagined through the interlocking correspondence of stem and branch signs emblematic of time, space and personal history.

Superimposed upon these abstract cosmological coordinates of "number" was the less symmetrical but powerful influence of Chinese astrology: of stars, wandering planets, comets or meteors, and the sky spirits from archaic myths that populated the Chinese zodiac. Thus the moon in the course of the solar year inhabits twelve distinct "palaces," each the site of a specific conjunction with the sun. Thirteen potentially malevolent star spirits, such as Thunder Lord, Heavenly Dog or White Tiger, dwell in the lunar palace in turn, marking the direction the parturient woman must avoid or risk offending spirits capable of harming her and her child. On the other hand, auspicious sky spirits were thought to dwell in the opposite and complementary direction, as a yin yang pair in celestial geography, marking the desirable orientation of her body for spiritual aid in safe delivery.[27]

In addition to gods and celestial spirits, the discontented spirits of the dead on earth could bring harm. For pregnant women in particular, the spirit world was populated with ghostly fetuses, those which had miscarried or aborted or been stillborn or killed at birth. These might haunt the gestating woman, as an evil doppelgänger to the child within or as a spirit from an earlier failed birth returning to blight her later pregnancy, inflicting agony in labor or delivering monsters.[28] In another

26. Huizong, *Sheng ji jing*, 30–31, explains it this way: the moment of conception is marked by the first of the twelve Earthly Branch signs, *zi*. It is identified with due north and the moment of creation, and each month of life thereafter proceeds through the sexagenary sequence in order, males proceeding left (counterclockwise) and females right (clockwise). *Zi* also is the ideograph for "child" in the sense of son and descendant.

27. *Taiping sheng hui fang*, 2422–25; Chen Ziming, juan 16, 448–50.

28. Liu Jingzhen 1995 discusses Song popular beliefs about infant abandonment, infanticide (*sun zi*), and fetal spoilage intentional and unintentional. In the Buddhist morality tales Liu cites, no distinction is drawn between the spirits from early and late abortion, or between these and dead infants. Buddhism in valuing reverence for life does not bound its form, and also implies that no death is final.

construction, a "wandering fetus killer" (*you tai sha*) shadowed the pregnant woman at home, taking up lodging about the house in a set itinerary, moving from bed to door to window to privy and altar. It was important to take precautions to avoid injuring this spirit, and to use "positions and directions" to evade it.[29] In a world where damage and spoilage threatened fetal life and where infants were often abandoned or killed at birth, fetus ghosts had a special place in the supernatural transactions of karma. In popular lore such karmic debt operated impersonally, independent of questions of human blame. Nonetheless, retribution worked through the mother's body.[30]

Chen Ziming and other Song authorities on obstetrics did not need to explain to their clients the deep structure of ritual calendars or of supernatural agency. They simply gave women practical instructions on how to determine their auspicious "positions and directions" by consulting a set of birth charts (*chan tu*). (See figure 5.) Twelve monthly graphs identified the auspicious and inauspicious directions, including the month-by-month position of the thirteen malevolent sky spirits (*shisan sha shen*). The chart specific to the month of birth itself guides the placement of couch, curtains and even the door of the room where a woman lies for labor and delivery, while the auspicious event of the burial of the placenta should be oriented in the opposite and complementary direction. In addition, a woman's personal calendar, determined by the time of her own birth, would identify further highly inauspicious days of unfavorable months when she should take special care to observe every precaution. Using these calculations she was urged to make sure that the sight of her laboring orifices not offend the spirit world, and that the blood, feces and urine evacuated during postpartum recovery not defile the ground.

29. See Chen Ziming, juan 11, 322–24. Chen gives three systems for tracking the location of the wandering fetus killer—one according to lunar seasons, one according to Heavenly Stems and Earthly Branches, and one attributed to the Grand Astrologers' Office (*Tai shi ju*) at court. Twentieth-century ethnographers have observed similar beliefs in a *tai xin* or *tai shen*, which shares the house with a pregnant woman and can seek revenge for injuries inflicted on the structure by careless use of knives, hammering a nail in the wall, etc. Chen Ziming's list of precautions are virtually identical.

30. Liu Jingzhen 1995. The Japanese *mizuko* sacrifices to the spirits of dead fetuses are an old popular Buddhist expression of the workings of karma and of the tie between mothers and unborn young. *Mizuko* today are rituals of atonement for abortion that also propitiate potentially vengeful ghosts. The complex of folk beliefs about fetuses found in these Song settings suggests similar Buddhist orientations in traditional China, although there is no Chinese Buddhist ritual parallel to the *mizuko*, and the Bodhisattva Ti Tsang in China is not, like his Japanese counterpart Jiso, the patron deity of fetus ghosts. See LaFleur 1992.

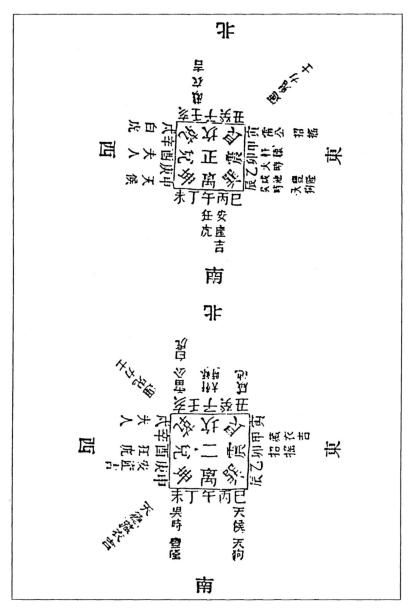

Figure 5. This chart shows the positions and directions for a birth that takes place during the first two lunar months. In the first month (the top figure) the auspicious direction for parturition is facing south, with the burial of the placenta oriented toward the north. Other signs mark the location of stars and planets identified with such spirits as "Heavenly Dog," "Thunder Lord" and "White Tiger." From Zhu Duanzhang, *Weishengjia bao chanke beiyao* (Essentials on Childbirth Preparedness from the Treasury of the House of Good Health), first published in 1184.

All of these instructions marked birth as a dangerous and polluting event that should take place in a carefully segregated space, paying attention to external influences identified with the supernatural world. The risks to the mother extended to the child, and to persons who might come into contact with her at this time. Throughout the entire postpartum month of seclusion and further precautions, the new mother's blood and body wastes continued to be sources of pollution, liable to offend the gods, bringing retribution on her head. The ritual segregation ended only as her afterbirth blood flow ceased, with the burial of the newborn's placenta, also according to the appropriate positions and directions. Its careful storage and disposal protected the child from harm that might result from violence done to this physical residue of its fetal tie with the mother's life. The complementary relationship of the "positions and directions" of the birth and the placenta burial figured the mother-child interdependence and gradual separation. From beginning to end, this was the month of birth (*zuo yue*) — a period of ritual liminality and danger strongly shaped by the taboos surrounding birth blood and newborn infants. Doctors advised one hundred days' rest for full physical recovery, rationalized in terms of the mother's physical health, and complained that women considered thirty ritually charged days "enough."[31]

How do we explain the complex ritual obstetrics that is such a striking aspect of Song medical lore? One possible reading is to consider these as obsolete practices preserved in writing in a spirit of pious conservatism. Certainly it is clear that the paper trail on birth rituals was very old. Chen Ziming, Yu Chong, Zhu Duanzhang and others cited not only the *Imperial Grace Formulary* but also pre-Tang traditions preserved in Wang Xi's eighth-century medical encyclopedia *Essential Secrets of the Palace Library (Wai tai mi yao)*. Today we can trace the ritual burial of the child's placenta back to texts on birth from the second century B.C.E., recently discovered in the Mawangdui tomb complex in Hunan province. There the placenta-burial site, named Yu's storehouse (*Yu zang*), refers to an archaic legend in which the legendary sage emperor taught the ritual to a woman whose babies had all died in infancy.[32] Notwith-

---

31. See Ma Dazheng 1991: 62, quoting the *Xiao pin fang*, an early pharmaceutical work. A full month's postpartum rest is still commonly recommended for new mothers in China today.

32. *Mawangdui Han mu bo shu* 4:126,134. The editors say the text is close to that of the *Chanjing*, known today from its excerpts in the *Ishinpo*. The legend concerning Yu is repeated in this latter source.

standing this antique legacy, the flexibility of Song *chanke* in itself is evidence that texts were written down for use in a variety of ways. Yu Chong instructed women to write out the appropriate birth chart data and post it on the north wall of the birthing room, arranging bed, curtains and door accordingly. He included a "twelve-month chart for auspicious and inauspicious directions for birth, for bed, and for placenta storage."[33] Chen Ziming's instructions allowed for simplifying the positions and directions using short cuts of a certain Master Ti Xuanxi. At other times he reminded his readers to take special pains, such as making extra computations if they faced birth in a "intercalary period" of the lunar year.[34]

It was a practical matter, then, this organization of obstetrics around ritual time and space, controlled through attention to "positions and directions." As practice it existed side by side with more purely social rituals surrounding birth. Among these were the labor-hastening gift (*cui chan li*): flower-covered baskets crammed with good luck buns and auspicious painted duck eggs, sent to the expectant mother by her natal family. There was also the third-day bath, where the infant was ritually cleansed and presented to kin, and—most elaborate in rich families— the one-month washing ceremony (*xi er hui*), in which, after the infant was bathed in a silver basin, older women threw trinkets in the water and urged the girls present to retrieve them as fertility charms.[35]

Like the childbirth *fang wei,* these women's rituals surrounding the new infant could be understood medically as well as socially and religiously. Good luck buns were narcotic, easing pain by inducing sleep; the baby's first washing in medicinal water warded off skin eruptions; the one-month bath cleansed the child of its residual fetal hair. Altogether they constructed a complex passage leading through the polluted and dangerous trial of birth to brighter celebrations as the infant matured enough to discard the bodily remnants of its fetal stages and be recognized by kin as a social descendant. Like the social ethos built around gift-giving and feasting among kin, the cosmology underlying divination and geomancy was "popular" in a catholic rather than folk sense—the cultural property of elites as well as masses. Song medical

33. Yu Chong, 2a, 13b/14b.

34. Chen Ziming, juan 16, 448–49, 457. To reconcile the lunar and solar years, the old calendar introduced seven intercalary periods over nineteen years. I am guessing that the thirteenth star spirit may have presided over these intercalary periods. Chen warned that the standard charts by month are inaccurate at these times.

35. See Wu Baoqi 1989: 39–45.

experts in obstetrics were conversant with this world of belief and contributed to it, less by a rationalistic medicalization of procedures otherwise understood in religious or ritual terms than by including health among the benefits that ritual confers.

In thinking about birth and rituals, Chen Ziming and other literate healers were seeking a middle path. They were students of the subject in order to discriminate between alternatives: "The teachings on fetal education and the birth charts are not to be dismissed, nor are they to be followed dogmatically."[36] Some practices met with their disapproval. Yu Chong warned that "old ladies have many different customs in connection with delivery," which he advised his readers to ask about in advance,[37] while Chen Ziming observed that "when the wandering fetus killer is inside the house there is no need to position bed and curtains according to the positions and directions or to sweep out the dwelling."[38]

All this showed that "among the common people and those who follow unorthodox ways the practice of avoidances and prohibitions is not according to decorum." Beyond proper ritual lay a penumbra of more dubious customs, to which doctors alluded in order to reject them. The darkest shadows were cast by practices which appear to have segregated birth from society. Some women "may give birth exposed to rain and dew. . . . or may sojourn away from home too much, and if they decline to move they are certainly to be blamed."[39] Wang Jingyue complained that it was unwise "to remove to a second dwelling, or to change beds and screens."[40] I think that "sojourning away from home" was an aspect of old customs that relegated birth, like death, to the margins of social space. These customs, alluded to in scattered sources, must be teased out of their traces in narratives that either took them for granted or ignored them. An early exception was Wang Chong, the Han dynasty philosophical rationalist, who wrote that in Jiangnan "families of women giving birth consider it taboo [ji'e] and set up grave mound huts along the roadsides and embankments. After passing the month there, the woman comes indoors again."[41] The *Birth Classic* among oth-

36. Chen Ziming, juan 10, 308.
37. Yu Chong, 3b.
38. Chen Ziming, juan 11, 324.
39. Chen Ziming, juan 10, 308–9. Chen is quoting one Ma Yiqing, who is remembered today for a text on external medicine (*waike*).
40. Okanishi Tameto 1948: 512, quoting the preface to the anonymous *Chan bao zhufang* of 1167. Wang was a *jinshi* of 1165–74.
41. Wang Chong, *Lunheng* (Contrarian Eassays), juan 23, "Si wei pian," 355–60.

ers had referred to methods for the "placement of the [birth] hut" (*an lu fa*) using the words also found in classical texts for the makeshift dwelling in which pious sons kept vigil beside a parent's grave.[42]

In this context Song *fuke* experts, while acknowledging the pollution of birth, understood it as detached from death and as manageable within the social space of the home. Doctors encouraged more convenient methods for "respecting the spirits while keeping them at a distance"[43] from the domestic hearth where normal birth could most safely take place. The option of "borrowing a place" (*jie wei*) — a method attributed to Master Ti Xuanzi — may have originated as just such an alternative: "Mark off ten paces in all six directions . . . in the center, place the birth couch according to the favored directions. Here the parturient woman may safely lie without offending the spirits and without fearing evil. All spirits will protect her and the hundred ghosts will depart."[44] Among Song authorities, Zhou Dun, Yu Chong and Chen Ziming all suggested in their writings that this was their preferred method. Moreover, their medical strategies supported ritual notions of birth's defilement. After delivery one should look to cleansing the "noxious dew" (*e lu*) of the afterbirth first: the mother should be propped up sitting for three days, submit to belly massage with a roller, and drink vinegar mixed with ink powder to break up blood clots, said Chen Ziming.[45]

Therefore I do not interpret Song medical writings on birth ritual as rote repetition of old formulas and perhaps outmoded beliefs. Rather, I think that in their respect for *fang wei* these Song authorities demonstrated greater intimacy with the activities surrounding ordinary birth than did the medical masters of the Tang like Sun Simiao. The evidence for rationalization may be less in any medical criticism of ritual than in the open involvement of doctors in these matters. By the thirteenth century, when Chen Ziming lived, the campaigns against *wu* shamanism had been going on for almost two hundred years, with the support of the state, the courts and to a considerable extent the scholar class.[46] When the learned man of medicine assumed the role of ritual advisor side by side with his role as practical therapist, he was participating in

42. For Han-to-Tang evidence of these customs, see Lee Jen-der 1996: 542–46.

43. This was Confucius's classic advice on how a scholar should deal with the supernatural.

44. *Taiping sheng hui fang*, 2426; Chen Ziming, juan 16, 457–58.

45. Chen Ziming, juan 18, 485. Here again Chen took a middle path, objecting to the "custom" of requiring the postpartum mother to spend the first three days on the ground, exposed to the "*qi* of Earth."

46. Chen Yuan-peng 1995.

this project by reimagining the world of the spirits rather than simply rejecting it. Like his neo-Confucian literati counterpart, he saw his role as fostering beneficent rituals while discouraging unwholesome ones.

Overall, there is a sharp contrast between the "ten months of pregnancy" as a cosmographic map and calendar of gestation and the divinatory and geomantic birth rituals based on *fang wei*. One is associated with the most celebrated medical masters and philosophers, presents gestation as an enactment of cosmic creativity, and sees "Heavenly True *qi*" flowing with menses and forming the fetus.[47] The other constructs an impure body of birth, symbolically juxtaposed to death; here blood, rather than embodied generative *qi,* incorporates the "power of pollution" of the anthropologists.[48]

Thus, conflicting images were available to construct the gestating medical body and the meaning of medical practice for those who occupied themselves with it. From the time of Sun Simiao on down, male healers engaged in ritual therapies were taught that efficacy depended upon the healer's purity, requiring not only moral sincerity but also the avoidance of contact with corpses, mourning, menstrual blood and the defilement of birth.[49] If there were prohibitions warning some healers to avoid contact with female dirt, similar prohibitions barred polluted persons — those tainted by mourning or "filth" (menstrual blood) — from the birthing room.[50] Chen Ziming's account also hints at how

47. Qi Zhongfu, question 53.

48. Modern ethnographers have recorded many folk practices based on beliefs about the pollution of menstrual blood and the blood of childbirth. In Taiwan and in many other parts of China, menstruating women were not to visit temples, touch images of the gods or (male) tools and weapons, be present at funerals or enter the rooms of women recovering from childbirth. To wash bloodstained cloth or garments in the running water of streams was also deemed inauspicious (Ahern 1975, Furth and Chen 1992). These taboos can be linked to old teachings about the pollution of birth in popular Buddhist sutras (Overmyer 1976, Grant 1989) and to the uniquely Chinese Buddhist belief, illustrated in many temple wall paintings and incorporated into funeral ritual, that mothers must atone for the pollution of childbirth by suffering after death in the "bloody pond" of purgatory (Seaman 1981). James Watson (1982, 1988) and Emily Martin (1988) have looked at ways in which symbolism linking the pollutions of birth and death has shaped south Chinese funeral rituals and the tasks assigned female, as opposed to male, mourners.

49. Sun Simiao, *Qianjin yi fang,* juan 29, 341, quoting an anonymous *Jinjing* (Classic of Prohibitions). The male ritualist was advised to "avoid the sight of corpses, the sight of the blood of executed criminals, the sight of childbirth, the sight of domestic animals giving birth, the sight of mourners weeping." He was also to avoid embracing infants or sleeping with females. For a late Qing version, quite similar, see the anonymous *Jiang hu yishu michuan,* juan 3, 26.

50. Chen Ziming, juan 16, 443.

midwives and birth attendants performed their own countervailing rituals of purification around the birthing room. In one scenario, when the woman began the month of birth and postpartum seclusion they summoned the spirits dressed in ceremonial garb of white, green, yellow, red or black depending upon which of the Five Phases was deemed auspicious. Buddhist, Daoist and Confucian imagery mingled in other prayers to be chanted over the matting and straw prepared to catch the birth blood, and over the water made ready to bathe the newborn. Since Chen Ziming says these other ritual dances, prayers and incantations were carried out by practitioners called *shi kan chan* and *shi po* — terms denoting midwives and female shamans — they suggest to me a women's sphere of healing.[51] It isn't necessary to believe that these last ceremonies were commonplace performances (some Song sources imply they are dying out) to interpret them as traces of a ritual obstetrics with deep roots in the ancient shamanism so intimately associated with medicine. Ma Dazheng speculates that rituals like the divination of proper positions and directions were the specialty of occult male technicians of healing and other arts known as *fang shi*.[52] Regardless of how male or female ritualists were involved in the full range of divinatory and other birth rituals, Song *chanke* emerges as one of the sites of negotiation between the diverging trajectories of shamanism (*wu*) and medicine (*yi*) spoken of by medical historians.

All this shows that Song learned experts in *fuke* were drawing closer to a sphere of medical practice that historically had been associated with female gender and ritual impurity. This helps explain why, in an era usually represented as one of increasing rationalism in both religion and medicine, authorities like Chen Ziming appeared to be more involved than their predecessors in the ritual management of childbirth. In this context, the Song theorization of the "ten months of pregnancy" as cosmogenesis harmonized with the construction of *fuke* based on a female body of generative Blood and *qi:* both served to tame the power

51. Chen Ziming, juan 16, 450–59. The prayer purifying the straw bedding used for birth quotes the *Book of Songs,* while the one purifying the washing water ends invoking the name of a Bodhisattva. The account of these rituals follows the *Taiping sheng hui fang,* 2426–27.

52. Ma Dazheng 1991: 132–34, discusses the ritual obstetrics of the *Birth Book* attributed to one Wang Yue, who may have lived in the middle ninth century. This book, he argues, shows the synthesis of medical and magical arts characteristic of the *fang shi.* It continued to circulate in the Song dynasty but disappeared thereafter, and is known today largely through corrupted excerpts in a fifteenth-century Korean compendium. He Shixi 1984: 60, also discusses this book, but gives different dates.

of pollution and to facilitate classical doctors' engagement with child-birth as a labor of humanity.

Clinical Obstetrics

When they assisted birth, healers practiced their craft in a world of popular belief and activity where biomedical distinctions between ritual and empirical efficacy had no place. A herbal medicine's potency was based on cosmological affinities inseparable from its somatic effects. The clinical encounter simply revealed spheres where the spirits actively intervene and those where they do not, leaving human agency at the fulcrum between fate and possibility. As one doctor put it, "It is certainly a correct principle to say that in difficult and abnormal deliveries malevolent spirits have been offended; but there are also natural cases of difficult birth, in which the child of itself assumes an abnormal position."[53] Here doctors were not contrasting ritual magic with empirical therapy but were giving each of the overlapping spheres of human action and the agency of the gods its due. Between what fate decrees and what human effort can influence, the wise Song doctor chose to find a balance. Discourse on these matters is illuminated by the issue of labor-hastening drugs, which addressed both the clinical emergency of protracted labor and the ritual danger of birth on an inauspicious day.

Chen Ziming profoundly believed that fortune and misfortune in human life are shaped by timing (*shi*), that is, by cosmological influences bearing on the circumstances of birth and determining fate; but he also thought that attempts to manipulate the timing of birth were foolish efforts to outwit destiny. He chided those who tried to achieve delivery on an auspicious day by the ritual magic of "horsepower," spreading donkey- or horsehide over the rushes normally laid out for the last stages of labor and substituting a horsewhip for a rope to pull on as an aid, and he also worried about the abuse of labor-hastening drugs for such purposes.[54] When famous doctors offered their prescriptions as better

53. Chen Ziming, juan 16, 449, quoting Wang Ziding.
54. Predicting the date of birth by divinatory means was an old technique, alluded to in now-lost Six Dynasties and Sui texts. See Ma Dazheng 1991: 208. In Chen Ziming's account the problem arose particularly when a woman's own ritual calendar (*xing nian*) showed an unlucky conjunction of her "fate" based on her own birth date and the approaching date of her delivery. See Chen Ziming, juan 17, 468–69.

solutions, they made a claim for a particular sphere responsive to human intervention in a world where sages shared in but did not dominate the powers of Heaven and Earth. If orthodox formulas to move Blood and *qi* might be used to force the timing of birth, difficult labor could also be a consequence of inauspicious timing. Purely ritual medicines like *fu* charms — esoteric written ideographs imaging the speed and power of horses, the supernatural presence of ghosts and the agency of the infants themselves — were praised as effective. (See figure 6.) The choice of efficacious materia medica like rabbit brain marrow (which Chinese doctors today praise as empirically effective due to its chemical oxytoxcins) was shaped by the symbolic associations of rabbits, the moon, and the incipient yang-within-yin forces of nature concentrating in the dead of winter, as well as by the logic of medical correspondences linking semen, marrow and the brain in the circulation of vital Essence.[55] In their entirety, the complex of clinical strategies available for birth did not separate the forces of nature from those of human action, and allowed human agency a limited role in influencing the outcome.

Beyond drugs and rituals, human agency also had a place in the physical interventions of birthing. Chen Ziming was responsible for the transmission and historical survival of the most concrete guide to the manual assistance of problem delivery found in the entire literate medical corpus. This was the "Ten Topic Discourse on Birth" (*Shi chan lun*), attributed to a shadowy Northern Song figure known as Yang Zijian.[56] Yang's "Ten Topics" featured instructions for several kinds of abnormal delivery: modern doctors would recognize transverse presentation

55. The most famous formula using rabbit brain marrow, *Tu nao cui sheng wan*, is first found in *Taiping sheng hui fang* and appears in major works of *fuke* thereafter. In Chen's version the marrow had to be from a "winter solstice rabbit" (presumably one caught and killed at that season) and mixed with expensive fragrances of musk, frankincense and clove. See Chen Ziming, juan 17, 471. For modern evaluations see Ma Dazheng 1991: 175–76.

56. The origins of the *Shi chan lun* are obscure, and there are no surviving versions as an independent text. Modern understandings come from the version transmitted in Chen Ziming, juan 17, 463–68. As for Yang himself, some commentators identify him as Yang Kanghou, a man said to have been alive during the Yuanfu reign of the Northern Song (1098–1101), but who may have been a Southern Song figure. *Medical Browsings* (*Yi yuan*), a rare late-nineteenth-century manuscript anthology held in the library of the Beijing Zhongyi Yanjiuyuan, includes copies of prefaces dated 1025 and 1198 that offer anecdotes concerning a Yang Zijian who lived under the Liao dynasty (which ruled the region around Beijing between 907–1124 C.E.). Unfortunately the attached obstetrical manuscript attributed to Yang is mostly prescriptions, quite unlike Chen Ziming's version. It is probably best to think of Yang Zijian simply as a name attached to a diffuse manuscript tradition of *chanke*. See Ma Jixing 1990: 221; Okanishi Tameto 1948: 494; He Shixi 1991, 3:34.

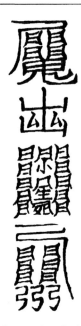

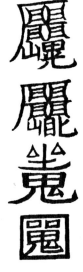

Marvelous *fu* charm for difficult childbirth, transverse and adverse fetal position or undescended placenta.

Marvelous four path *fu* for undescended placenta. Quickly write in red cinnabar ink and swallow.

If she feels disturbed, write this in red ink and paste it on the north wall of the birth chamber.

Marvelous *fu* for cases of transverse fetal positon. Quickly write this *fu* charm with red cinnabar ink, to be swallowed with water.

Figure 6. Song *fu* charms to facilitate labor. These fanciful characters incorporate ideographic elements for the words "child," "ghost," "horse" and (archer's) "bow," as well as the verb "to go out." Based on Chen Ziming, *Furen ta quan liang fang* (All-Inclusive Good Prescriptions for Women), first published in 1284.

(shoulder or arm present first), breech birth (feet first), brow presentation (head twisted to one side), and cord presentation (cord wrapped around child's shoulder). Here is the account of this last complication:

> Topic nine: obstructed birth. The child's body and the mother's birth canal are both positioned normally; the child's head has crowned but it cannot emerge further. This is because as the child's body turned [earlier, to assume the birth position] the umbilical cord wound round its shoulder. . . . The method to assist this birth is to direct the mother to lie on her back and direct the birth attendant gently to push the child upward, and slowly to introduce a hand, using the middle finger to push the child's shoulder down below the cord. Wait for the child's body to straighten and then order the mother to give one push and deliver. This is called [delivery of] an obstructed birth. If the birth attendant does not have subtle and clever hands, don't employ this method, for it is to be feared that reckless stupidity may cause grave harm.[57]

Using passages like this one, modern clinicians have praised Yang Zijian's "Ten Topics" as a tribute to the high level of Song technical obstetrics.[58] The text represents the literate male physician as familiar with delivery and able to supervise the conduct of ordinary birth attendants (*kan sheng, shou sheng*). The "Ten Topics" was reported to have been included in the now-lost versions of Yu Chong's handbook, and in other vanished Song-era writings as well. It is the best evidence we have that Song learned physicians were more involved than their predecessors in the hands-on management of birth.

Gender and Healing Practitioners

The foregoing picture of Song *chanke* could suggest that expertise in obstetrics was gradually shifting from the control of folk midwives into the hands of elite doctors, as happened in parts of early modern Europe. But just as it is mistaken to bifurcate Song obstetrical practice into two independent spheres of ritual and empirical therapies, it is also dubious to think of healing as simply gendered around a male domain of pharmacy versus a female ritual sphere, or around male doctors and female midwives. Texts always represented literate male doctors

57. Chen Ziming, juan 17, 467.
58. Ma Dazheng 1991: 177, says Yang's topics were "revolutionary" in their use of manual techniques. See also Lee T'ao 1958: 481; and Ma Kan-wen 1983: 161–62.

as the superior authorities and spoke of childbirth as women's business. But as the foregoing shows, in the Song male specialists in *fuke* could also concern themselves with birth. Therefore one task for my account of Song dynasty medicine is to understand how gender boundaries were flexible and negotiable enough to account for the knowledge and practice about *chanke* that flowed across them. Another is to show how that same flexibility gave some female healers a place outside of midwifery.

Normally women managed labor and delivery, and the wealth of informal names given them — birth attendant (*kan sheng ren*), delivery woman (*shou sheng zhi ren*), auntie (*guniang*), delivery granny (*zuo po, wen po*) — suggest, like the English word "midwife," that humble but respectable matrons used skills acquired in daily life to negotiate women's childbirth experience. A conventional division of labor between these and state-educated doctors shows up in an eleventh-century anecdote recounted by the famous scholar official Ouyang Xiu. A palace maid claimed (falsely, it turned out) to have been impregnated by the emperor, and several "medical officials expert on birth" (*yi guan chanke*) were summoned along with three midwives (*zuo po*) to await her delivery.[59] In other accounts female birth experts were called "doctor" in keeping with the old Han-to-Tang palace nomenclature. These were "childbirth doctors" (*ru yi*).[60] One such, "surnamed Hu," from the Pu river region in Shandong, told of her community's gratitude to the visiting official who made available a famous formula Black Dragon pill to expel bad postpartum blood.[61] Here it looks as if the official male expert in *chanke* was in fact primarily a herbalist, bringing supplies from the sophisticated pharmacopoeia of the Song state medical establishment to provincial districts. Still other "childbirth doctors" were clearly midwives, like the *ru yi* who delivered the scholar Gong Tao, travelling through the streets of Southern Song Hangzhou in the middle of the

59. See Ouyang Xiu (1007–1072), *Ouyang Wenzhong gong quanji,* juan 219, "Zou shi lu." See also Leung 1996: 7.

60. *Ru,* which means "breast" today, was an old classical term meaning to give birth as well as to nurse the young; a variant, *ru,* identical in pronunciation but using a different ideograph, referred to the rush matting used in childbirth.

61. Chen Ziming, juan 18, 493–95. Chen cites as a source for this story the narrative of one Guo Maoxun, writing in 1101. Black Dragon pill, still recommended by Chen himself, is not, as far as I can tell, in modern use in TCM. It involved a two-stage process of roasting herbs, including *danggui, chuanxiong, wulingzhi* and *dihuang* with "red earth," "salt mud" and other mineral ingredients, adding frankincense, amber, and other ingredients in the second stage to produce a granular black powder. It must have been quite expensive.

night and, after finishing her work and swaddling the baby, returning home again.[62] In sum, in Song discourse, if both males and females expert in birth were sometimes identified as "doctor," this did not mean that they had identical functions.

Chen Ziming's account makes clear that in his day male and female experts on birth performed different functions. In presenting himself as a teacher on labor and delivery, transmitting Yang Zijian's ten topics, he addressed women, not men: "All who give birth should first know these ten points. On the few occasions when there are labor difficulties the life of mother and child can suddenly hang by a thread. The only people who confront this calamity are birth attendants [kan shengchan]. Few delivery women [shou sheng zhi ren] have subtle and clever hands, and for this reason many are endangered. Because I grieve for their plight, I must offer assistance."[63] Moreover, although he presented himself as a teacher, a close reading shows Chen's involvement in childbirth was secondhand, mediated through female birth attendants whom he spoke of as fellow experts. He drew upon his personal experience to add an eleventh topic (on uterine prolapse) to Yan Zijian's list, but his narrative shows that in fact he had called in a midwife (zuo po) from the city who had administered a folk remedy: she splashed the mother's face with vinegar water.[64] As a teacher of such midwives, Chen Ziming also had to learn from them.

Did midwives and other birth attendants, then, also learn from doctors, particularly the pharmaceutical skills that were the doctors' forte and which were associated with literacy? Chen Ziming clearly hoped that his text would help women who were in charge of labor and delivery, but he also expected midwives and birth attendants to know how to prescribe herbal remedies. Consider the list Chen made of items a family should prepare in advance for childbirth. It included the paraphernalia of midwifery: a bed of ashes, dry rushes and thick felt for the ground over which the mother would be propped up in a squatting position for delivery; knives and string and cloth for cutting the cord; basin and water for bathing the infant; and the cooking equipment for preparing porridge for sustenance and hot steaming vinegar fumes in case of fainting. It also included a list of twelve ready-made prescription

---

62. This anecdote is in Hong Mai 1:338. I want to thank Reiko Shinno for bringing it and several others to my attention. See also Zhongwen da cidian 2:72.

63. Chen Ziming, juan 17, 463.

64. Chen Ziming, juan 17, 463.

formulas and fourteen additional individual materia medica. To compound and prepare infusions on the spot, a small brazier and long-handled pan for frying herbs were needed, plus cloth to strain the liquid, wine and boy's urine as liquid additives to the final decoctions as called for, and medicine bottles.[65] Here the birthing room was also to contain an apothecary's cabinet for use of the women in charge of delivery.

Case histories involving famous male doctors and childbirth were rare, and usually showed them as heroic practitioners of crisis medicine.[66] One example is a story told of Pang Anshi, a renowned hereditary physician of the eleventh century, who was called to the dwelling of a woman who had been in labor for seven days. "He personally patted and massaged her from top to bottom; she felt a slight pain in her belly and, in the space of a groan, delivered a boy." He claimed that acupuncture applied to the child's hand in utero had stimulated it to release its grip on its mother's bowels and give way to birth. This tale echoed a famous case of a Tang empress who valiantly died giving birth to the heir apparent, knowing that the acupuncture treatment that forced the infant to let go and be born would kill her.[67] Such stories, like the even earlier tale of Hua Tuo, portrayed acupuncture used by male masters in childbirth as radical and dangerous surgery with a touch of wizardry about it.

Another story of male intervention was more grittily prosaic. Zhang Congzheng (1156–1228), a renowned Northern practitioner active in the early thirteenth century, intervened in a case of abnormal presentation in which the midwife had accidentally broken the baby's arm, killing it. Zhang and the midwives together delivered the dead child manually, using a hook Zhang had improvised.[68] On the one hand these stories

65. Chen Ziming, juan 16, 458.

66. An important anthology of famous cases is the sixteenth-century *Ming yi lei an,* compiled by Jiang Guan, which has a number of examples from Song, Yuan or early Ming in juan 11. Chen Ziming himself is represented by a case in which he rejected the diagnosis of dead fetus, prescribed Purple Thyme infusion (*Zisu tang*) to stimulate labor, and saved the baby. See 334.

67. Pang (1043–1100), a hereditary physician from Hubei with a wide practice and many disciples, was most famous for his clinical work with Cold Damage fevers, not *fuke.* This story about him appeared in Hong Mai's collection of tales of the strange and marvelous, *Yijian zhi,* juan 10, and made its way into Pang's biography in the Song dynastic history. See Chen Bangxian 1982: 279. For the Tang empress, see Lee Jen-der 1996: 569, quoting Zhou Mi. Several similar tales are found in *Ming yi lei an* and its successor, Wei Zhixiu's *Xu ming yi lei an,* the latter with skeptical editorial comment. See juan 25, 626.

68. See Wei Zhixiu, juan 25, 634–35: "Zhang said, 'Her life is in imminent danger; needles and drugs won't help her.' Quickly he took a hook from a yardarm scale,

suggest how acupuncture as an emergency method was romanticized in medical literature on birth, perhaps to mask the brutal expedients of fetal dismemberment that were sometimes resorted to. On the other hand, these doctors also appear familiar with the more ordinary hands-on techniques of massage and moxibustion used by midwives, and in passing, as collaborators with them in medical emergencies.[69]

If a Song healer addressed as "doctor" could on occasion be a practitioner of midwifery, other female "doctors" were not identified as midwives. I have already mentioned the matriarch of the Guo lineage, honored with titles by the emperor and ancestress of a long line of *fuke* practitioners. Less praised, but no less interesting, is the woman from twelfth-century Hangzhou who caught the attention of the medical essayist Zhang Gao:

> There was a woman in the capital named Bai; she was beautiful and the city people all called her Peony White. She sold abortifacients for a living. All of a sudden she was afflicted with brain sickness. [Her head] daily swelled larger and none of the famous doctors of the city could cure her. By day it suppurated and stank unbearably, and nightly the neighbors heard her groans. One day she called her household together and said, "You are to burn my entire collection of abortion prescriptions; I warn you, my children and disciples—you cannot carry on this calling." The sons said to their mother, "Our mother has made the family livelihood from this. How can we throw it away?" The mother said, "Every night in my dreams hundreds of infants gnaw at my skull, making me cry out in pain. This is all retribution because I used poisonous drugs to ruin fetuses." Having spoken thus, she died.[70]

Zhang Gao included this woman in his chapter on "Doctors Recompensed for Their Deeds." Although presented as negative moral example, she ran a medical shop as a herbalist, headed a family of practitioners, and commanded the resource of literacy in the practice of her craft. By standards applied to many males at the time, she was a doctor.

In sum, in the Song the boundaries between male and female spheres

---

attached a rope to it, lubricated it with grease, and ordered the mother to spread her feet. When she was propped up on either side by attendants with her feet braced, he attached the hook and ordered a strong woman to use the full weight of her body to pull the fetus down." Ma Dazheng 1991: 171–79, 188–89, discusses this and similar cases.

69. Moxibustion treatments stimulated *qi* circulation with heat, produced by aromatic herbs burnt on the skin at approved acupuncture points. See also chapter 8, pp. 290–92.

70. Zhang Gao, juan 10, 35a/b.

of medical expertise were permeable in several ways. One was medical emergency, which in *chanke* made doctors and midwives participants in a common enterprise; a need for cooperation placed a premium on knowing about one another. Second was the gender permeability of family relationships. Women in medical families sometimes had the potential to become experts, and a few families even got a foothold in medicine through their matriarchs. Here the example of Mistress Bai the abortionist is structurally identical to that of the mistress of the Guo family who doctored an empress. Finally, the linguistic blurring of boundaries between what in English would be rendered "doctor" and "midwife" suggests that the gendered division of medical labor concerning birth was not always perceived as marking an important distinction of status.

These few examples deal with practitioners who were service providers in a pluralistic medical world where, in spite of the imperial medical offices and academies at the top, the ideal of the classically trained "literati doctor" (*ru yi*) had not yet become a hegemonic model of good medical practice. As Angela Leung and Robert Hymes have argued, most doctors in the Song were still "not quite gentlemen." Their fraternity might include itinerant acupuncturists or Buddhist and Daoists claiming to have been taught by immortals themselves, while even the shamanistic *wu* often survived state and elite censure and repression. In such a heterogeneous setting the social distance between female and male healers, while always present, was less marked than in a later medical world with more highly stratified medical statuses and a more marked distinction between religious and other modes of healing practice. During the Song the social separation between the sexes was also less strict than it was to become in the thirteenth century and after. All of this may help explain how female healers, including midwives, carried out their business without attracting negative comment. The Song record on them may be sparse, but it is also comparatively free of the misogynistic rhetoric that became commonplace later.[71]

Chanke and the Domestic Sphere

The study of *chanke* is a valuable window on the social relations between males and females who practiced medicine as workers,

---

71. Hymes 1987, Leung 1996. I am grateful to Angela Leung for allowing me to see her work in progress.

providing services on demand. However, *chanke* also provides a look at medicine as an expertise accessible to cultured amateurs and practiced at home among the social elite. The ideal of filial piety rationalized the pursuit of medicine among gentlemen by encouraging them to care for their families — a pursuit also fostering the vogue for medical publishing by "gentleman admirers of medicine." Literary sources speak of virtuous gentlemen who read works of pharmacy to cure their mothers' illnesses. (See figure 7.) But several childbirth handbooks suggest a different kind of relationship among upper class men and their social equals, the women of their families.

Over the course of the Southern Song, several handbooks on obstetrics produced by private gentlemen versed in medical matters made their way into print. These texts by literati householders offer glimpses of a female sphere through the eyes of males who took an interest in the health of their own families.[72] These authors focused on the family event of delivery and offered advice on procedures and equipment similar to that reported from Chen Ziming above. They recommended that herbs be stocked and prescriptions be compounded in advance, and that instructions concerning "positions and directions" be prepared and posted on the wall. They had suggestions about the birth attendants (employ no strangers; stable, clean, calm women of mature years are best, and to assist them use reliable maids of the household). They wanted the room to be free of drafts and not too crowded, and for its images of gods to be covered respectfully before the mother stripped down for delivery. They had views about diet (heating foods stagnate Blood), about home remedies during labor (try raw egg white, or rice porridge with honey syrup), about postpartum restoratives (have her drink boy's urine mixed with wine, or inhale vinegar fumes), or about postpartum belly massage (use a wooden roller with downward motion from above to below the navel). Their remedies for a difficult labor were confined to herbal prescriptions, with a liberal admixture of more purely ritual medicines involving masculinist magic (bind her waist with the skin of a male snake; have her swallow a large bean on which the father's name has been written).[73] These authors wrote in a plain style; the material

72. Yu Chong and the anonymous authors of the *Chan bao zhufang* and of *Chanru beiyao* wrote of the affairs of their own households.
73. Yu Chong explained that male snakes are found in high places, females in low ones (33a/b). Lee Jen-der 1996 found many pre-Song ritual therapies for difficult labor that drew upon the power of the father, by implication actively involving him in childbirth. The child in turn was imagined to be capable of filial response. See 568.

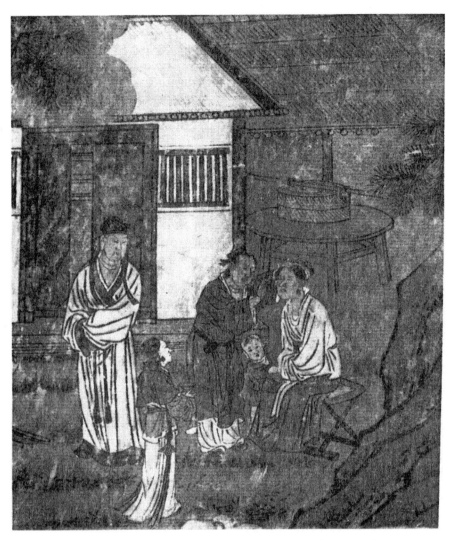

Figure 7. A gentleman cares for his mother's health. In this thirteenth-century temple wall mural a Daoist healer restores an old woman's sight, watched over by her adult son at left. From the Yongle Gong, a Daoist temple in Ruicheng county, Shanxi province. Reproduced from the *Yongle Gong pihua*.

resources needed were those commonly at hand; even the recommended prescriptions used only a few well-known ingredients and stressed the role of food as medicine. Yu Chong's remedies came from family recipes, fleshed out with a few formulas identified with famous names. One such was a labor-hastening preparation known locally as Shen Family Five Accumulation powder (*Shen jia wujisan*), named for Shen Gua, an eminent scholar-official learned in medicine and other sciences. Other formulas were added to his text by a more obscure associate, "Scholar Xu."[74]

Here the art of prescribing appears as something educated householders felt competent to do for themselves. Boundaries between professional and lay expertise were blurred and so were gender boundaries concerning appropriate knowledge. "Women need to know prescriptions," said Yu Chong, but he did not present such knowledge as abstruse. The anonymous author of *Prescriptions from the Birth Treasury* (*Chan bao zhufang*) elaborated further:

> In my household all the women and girls are taught personally how to doctor themselves. Then in childbirth they all know how to save the situation. It is proper for families to instruct orally [*yu*] so that households know this. In the fifth month and afterward, pregnant women take a decoction of bitter citrus peel [*zhike*] to shrink the fetus.[75] For postpartum pain they take Four Ingredients infusion. To close the womb and discharge blood they supplement with [donkey-hide] glue and artemisia [*jiaoai*]. For difficult labor they take Black Spirit powder [*Hei shen san*]; as delivery is imminent they take Regulate Center pills [*Li zhong wan*] to boost fetal *qi*. In the first three days after birth they take Four Ingredients. To dispel birth blood and clots they take lamb meat cooked with Four Ingredients. After three to five doses all grief is vanished.[76]

In this way the scholarly gentleman offered the women of his own family as a model. In his report I read traces of healing strategies well known and informally taught among women themselves. In such gentry

74. This text fits into a pattern of works published by "gentlemen admirers of medicine" analyzed by Chen Yuan-peng (1997: 130–158). Chen identifies 106 titles authored by scholars living under Northern and Southern Song rule. Few of these authors had formal teachers or wrote on theory or classics; a majority offered family collections of prescriptions stressing self-cure and using common, easily available ingredients.

75. Citrus aurantium or other sour citrus. The peel was considered bitter and cooling, appropriate to repress the vigorous yang growth of the fetus.

76. *Chan bao zhufang*, 20/b.

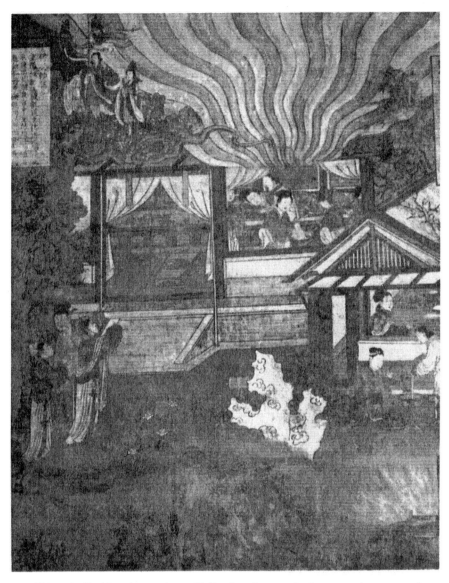

Figure 8. Bathing the newborn. Following the popular iconography surrounding the Buddha's birth, this Yongle Gong wall painting celebrating the Daoist immortal Lu Dongbin depicts his birth in a domestic setting. An older woman attends the mother, while maids bathe the infant and down below other servants work in the kitchen and draw water.

households medical knowledge was a domestic skill, and males versed in medicine related to the women's sphere of childbirth (as seen in figure 8) as kinsmen. The textual knowledge produced here, arising from a spreading amateur ideal of medical learning as a gentleman's family duty, fit in comfortably with medical knowledge as a household practice involving women as well as men in self-cure and the tending of ill family members. While on the part of males there was paternalism and aspiration to control socially critical skills, there was also a degree of intimacy between a family's men and its women. Although an informal female sphere of knowledge and practice is only indirectly revealed, this says more about male monopoly of the emerging technology of print communication than about the gendered structure of that knowledge itself, or its oral or handwritten forms in its domestic setting.[77]

Gender, Medicine and Society

Although I have treated them separately here, Song gynecology (*fuke*) and Song obstetrics (*chanke*) were actually in the larger sense linked discourses focused on women's reproductive functions. The "leadership of Blood," in its most sophisticated manifestations of diagnosis based on pattern analysis, constituted a holistic approach to internal illnesses and to all generative and gestational processes where Blood was deemed the leading factor. But as classically trained doctors came closer to obstetrical matters, they faced the problem of bridging both a gendered social gulf and the gulf between ill-fitting medical paradigms.

Theorizing gestation did not easily accommodate pattern diagnosis. Although conception and gestation could embody cosmogenesis in evocative ways, therapeutic strategies for pregnant and postpartum women were named in the language of symptom relief and not according to the constructs of yin yang and the Five Phases. Though doctors did not identify pregnancy as in itself an illness, birth was potentially life-threatening, and in birth a woman's blood was defiling and dangerous. Menstruation may have been understood as an ideal normality integrating the spheres of generation and gestation. But representations of the mother in childbed as weakened coexisted uneasily alongside rep-

---

77. For passing mention of Song gentry women literate in medicine see Ebrey 1993: 84 and Bossler 1996: 15–16.

resentations of her as unclean. Unlike the Yellow Emperor's androgynous body of generation, the gestational body of pregnancy and delivery resisted the symmetries of homologous gender difference and brought doctors in contact with an essentialist model of the female body as impure. In this situation the rule of Blood as a gynecology constructing female difference around a generalized functional sickliness operated as a medicalized alternative to pollution beliefs, allowing doctors to overcome an unspoken aspect of the "difficulty" of curing women and to assume the role of healers protective of them in a paternalistic Confucian order. However, the multivalence of Blood as a symbol, expressed in both pharmacy and ritual, made this resolution an incomplete one.

One way to try to understand the patterns of thought and practice in Song *fuke* is to look for links that reveal a functional relationship between medicine as a cultural domain constructing human subjectivity and the social system. Can we see the Song medical female body and the Song concern with obstetrical practice as functionally related to changing gender norms in the larger society? Certainly the medical engagement with reproductive rituals and the subordination of the erotic body to the maternal one encouraged enhanced respect for women's social roles as mothers, while the medical emphasis upon female frailty supported paternalism within the enclosure of the gentry family. Recent studies of Song upper class women have talked about the decline of erotic representations of gentry marriage and about the shift to a frailer feminine ideal as masculinity came to be defined in terms of Han literati refinement as opposed to barbarian martial vigor. They have also talked of higher birth rates and high rates of infant mortality among the Song elite in the context of a culture favoring large families.

Some note that along with the growth of neo-Confucian familism went increased state and religious censure of the prevailing high levels of abortion and infanticide.[78] Francesca Bray has argued for a long-term historical trend toward a social emphasis on women's reproductive roles, as opposed to productive ones, stimulated early on by the Song spread of neo-Confucian agnatic lineages, which allowed commoners as well as

78. See Liu Jingzhen 1995, Birge 1995 and forthcoming, and Ebrey 1993, 1995. Ebrey studied 189 couples for whom funerary biographies supplied demographic data on both husband and wife. In this she found that women who survived to age forty-five without being widowed gave birth to an average of 6.1 children (1995: 24, 32). She reports infant mortality of fifty percent among daughters born to Song emperors. See 1993: 172–76.

aristocrats to set up household shrines and made every husband a potential ancestor of his own descent line.[79]

Medicine, then, seems to support a picture of the emergence of a neo-Confucian emphasis upon the social value of maternity. *Fuke* and pediatrics were complementary disciplines supporting the well-being of the family as a multigenerational collective. However, like functionalist explanations generally, this account minimizes the ambiguities of a complex social field. At stake are the meanings that were assigned to maternity itself, as well as the implications for women of the shifting practices of family life. In the ideology of agnatic kinship according to neo-Confucian philosophers following Zhu Xi, moralists wrote about social motherhood more than bodily maternity. They encouraged respect for the first wife — matriarchal ritual partner, teacher and domestic manager who was owed filial piety by her adult sons — over the young woman with a nursling at her breast.[80] Moreover, over the course of the Song there was also an expansion in the commercial market in lower class women as prostitutes, or as maids and concubines whose incorporation into households complicated the micropolitics of gender there. And it was in the Song era that the bound foot began to spread as an aesthetic of erotic allure based on fragility and concealment. Footbinding, a practice that developed largely outside Confucianism, spread from aristocratic palaces and brothels to the houses of the gentry, splitting off the body of desire from the body of reproduction. Medicine's concern with maternity, then, was only one of a multiplicity of Song discourses surrounding gender and the body.

None of these accounts of the reproductive domain fits easily into a pattern of either progress or decline in the status of women during the Song. As social history, changes in the gender system fit better into a narrative of the emerging cultural politics of neo-Confucian familism. Here the long-term trend was toward the tighter incorporation of women into the multigenerational agnatic households into which they married as wives, where the respect accorded them as mothers within that domestic domain was counterbalanced by greater limitations on their kinship ties, property rights and legal prerogatives outside of it.

An alternative way to think about Song *fuke* and gender in society

79. See Bray 1997: 150–55. Her argument, which looks also at shifts in the technology and economics of the "womanly work" (*nü gong*) of cloth production, surveys late imperial history from the Song to the end of the eighteenth century.

80. Birge forthcoming; Bossler 1998.

may be to look at the internal dynamics of the development of medicine itself. Certainly the emergence of a literate tradition of *fuke* and of a more engaged obstetrics had much to do with the development of medicine as a science beginning in the Northern Song—stimulated by state patronage and supervision, by the growing population of medically literate gentry, and by the spread of printing. In gynecology the "leadership of Blood" may be read as an effort to interpret medicine for women within the framework of the new diagnostics. The more engaged obstetrics may also be read as an aspect of the gradual encroachment of literate medicine on the spheres of practice of shaman healers (*wu*) and of "medical craftsmen," including—to a limited degree—female healers.

Historians of Chinese medicine have conventionally equated these, like other Song innovations in diagnosis, pharmacology and medical theory, with empirical achievements (the modern biomedical standard) against which later medical history has appeared as a decline, measured most visibly by a diminished activism on the part of the state in Ming-Qing times. In this reading, as offered by Ma Dazheng, Fan Xingzhun and others, Song empirical advances in gynecology and obstetrics were undermined by "feudal customs" of the subsequent Yuan and especially Ming dynasties. However, historians of medicine have been less likely to find seeds of decline in evolving norms of learned medicine itself, which increasingly constructed knowledge on a literati model involving reverence for canonical texts in competition with the practice-centered authority transmitted by master to apprentice or the family wisdom of the domestic domain. The gradual ascendancy of the art of prescription itself can be seen as part of the picture, as this most refined and literary of medical skills became the hallmark of the "literati doctor," marginalizing other techniques like acupuncture, moxibustion, massage and rituals.

Gender boundaries between doctors and women patients were certainly also exaggerated by such learned norms, which kept the suffering body at a greater distance from the elite healer's contact. Similarly, the complex shifts between orality and literacy set in motion by the invention and spread of printing gradually challenged the centrality of those domestic spheres of medicine as a practice where elite women could command resources more nearly equivalent to those of elite men. Among professional healers, the emergence of printed sources as a public resource may have democratized medicine by breaking the monopoly of master-disciple lineages ritually transmitting texts as craft secrets. But this kind of democracy, privileging literate skills, also placed female healers at greater disadvantage compared with males. One's evaluation of medical progress in *fuke* will depend on whether one concludes that the new diagnostics' textual bias, and its formal rigor and elegance, brought also an improved ability to heal. One's evaluation of Song obstetrics in particular will be negative only if one assumes that the ritual management of childbirth offered women less ease of passage than the manual and pharmaceutical remedies available.

Finally, the leadership of Blood itself was an ambiguous construction. It veiled the pollution beliefs that ritual medicine acknowledged and accommodated. Evidence of closer male involvement with matters of reproductive health, it revealed by contrast how far the Yellow Emperor's classic androgynous body had repressed maternity. Imagining an integrated generational and gestational body of Blood and *qi*, Song gynecologists tried to reinforce androgyny and disguised the theoretical and practical problems that gestational functions posed for doctors. They did so by accommodating female weakness and male paternalism. To be led by Blood, to be subject to illnesses that are deeper and more difficult to cure than those of males, was a functional product of a woman's body history over time. It went with her body's dedication to the socially necessary task of producing young. The Song gynecologist's medical body was not weak due to the Greek's hysteria or the Victorian's neurasthenia. Nor was it an essentialized body of female inferiority in the manner of nineteenth-century bioscience. Rather, it was a body in use over the years of a woman's adult life — one dedicated to a specific labor in service of the family and descent group. Like the chaste widow, the good wife suffered bodily damage which both de-eroticized her person and ensured her entitlement to filial respect in old age. Is it a coincidence that this ascendancy of a sacrificial reproductive body as a medical paradigm of the female occurred around the same time as the bound foot was beginning to gain ground as a sign of female eroticism? Displaced downward, this fetishist signifier of woman as desirable was not identified with any part of the body associated with a reproductive function. On its relation to health, medicine was silent.

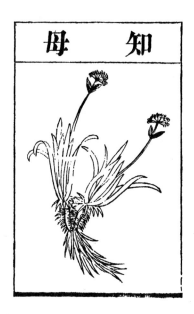

CHAPTER 4

Rethinking *Fuke* in the Ming Dynasty

In Chen Ziming, *fuke* had produced a medical master whose written work stood as a summation of the Song dynasty's clinical achievements. Even during his own lifetime north China was already cut off from the Song imperium, controlled by Jurchen conquerors from inner Asia, who ruled as the foreign Jin dynasty (1125–1234). When he died in 1270 the partitioned Southern Song state was about to be swept up in the Mongol conquest—a vast upheaval that disrupted first north China and then all of East Asia for over a hundred years (1225–1368). This historical rupture, still imperfectly understood, worked on medicine and on the gender system in contradictory ways. Foreign conquest and occupation encouraged an intensification of Han female seclusion, while the calamitous medical byproducts of war—famine and epidemic, especially in north China—fostered medical revisionism and a search for new paradigms for understanding disease process. Song approaches to *fuke,* along with much else in Song medicine, dropped out of fashion, even as women became less visible in public social space. Medical culture, on the other hand, was enlivened as the Song state domination of published discourse weakened and as learned physicians struggled to cope with new epidemiological threats. Chinese medical historians identify the Jin and Yuan dynasties as a creative period when "contending schools of thought" on medical matters emerged for the first time. Gradually over the thirteenth and fourteenth centuries thinking about *fuke* was realigned to fit emerging new paradigms of the medical mainstream. By this path the legacy of Chen Ziming was reshaped and the theoretical "leadership of Blood" in *fuke* ceased to guide the most learned pharmaceutical strategies.

First the Jurchen invasions of the north, and then the Mongol conquest of all China, were associated with a many-sided retreat of Han literati culture. In the south, elite families retired further into their local communities, while Zhu Xi's "philosophy of the Way" (known as *Daoxue*) and its lineage ideals gained ground, mandating female withdrawal to an even more bounded "inner" sphere of domestic life. The concurrent spread of footbinding from the elite to commoner classes may ambiguously relate to the same issues of bondage and concealment of both the social and the physical body. Patricia Ebrey and Dorothy Ko have argued that by the fourteenth century the tiny, bound, elegantly shod foot was well understood as a sign of civilization, marking Chinese female refinement as opposed to the crude natural feet of "barbarian" women, and Han civilian culture as opposed to the militarism of the conquerors.[1] Moreover, it advertised an aesthetics and erotics of concealment. Whereas *Daoxue* served as a elite strategy for repressing the erotic domain, through the bound foot a woman's sexualized body reappeared in an even more secret and private form, hidden from all but the most intimate gaze.

Under Mongol rule many domains of Han literary production narrowed, if the thinning out of the print record is any guide. As scholarly voices fell silent, many works were lost and traditions of textual transmission were interrupted. Medicine partially participated in this pattern of involution, but benefitted from the alien rulers' pragmatic, decentralized and cosmopolitan perspectives, which encouraged patronage of the practical arts. Ironically, the epidemiological crises afflicting north

---

1. Ebrey 1993: 33; Ko 1997.

China from the late twelfth to middle thirteenth centuries contributed to innovation by challenging confidence in the standard approaches to acute fevers derived from Zhang Ji's classic *Treatise on Cold Damage Disorders (Shanghan lun)*.[2] Leaders of new medical "schools of thought of the Jin and Yuan" came to question Zhang Ji's model of etiology, which led them to reevaluate Song state medical orthodoxy and to historicize the concept of disease itself. Particularly important were views attributed to Liu Wansu (1120?–1200) and Zhang Congzheng (1156–1228), physicians who practiced at the Jin court after the military conquest of the north, and Li Gao (1180–1251) and Zhu Zhenheng (1281–1358), who lived under the Yuan dynasty. The break in the documentary record of Song state medicine becomes a silence filled gradually by new voices with different things to say.[3]

Text and Context:
Visible Plagues and Hidden Women

The medical records of the twelfth and thirteenth centuries are scattered with fragmentary stories of war, famine and pestilence—the setting for Jin-Yuan revisionism. Medical classics had long emphasized seasonal types of climactic *qi* in the etiology of Cold Damage fevers. Liu Wansu, Li Gao and Zhang Congzheng interpreted the crisis-ridden clinical landscape of north China as evidence for a more profound mutability of disease itself. Adopting the slogan that "ancient and modern times follow different patterns [of seasonal *qi*]; old prescriptions are less effective on today's disorders,"[4] these reformers sought the etiological key to devastating fevers and epidemics like small-

2. Fan Xingzhun 1985: 161–88, argues that a series of epidemics between 1138 and 1232 shook North China, and that they may have included outbreaks of bubonic plague. State records of epidemics tabulated in Liang Jun 1995: 92–93, 116–17, suggest a more long-term epidemiological shift, perhaps related to population growth and urbanization. The emergence of smallpox in the Song as a recognizable and universal childhood disease was another aspect of the picture.

3. In modern histories of Chinese medicine these four men are identified as the "Four Masters" (*si dajia*) of the Jin and Yuan. During the Ming and Qing periods, writers on medical history understood the Four Masters as consisting of Zhang Ji and his Jin-Yuan critics, Liu Wansu, Li Gao and Zhu Zhenheng. See Chao 1995: 241–49.

4. This saying is attributed to Zhang Yuansu (fl. c. 1180). The story was that his insight into "today's disorders" enabled him to cure the fever of his more famous contemporary, Liu Wansu. He later became the teacher of Li Gao. See Zhang's biography in the Jin dynastic history, in Chen Bangxian 1982: 296.

pox in ever more elaborate understandings of environmental season-
ability, theorized loosely (after the *Inner Canon*) around "five cycles and
six *qi*" (*wu yun liu qi*).[5] They debated the changing nature of such seasonal *qi*, the role of inner and outer causal factors, and of warming or
cooling therapeutic strategies, but without arriving at a firm new consensus. Over the long term, Jin-Yuan revisionism made physicians pay
more attention to local and regional environmental factors independent
of year or season. But it also led them increasingly to emphasize internalist etiologies, focusing on Fire and other pathogenic *qi* independently
of the influence of land, wind and weather, and on organ system physiology.

Paul Unschuld believes that the complex innovations associated with
the Jin-Yuan masters produced a theorization of pharmacy that broke
fundamentally with older *bencao* technologies, which had been both
more pragmatic and more intertwined with magical beliefs.[6] Certainly
the revisionists elaborated a classification of materia medica begun by
earlier Song authorities, whereby each ingredient in an herbal prescription was identified in terms of its action on one or more of the twelve
channels and associated organ systems, while its flavor (*wei*) was linked
to the correspondences of the Five Phases. Drugs became more tightly
integrated into medicine's cosmological framework, and crafting prescriptions could take on new layers of formal complexity. While these
innovations were less important for the use of medicinal ingredients
than for the meanings given them, the Jin-Yuan masters and their followers also pushed for different, often mutually conflicting, therapeutic
strategies that had as a common theme criticism of the standard formulas
of the Song state medical establishment. These were too heating and

5. According to the *Inner Canon* the six environmental *qi* were Wind (*feng*), Cold
(*han*, associated with winter), Summer Heat (*shu*), Damp (*shi*, associated with
spring), Autumn Dry (*zao*) and Fire (*huo*). Building on the old belief that seasonal
change and unseasonable weather are keys to disease patterns, Song theorists combined the six *qi* first with Five Cycles (*wu yun*, correlated with the Five Phases) and
then with the sixty-year stem and branch system of calculating the calendar. Plotting
all of these factors together, they offered calculations whereby irregular and unseasonable phenomena of past years could be read to predict the timing and nature of
outbreaks of recurring epidemics like smallpox. This essentially divinatory method
presumed to reveal deeper levels of correlative correspondence than could be dis-
cerned with yin yang Five Phase reasoning alone. Porkert 1974: 55–106 describes the
system, which he dubbed "phase energetics," but its place in the history of Chinese
medicine is still relatively unexplored. My own account comes from Fan Xingzhun
1985: 126–34, and Despeux, forthcoming. For the place of *wu yun liu qi* in medical
thinking about smallpox, see Chang Chia-feng 1996: 60.

6. Unschuld 1986: 81.

acrid, addressing Wind rather than Fire; they reflected court fashions for fragrant and warming ingredients that were often no more than exotic, expensive palliatives for luxurious living. From a biomedical point of view, such revisionism could seem woefully inadequate in the face of the health catastrophes of a turbulent era; but its rhetoric echoed in medical discourse long after the dynastic crises were over. Clinically, many Ming lineages of practitioners claimed to follow distinct pharmaceutical strategies based on some combination of Jin-Yuan medical "schools of learning" (*xuepai*). Overall, pharmacy became a more refined art, as the ideal of the well-crafted prescription gradually came to favor a larger number of individual ingredients, each in smaller quantities, the whole tailored to a specific client's condition.[7]

In sum, by the end of the thirteenth century a significant paradigm shift had occurred in medicine that left the disorders of women on the sidelines, while much in the pharmaceutical repertory of Song *fuke*, along with the rest of Song state medicine, was declared outmoded. The *Imperial Grace Formulary*, for example, ceased to be of clinical interest and was not reprinted after the twelfth century, surviving—like many other Song works used in the previous chapter—only in the form of a rare manuscript or bibliophile's antique. Other works were preserved in the archives of ancient literature gathered in Ming-Qing imperial encyclopedias. Consider, for example, the later history of the twelfth-century *Childbirth Treasury Collection* attributed to Li Shisheng and Guo Jizhong. Within a few decades of its publication, the distinguished pharmacologist Chen Yan produced a revised edition with his own withering commentary on its theoretical crudity and pharmaceutical limitations. The version preserved in the imperially sponsored fourteenth-century *Yongle Encyclopedia*, and in the even grander eighteenth-century *Complete Collection of the Four Treasuries*, was the one that incorporated Chen Yan's critique. Only Chen Ziming's *fuke* text enjoyed a continuous history of transmission for practical use. It escaped becoming an archival museum piece but not, significantly, the process of revision through

7. Unschuld 1986: 85–118; Fan Xingzhun 1985: 161–190; Ren Yingqiu 1980: 39–79. Scholars trace the overall origins of this complex movement to the twelfth-century Song physicians Zhang Yuansu and Kou Zongshi, and divide it internally between regionally based groups in Hejian and in Yishui. However, Wu Yiyi 1993–94 shows that the framework of medical "schools of learning" used by historians overstates the cohesion of the networks of disciples who over time adapted teachings traced back to Liu Wansu to their local lineages of practice. No text by any of the Jin-Yuan masters was codified as an authoritative classic (*jing*) rivalling the *Inner Canon*. Rather, many of their teachings were passed along through local manuscript traditions and personal apprenticeship.

critical commentary. In the mid-Ming it too was edited to accord with later generations' standards of erudite practice.[8]

Further, the links between *fuke* and court medicine became more tenuous. In the Ming and Qing, no renowned *fuke* experts emerged from palace ranks, while for physicians in general imperial patronage and court office gradually lost importance. The main textual witness to the continuation of the clinical traditions of Song court *fuke* lies in a few surnames: Guo, Xue, Cheng, Chen. These were lineages of hereditary family practitioners of *fuke* in Ming-Qing Zhejiang, the former home of the Southern Song capital of Hangzhou. They claimed that their practices had been handed down from ancestors who were Song court physicians, both male and female. Such pedigrees were mentioned in local histories and in rare surviving handwritten manuals, but their possessors were not associated with published authorship.[9]

Learned *fuke* in the Yuan and early Ming dynasties was first of all a discourse shaped by new directions in medical learning and the shape of medical textuality, framed by master healers for whom illnesses of women were secondary concerns. It is more compelling to see it as a return to the androgynous body of classical precedent, rather than as a reinscription of sexual difference based on emerging neo-Confucian norms of sex segregation. However, *fuke*'s reduced medical visibility during this period does correspond with a reduced visibility of women in society. A social key to the construction of discourse was the increasingly distant relationship between male healers and the female sick. The twelfth-century pharmacologist Kou Zongshi was the first I know to have recorded a complaint about the physical seclusion of high-ranking women, whom the doctor could neither see nor easily address to question:

> Though the treatment of women is a medical specialty [*ke*] of its own, [doctors] can't always make full use of the ancients' skills. In today's high-ranking families, [women] dwell in remote chambers, behind curtains and screens. Further, they cover their arms and hands with a cloth, so one cannot practice the art of examining their appearance or exercise the craft of pulse-taking. Of the four methods of diagnosis, two are lacking. The Yellow Emperor says that in treating illness one must investigate physical form [*xing*], movement of *qi* [breath], skin color and animation [*se*], and moisture . . . If a sufferer's pulse does not correspond with [other signs of] illness, and one cannot observe the sick person's physical

8. See the 1985 edition of Chen Ziming, editors' preface.

9. See Chen Menglei et al. 1962, 12:168–74, for lineages of medical practitioners of *fuke* in Ming Jiangnan. See also Ma Dazheng 1991: 232; Zheng Jinsheng 1996. Qing era Jiangnan *fuke* is discussed in Wu 1998.

form, the doctor must prescribe according to pulse alone. Can he succeed this way? . . . Doctors must ask substantive questions, based on thorough reasoning. Seeing that his questions are complicated, his clients think him unskilled and often are not willing to take the prescribed medicines. Bianque could observe the appearance of the Duke of Ji, and still [his diagnosis] was doubted![10]How much worse it is when the doctor cannot observe. Alas, [curing women] may well be said to be difficult.[11]

There was some exaggeration here, since Kou's own case histories show him taking his female clients' pulses as well as speaking directly with them. Nonetheless Kou's lament must have struck a nerve among practitioners, for it became a narrative trope in later writings on *fuke*. In Southern Song Nanjing, 150 years after Kou first wrote, Chen Ziming took for granted the following clinical situation: "Mistress Du had been in labor for several days without delivering. Midwives [*zuo po*] and shamans [*hun tong*] had all failed and I was summoned. I said, 'I could not take her pulse before she began to labor, but I will need to observe her appearance now.' They drew aside the curtain and brought a lamp. Her face was red and her tongue was dark. From these signs, I knew that the child was already dead and that the mother was not in danger."[12] Chen followed this case with instructions on recognizing advanced labor from pulse readings, the diagnostic technique most respectful of emerging elite ideals of female modesty. A fourteenth-century temple wall painting of a stillbirth (figure 9) shows the decorum expected of a literati physician. As the late Song cult of female chastity spread in the Yuan and early Ming, virtuous widows might burnish their saintly reputations by refusing the attentions of male physicians.[13] In popular Yuan drama, doctors were satirized for bungling the diagnoses of their invisible female clients; doctors baffled by a cloth-covered hand

10. An allusion to a case of the semilegendary doctor, Bianque, narrated in the Han dynasty history, the *Shiji*, juan 105.

11. Kou Zongshi, juan 3, in ZGYXDC 2:56. This passage is paraphrased in Chen Ziming, juan 2, 64–65. See also the eighteenth-century encyclopedia *Yi zong jinjian* (Golden Mirror of Medicine), compiled by Wu Qian et al. See 3:29. For a seventeenth-century doctor's comment, see below, chapter 7, page 249.

12. Chen Ziming, juan 17, 482.

13. See Chen Bangxian 1982: 333, for two fourteenth-century examples from the New Yuan dynastic history. Mistress Fan, after being widowed for twenty years, refused all medicines because it was time to die, while Mistress Ma would not let the doctor examine her inflamed breast: "I am a widow, how can I let a male see this?" In the late Ming the famous literatus Gui Youguang commemorated a widow who would not let doctors inspect her hands, an extreme stance. See the *Kunshan xianzhi* 1576, juan 7, 176. My thanks to Katherine Carlitz for supplying this reference.

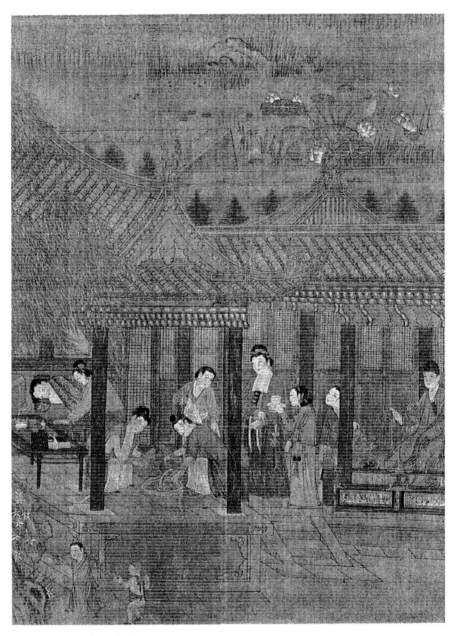

Figure 9. This early Ming wall painting from the Baoning temple in Shaanxi province portrays the medical emergency of a stillbirth. The caption—"aborted fetus and dying mother"—calls attention to Buddhist themes of retribution for the sins of former lives, but the painting shows the newborn's bath in the style used for pictures of the birth of saints. The doctor, seated at the far right, prescribes from a respectful distance, while a senior woman supervises the care of mother and child. Reproduced from the *Baoning si Ming dai shui lu hua* (Ming Dynasty Wall Paintings of the Baoning Temple).

or pretentiously claiming to read a pulse through a string tied around a woman's wrist were the stuff of stage comedy.[14] Such burlesques exaggerated real dilemmas. Whereas in the early years of the Ming dynasty suitably chaperoned palace women could still consult a male doctor directly, later regulations forbade face-to-face contact between them.[15] Gentry customs must have evolved in a similar direction, producing situations like the ones prompting this outburst from a doctor writing at the end of the dynasty in 1640: "Their syndromes are about menstruation and birth or else they are a matter of vaginal discharges [*dai*] and urinary difficulties [*lin*]. . . . If you ask [about such symptoms], the doctor is in danger; if you don't ask, the patient is in danger. However, if you do ask, then the sick woman speaks to her maid and her maid speaks to the master. Before the master says a word his face is crimson and when he does speak his language is roundabout. Having gone through three changes, how can [the account of the symptoms] be clear?" To this doctor the newly published text of Qi Zhongfu's four-hundred-year-old *One Hundred Questions on Medicine for Females* appeared to be a clinical godsend. "It asks what cannot be asked, and answers what is inconvenient to answer."[16]

Social barriers like these, further estranging male physicians from sick women, had something to do with the silencing of physicians' textual voices as well. However, the stricter sex segregation that complicated the social relations of healing did not make Ming doctors more committed to the primacy of Blood and its constructions of bodily gender difference. Instead of reaffirming a holistic bodily female difference that matched their social experience of female seclusion, in thinking about *fuke* they followed a revisionist Ming mainstream of theory, returning to the classically androgynous body. Accordingly they narrowed rather than broadened the scope of "separate prescriptions" for women and questioned the sweeping nosology of Song state medical theory. Rather than displaying a functionalist harmony between dominant social structure and medical construction of the gendered body, Ming *fuke* is evidence for the elusiveness of such models of cultural coherence in the face of the internal complexities of medical discourse itself.

14. Lee T'ao 1950: 34–43.
15. Zheng Jinsheng 1996, quoting the *Ming hui yao*. See also Souliere 1986: 284.
16. See the 1983 edition of *Nüke baiwen*, preface dated 1640 by Min Qiji. In this situation, the Song work's question and answer format particularly recommended it.

Xue Ji and the Legacy of Chen Ziming

Almost exactly 250 years after the death of Chen Ziming, Xue Ji (1487–1559) offered a new version of Chen's *fuke* classic to the world. Xue was the son of an imperial medical officer who followed his father in government medical service in Nanjing before retiring to private practice and authorship in middle age. In the sixteenth century the government rank of *Taiyi* was no longer particularly prestigious, but it did give Xue access to a large medical library, facilitating his work as compiler of new editions of Song texts in many fields, including acupuncture, materia medica, external medicine, dentistry and eye disorders as well as pediatrics and *fuke*. Xue's *Revised Good Prescriptions for Women* (*Jiaozhu furen liang fang*),[17] completed in his sixty-first year, offers an excellent perspective from which to begin to assess the orientations of learned *fuke* in the Ming period. Xue emerges as an eclectic follower of the Yuan revisionists Li Gao and Zhu Zhenheng. Following Li he subsumed the reproductive body under a metabolic one, privileging digestion and the Spleen-stomach organ system as the key to health in females and males alike. Following Zhu he stressed a new interpretation of Fire as a primordial vitality susceptible to pathological transformations under the influence of emotions. His revisions of *Good Prescriptions for Women* bring a subtly altered Ming medical body into view.

Xue honored Chen Ziming as an authoritative ancient master — but his work shows how the conventions of classical commentary worked to reorchestrate an original, repackaging it according to the wisdom of an editor's own experience. The medical text continued to be a malleable product, relocating ancient authority in the stream of changing practice. While respectful of the nosological categories used in Chen Ziming's sections and subheadings, Xue abridged narrative passages, eliminated about six hundred of the original's repertory of prescriptions, and substituted over two hundred of his own formulas. He justified these changes in his own commentaries to each section, illustrated further in over four hundred of his own case histories. Thus altered, Xue's edition became the standard version of Chen Ziming, and the most frequently reprinted and quoted in late imperial times.[18]

17. Xue Ji, *Jiaozhu furen liang fang*, first published 1547. Seventy juan of cases survive, of which his *fuke* is only a fraction.
18. For the history of Xue's revision of Chen, see the preface to the 1985 edition of Chen Ziming, edited by Yu Ying'ao; see also Ma Dazheng 1991: 227–29. Xue also

From the first chapter on menstruation, Xue signaled his approach by his comment on the nature of Blood: "My humble judgment is: Blood is the vital *qi* [*jing qi*] *produced by the digestive process*, which harmonizes the five *zang* organ systems and infuses the six *fu* organ systems. In males it makes [seminal] Essence and in females it makes breast milk and descends to make the Blood sea. So though Heart leads Blood and Liver stores Blood, for both *the controlling function lies with the Spleen system*. Replenish Spleen and harmonize stomach and Blood will grow naturally."[19] Here I see one of the therapeutic consequences of post-Song paradigm shifts. Even though all aspects of function are interrelated, doctrine justified a variety of approaches to the root of an illness: the root might be found in the energy channels, or in one or more organ systems, particularly the five *zang* organs understood as activated in accordance with the Five Phases of bodily and cosmological function. When doctors said their craft was based on "opinion," as they often did, they were recognizing that the act of naming a root dictated their choice of therapeutic strategy. Such names also carried the semiotic messages by which the body was actively imagined.

For Chen Ziming, female disorders were typically rooted in Blood-*qi* malfunction, often from the action of Cold or Wind. Therefore he privileged action on the cardinal channels and their pulses (*jingmai*), revealing the state of Blood and *qi* as energy flows. Xue Ji, on the other hand, privileged the organ systems over circulation channels as the likely root of a problem, and among them the Spleen-stomach system controlling digestion was primary, closely followed by the associated Liver and Heart functions. When he mentioned the Kidney system it was more often with reference to the function of discharge of body wastes. Thus, in cases of menstrual disorder, while Chen's named strategy was to adjust the flow of Blood and *qi*, Xue recommended prescribing to correct Spleen or Liver function. In thinking about "all-purpose prescriptions" like Four Ingredients infusion, Xue commented that all Blood depletions may be traced back to underlying Spleen or Liver malfunction. In all these ways his *fuke* saw reproductive processes dependent upon the metabolic functions of key *zang* organ systems.

When considering "miscellaneous disorders" of women Xue reiter-

---

was the physician most frequently cited (seventy cases) in the *fuke* section of Jiang Guan's *Ming yi lei an*, published in 1591, not long after Xue's death.

19. Xue Ji, juan 1, in ZGYXDC 5:479. Italics mine for emphasis. The term *jing* paired with *qi* calls attention to the way *qi* acts to create new bodily vital substances, here what we could call energy from food. See Sivin 1987: 52.

ated similar themes and added another that had been missing in Chen Ziming. His case histories highlighted a complex of problems rooted in a functional pattern of Liver Fire (*ganhuo*). It produced symptoms of heat (*re*) or was experienced as stasis (*yu*), the latter often coupled with anger (*yunu*) and with congestion (*yujie*). Menstrual disorders and miscellaneous disorders such as Wind attacks (*zhongfeng*) or "depletion fatigues" (*xulao*) also often were traced to a root in Liver Fire.

Behind these accounts of syndromes and their roots lie the views of the Jin-Yuan masters Li Gao and Zhu Zhenheng.[20] Li Gao had argued that "stomach *qi*" derived from food and drink was essential for the nourishment of all primordial *qi* (*yuan qi*), mandating a therapeutic strategy of "warming and replenishing" drug actions to aid digestion. His favorite formulas had names like "replenish center and boost *qi*" or "restore Spleen function," and modern practitioners of TCM read this as a straightforward focus upon the metabolic function of digestion as essential to health and life. Xue Ji's reading of the function of Blood was a direct application of Li Gao's views. Accordingly, in his case histories the preferred therapies for menstrual disorder were prescriptions to "restore Spleen function" (*gui pi*) or to "replenish center and boost *qi*" (*bu zhong yi qi*). To understand Xue Ji's revisionist clinical emphasis upon the syndromes of Liver Fire and "stasis," one must turn to the more intricate reasoning of Zhu Zhenheng (Zhu Danxi), the last of the Jin-Yuan masters, whose synthetic approach made his followers the most widespread Ming interpreters of their teachings. When Ming clinicians of *fuke* looked back to Jin-Yuan teachings, like Xue Ji they were particularly likely to turn to Zhu.

The Body of Yang Surplus and Yin Deficiency

Zhu Zhenheng was important to the rethinking of bodily gender in the Ming dynasty because he was the creative synthesizer of new interpretations of the Yellow Emperor's body of yin and yang. His

20. The other two of the four masters, Liu Wansu and Zhang Congzheng, were less important for *fuke*. They were better known for their environmental interpretation of epidemic fevers, according to *wu yun liu qi* patterns of latent seasonal influence. In pharmacy Zhang was associated with purging "attack" therapies ("sweating," "purging" and "vomiting") and Liu with "bitter cold and cooling" formulas. These strategies were sometimes identified with Northern and lower class practices, while *fuke* owed more to Southern and gentry traditions. See Fan Xingzhun 1985: 166–73; Ren Yingqiu 1980: 39–50; Ma Dazheng 1991: 184–200, 227–230.

characteristic approaches to *fuke* were no more than secondary applications of a theory that reimagined androgyny itself. Medical authorities praised Zhu as the last and greatest of the Jin-Yuan masters, whose integration of Northern and Southern regional styles of diagnosis and prescription was widely influential in the reunited Ming polity. He was also admired as a genuine scholar (*ru*), student of one of Zhu Xi's latter-day disciples and respected member of the elite in Jinhua prefecture in Zhejiang, one of China's centers of *Daoxue* learning.[21] In fact, as a "literati physician" he was also a fashioner of a literati body.

Zhu's motto "Yang is always in excess; yin is always deficient" (*yang chang you yu; yin chang bu zu*) encapsulated his criticism of Song court pharmacy and its official "[Medical] Bureau prescriptions" (*ju fang*), which he blamed for bias toward heating, acrid and drying drug action, and for overemphasizing external etiology based on Wind and Cold. But his theoretical model of bodily functioning went deeper, reinterpreting the *Inner Canon* and the earlier Jin-Yuan masters' discourse on Fire in the light of the neo-Confucian metaphysics of Zhu Xi and Zhou Dunyi.[22] Zhu Zhenheng imagined a yin yang body out of balance, where rather than encompassing yin in a benign hierarchy, yang power was always a potential source of destructive instability. This was a more feminized Southern body, Han, not "barbarian," naturally delicate, in which yin Water — fluids associated with generative centers — needed protection from being overwhelmed by desire's assaultive heat. In opposing the dynamic yang energy of Fire with the tranquil yin realm of Water, Zhu named the bodily basis for a naturalization of ethics, making him a theorist of the body's passions well suited to the sober morality of *Daoxue*.[23]

In Zhu Zhenheng's imagination the human body was animated by

21. Like many "literati physicians" Zhu tried and failed the civil service examinations before turning to medicine. His Confucian teacher, Xu Wenyi, was a fourth-generation disciple of Zhu Xi. It was said that Zhu began to study seriously when Xu instructed this talented pupil to research his master's own chronic illness. For Zhu's life see pp. 1001–41 of the 1993 edition of his collected works. See also Fan Xingzhun 1985: 176–81, and He Shixi 1991, 1:249–57. For *Daoxue* see Bol 1992: 300–341.

22. Zhu Zhenheng's criticism of Song pharmacy was laid out in *Ju fang fahui* (An Exposé of Official Prescriptions). His other major theoretical essay was *Ge zhi yu lun* (More on the "Natural Knowledge" of Phenomena). This title shows that he saw his ideas as building upon Zhu Xi's natural philosophy.

23. According to Bol 1992, *Daoxue* philosophers taught that there is a direct relationship between cosmology and ethics, and that human beings could apprehend their principles directly. Thus the deeper meanings of the teachings of the ancient sages were to be found in nature itself rather than in the literary heritage of the classics.

the unstable interdependence of Water and Fire. "Fire," which played a fundamental role in his thought, was not in itself a pathogenic phenomenon but rather the yang energy driving living functions — or, as he put it, movement through all Five Phases of bodily activity. But as the vitality governing the corresponding five inner *zang* organ systems, including the generative centers of Liver and Kidney, Fire was "yin within and yang without," dependent upon yin primal Water for the healthy functioning of the primordial *qi* of life and death. In this fundamental aspect, freighted with power and danger, it became Ministerial Fire (*xiang huo*), evoking old political metaphors from the *Inner Canon*. Princely Fire (*jun huo*) joined it to constitute a yin yang pair constructing a body of living functions, governing the play of human emotions, and patterning the relationship of the bodily microcosm to the macrocosmic universe.[24]

Through his interpretation of Fire Zhu Zhenheng brought the medical body into correspondence with neo-Confucian metaphysics. No longer a pathogenic environmental *qi*, his Fire had become the active yang principle of motion generated out of the vacuity of the Great Ultimate as described in the philosophy of the neo-Confucian master Zhou Dunyi.[25] This principle was at work in Heaven and Earth as in the human body:

24. The terms *xiang huo* and *jun huo* appear only in passing in the *Huangdi neijing* (*Su wen* 66.3, 68.2.1) as some kind of environmental *qi*. Some said that *jun huo* was the summer heat responsible for fevers in that season, and that *xiang huo* referred to the blazing heat of the direct sun. Looking at Song versions, Catherine Despeux (forthcoming) argues that in *wu yun liu qi* theory Fire was divided into these two aspects in order to have six Cycles to match the six environmental *qi*. The pair also gained internalist readings in Song discussions of the Kidney system as structurally double (left and right Kidney), aligned with both Fire and Water. *Xiang huo* became the name for Kidney's hidden Fire, sometimes identified with the Vital Gate. On the other hand, *jun huo* became a vitality of the Heart system, following Buddhist associations of a physical heat with consciousness (*yijnana*) localized in the Heart. Although this last would seem the closest antecedent to Zhu's reading, Fan Xingzhun 1985: 167–69 points to the influence of Liu Wansu, who promoted cooling formulas for epidemic *shanghan* fevers on the grounds that Fire is both a predominant pathogenic *qi* in the environment and the internal governor of all Five Phases of body function. At the very least Zhu lived at a time when Fire had become a symbolically charged metaphor in representations of the medical body.

25. For Zhou Dunyi's philosophy see the translations in Chan 1963: 460–80. Chan's commentary points out that Zhou's cosmology was novel to his Song followers because it relied on the *Book of Changes* in combination with Five Phase theory rather than using the *Changes'* own Eight Trigrams. This combination, even more than the presumed Daoist inspiration for the concept of the Great Ultimate (*Taiji*), would make a student of the *Huangdi neijing* conclude there was an affinity between the

Fire is dual: there is Princely Fire and Ministerial Fire. Princely Fire is the Fire of man; Ministerial Fire is the Fire of Heaven. Thus Fire is yin within and yang without, and since it governs movement, all that moves is dependent on Fire. To speak of its name, it is called Princely because visible phenomena of the world are produced in succession according to the Five Phases. To speak of its position [i.e., its point of origin], it is called Ministerial because it is generated out of vacancy and nothingness and it guards the place of the human being's primal endowment [at the Vital Gate]. In creating things, Heaven relies on movement, and since human beings enjoy this life they too are in constant motion. Ministerial Fire is that by which this unceasing activity is fostered. . . . Without this Fire Heaven would not be able to create; without this Fire man would not have the wherewithal to be born.[26]

Here Ministerial Fire is constructed as an overarching vital energy manifest as cosmogonic yang in Heaven and as generative yin in the earthly function of reproduction. However, when manifest in the form of embodied emotions Fire assumes a potentially destructive aspect, pointed out in Zhu's famous warning that "Ministerial Fire is the thief of primordial *qi*."[27] To explain how the creative foundation of life can also be a force of destruction, Zhu drew on ideas of creation and the problem of desire in Zhou Dunyi's metaphysics. In the cosmogonic sequence Heavenly Fire activates and arouses consciousness, producing the world of phenomena; on earth human feelings respond to the stimulation of the world of external things, and so desires are born. "Master Zhou [Dunyi] said, 'One's psyche [*shen*] becomes aware, the five human feelings [*wu xing*] are moved in response and all phenomena arise [in one's consciousness].' "[28] Fire here becomes the bodily vitality driving human emotion and all the restless cravings of the desiring self. Such Fire is both Princely and Ministerial, identified with the faculty of consciousness (*shen*) ruled by the Heart system above, and animating the sexual drives of the generative Kidney system below. When this govern-

---

two. Zhu Zhenheng's friend, the Jinhua scholar Dai Liang, summarized Zhu's thought as combining "the discourses of the three [Jin-Yuan medical] masters . . . the ideas of the philosophy of the Great Ultimate, the *Book of Changes*, the *Book of Rites*, the *Tongshu* [of Zhou Dunyi] and the assorted works of the orthodox [neo-Confucian] philosophers." See Dai Liang's biography of Zhu in He Shixi 1991, 1:249–53.

26. "Xiang huo" section of Zhu Zhenheng, *Ge zhi yu lun*, in SKQS 746:667.

27. This aphorism originated in a cryptic saying of Li Gao.

28. Zhu Zhenheng, *Ge zhi yu lun*, in SKQS 746:667. The "five human feelings" are conventionally understood as emotions—joy, anger, desire, fear and sorrow—but in this context something broader seems to be meant, closer to the affective capacities fundamental to *xing* as human nature. Zhu aligned these "five feelings" with the "five Fires" of the *Huangdi neijing*.

ing Fire was destabilized, producing restless, chaotic and wayward movement, yin Water was threatened and illness arose. Zhu explained this psycho-physical dynamic in a critical passage about Sun Simiao's classic advice to males on the art of the bed-chamber:

> In living persons the Heart system produces Fire and dwells above, and the Kidney system makes Water and dwells below. Water can ascend and Fire can descend in ceaseless movement, sustaining life. Water in essence is tranquil and Fire in essence is active. Activity is easy and tranquility is difficult: the sages have never been wrong about this. When the scholars [*ru*] say, "Rectify your Heart, guard your Heart, nourish your Heart," they are teaching how to keep this Fire from random activity. The physicians' teaching that "mild habits and meditative practices guard one's spirit within"[29] is also a means to curb Fire's random activity. Now Ministerial Fire is stored in the yin regions of the Kidney and Liver systems; and when Princely [Heart] Fire is not moving randomly about, Ministerial Fire will simply keep one's innate foundation [*bing ming*] secure. How then could there be fierce blazes and madly dashing flames?[30]

As a moral psychology of emotions, this was not a dualism of reason and passion but a complex mode of embodiment whereby Heart, seat of consciousness (*shen*), impressionable and easily stirred to sensuous heat, could flare up and go astray, igniting the fires of sexual desire and turning generative vitalities into self-destructive forces. The warning that "Ministerial Fire is the thief of primordial *qi*" called directly for sexual control in males. However, restraining lust was not a matter of abstinence; rather, the management of desire was a moral enterprise of self-cultivation, channelling the sexual powers of the body according to a telos of human reproduction in a universal continuum of life linking progenitors and descendants. "When man's Heart assents to the will of Heaven according to the Way, it is governed by tranquility. The motions of the five Fires will be controlled within and one's Ministerial Fire will simply support the creative principle [*zao hua*] enacting the succession of human lives without end [*sheng sheng bu xi*] in their cyclical functioning."[31] Here the control of sexual desire was linked to higher forms of sagely self-cultivation, and the virtuous body was dedicated to the ancestors. In turn self-cultivation was also somaticized as bodily health.

---

29. The aphorism is from the *Su wen* 2:8.

30. See the subsection entitled "Fang zhong bu yi lun" (On [Sun Simiao's] "Replenishing Benefits of the Bed-Chamber"), Zhu Zhenheng, *Ge zhi yu lun*, in SKQS 746:671–72. See also Song Shugong 1991: 356–58.

31. Zhu Zhenheng, *Ge zhi yu lun*, in SKQS 746:668.

However, Zhu Zhenheng imagined the dialectic of Fire and Water in the human body as a relationship of unequal forces. The inevitable deficiency of yin is a vulnerability of body fluids to the heat of external pathogens, and a vulnerability of generative vitalities to sexual depletion from uncontrolled desires and reproductive use. Yin's innate vulnerability is revealed in the limited span of reproductive years ("thirty years of use") in a human life bounded by age and death. Yin's deficiency is recognized in the gap between the primal Kidney's finite powers of generative vitality, which wane with age, and the boundlessness of the Heart/psyche's desires. Thinking of Heart and Kidney, Fire and Water, as yin yang pairs in the human body as opposed to the realm of the Great Ultimate, Zhu Zhenheng did not ground Fire in Water's inexhaustible creative source but represented the latter as prone to the instability of the human order of things. "When yin is depleted, Heavenly *qi* is exhausted; when yang is flourishing, the *qi* of Earth is weak." In this subversive reading of yin and yang, chthonic Earth is generative but weak, while lordly Heaven can be overbearing and destructive. Such an ambiguous inversion of the normal yin yang value hierarchy is striking for its moral pessimism. It shows the limits of a model of body balance based on the cyclical rhythms of yin and yang when applied to a human life path understood in terms of finite resources and fixed span of years. In therapy, it also called attention to Zhu's signature clinical strategy, "nourish yin and make Fire descend" to its proper hiding place in the Vital Gate (*ming men*) of the Kidney region, protecting vulnerable fluids against heat.[32]

With Zhu Zhenheng the medical body was aligned with distinctively neo-Confucian constructions of cosmological and moral order, and so with the *Daoxue* scholar's project of self-cultivation. In this revision textual fragments of the Yellow Emperor's body as preserved in the *Inner Canon* were deployed to highlight the problem of human desires in a bodily economy of finite resources. The ancient ideal of longevity was imagined as realizable through the internal moral discipline of the sage rather than through the kingly power to tap the energies of the cosmos itself. However, like the original, Zhu's body of yang Ministerial Fire and yin Kidney Water was an androgynous one. Its metaphorical pathos simply evoked a more feminine core—one that saw healthy bodily vitalities in terms of "yin within yang" as well as "yang within yin." This quietistic ideal of healthy function, where tranquil yin waters would be

32. Zhu Zhenheng, *Ge zhi yu lun,* in SKQS 746:640–41, 667–68.

protected against the activist assault of unbridled yang, was a revision of androgyny, not a negation of it.

Nonetheless, Zhu Zhenheng's body of Ministerial Fire was, like the Yellow Emperor's original, rhetorically male. If his words projected onto the body relations of power in society, these most likely were the postures available to Han men as southerners, scholars and subjects of the conquering Mongol Yuan dynasty. They evoked the literati ideal of letters (*wen*) over arms (*wu*), and a weaker body of yin culture over a stronger one of yang force. When his words addressed the problem of desire in the neo-Confucian movement of *Daoxue*, they most directly applied to the construction of a literati masculinity.

Ming *Fuke* and Ming Androgyny

Zhu Zhenheng's body of Fire and Water offered an important refiguration of the meaning of gender in the androgynous body, rather than a construction of bodily difference between the sexes. In fact Zhu was among the first to move away from Song *fuke*'s emphasis on Blood as a root in pattern diagnosis.[33] But Zhu's emphasis upon nourishing yin fluids did support distinctive therapeutic strategies for the gestational body. Focus shifted from pathologies of external origin—Wind and Cold, for example—to those arising from internal depletion often associated with emotions. Whether the problem was menstrual irregularity, miscarriage, lactation failure or barrenness, followers of Zhu blamed hot and acrid medicines, heating foods, or the Fire of desires in turn.[34] Concerning postpartum his revisions were particularly influential. The saying attributed to Zhu, "First give strong replenishers of Blood and *qi* and treat other illness symptoms as secondary," became the clinical standard among his successors.[35] Such a doctrine medicalized normal postpartum as depletion of both yin and yang, thus explaining diverse symptoms. It served both to criticize doctors who carelessly read postpartum symptoms as indicators of opportunistic diseases and also

33. This is observed by Ma Dazheng 1991: 191–92.
34. Zhu Zhenheng, *Ge zhi yu lun*, in SKQS 746:654, 661–63.
35. Zhu Zhenheng, *Ju fang fahui*, in SKQS 746:655, 695–96. For a late Ming interpretation, see Fang Guang, juan 20, 4:2252. For a modern summary of Zhu's *fuke*, see Ma Dazheng 1991: 191–92, 218. Ma emphasizes passages showing Zhu's observation of uterine anatomy and his construction of some types of vaginal discharges as "phlegm" disorders, the product of Damp Heat.

to cast doubt on formulas like "Black Spirit powder" that purged after-birth as bad or stagnant Blood.

Zhu Zhenheng summed up his construction of gestation as depleting in a widely reported case of miscarriage involving his sister-in-law. It made him realize, he said, that wealthy women of his own day suffered from the melancholy stasis of an idle life. "Their plump appearance is a sign of *qi* depletion; their prolonged inactivity shows in a lack of cir-culation [of the Five Phases of body activity] and in the feebleness of their *qi*." Instead of the "shrink fetus" doses with which Song gentle-women had sought to ease birth by repressing fetal *qi*, he recommended a well-known fetal tranquilizer, Purple Thyme (*zisu*) infusion, to "re-plenish *qi*."[36] In sum, the clinical traditions associated with Zhu Zhen-heng's views encouraged drug action on *qi* to move Blood, constructed gestational processes as weakening rather than polluting, and identified pathological heat as a bodily manifestation of the psyche's emotions and desires, a function of the Heart system. If nourishing generative yin in males meant protecting Kidney fluids, in females the corresponding *zang* organ system was Liver, whose function of Blood storage was threatened by depletion and heat. This led practitioners of *fuke* to the syndromes of Liver Fire and "static congestion" as pathological patterns damaging generative vitalities in women. Hot dry symptoms associated with negative emotion and menstrual irregularity revealed underlying depletion, expressed in weak *qi* flow, which threatened fluids and repro-ductive health.[37]

In a variety of ways, then, Zhu Zhenheng's views shaped the way Chen Ziming was read by his Ming interpreter, Xue Ji. When Xue Ji identified the symptoms of his *fuke* patients as manifestations of Liver Fire or of static congestion, he was placing the functions "where Blood is leader" within Zhu's model of disease process. In anger, unregulated Ministerial Fire might assault yin fluids and disrupt the storage function of Blood. The Liver system was the likely root of "depletion Heat"

---

36. Zhu Zhenheng, *Ge zhi yu lu*, in SKQS 746:654. See also Jiang Guan, juan 11, 333; Ma Dazheng 1991: 191–92; and Ren Yingqiu 1980: 52–54. For "purple thyme" see *Zhong yao da cidian* 2:2355–56.

37. The clinical traditions associated with Zhu's many disciples are traceable through a variety of Ming-era texts grouped under the generic title *Danxi xinfa* (Es-sential Art of Danxi). I have looked at two: Fang Guang's *Danxi xinfa fuyu*, 1536, and Chao Yingchun's *Danxi xiansheng zhifa xinyao*, 1556. They are essentially inde-pendent works on common themes. Liu Shijue 1995 says that all of the *Xinfa* texts may trace back to a set of notes compiled by Zhu Zhenheng's disciple Tai Yuanli, perhaps after the master's death.

triggered by such negative emotions. In his case histories of "miscellaneous disorders" in women, the diagnosis of Liver Fire was Xue's way of pointing to the role of heat and emotion in the etiology of depleted or congested yin Blood. Similarly, stasis (*yu*) was a commonplace Hot syndrome, identified with Fire, anger and congestion.[38] Although judging by his case histories Xue seldom used the term Ministerial Fire as a diagnostic category in clinical settings, Zhu Zhenheng's underlying model of the relationship between body function, generative vitalities, emotion and sickness underlay such diagnoses.

In Zhu Zhenheng's body of Ministerial Fire, broadly macrocosmic views of disease pathology linked to the environmental *qi* of seasons and Wind gave way to a discourse on internal weakness — the inherent instability of internal yin yang relationships in a body prone to age and decline. Fire, both creative and destructive, named the energy driving living functions and also the havoc resulting from uncontrolled desires. In this way Zhu Zhenheng's revision of the Yellow Emperor's body led the Ming imagination not only to locate the sources of disorder within a more bounded form, but also to focus on bodies of generation linked to sexual function calling for morally responsible management.

Some have argued that the competitive pressures of the Ming-Qing examination ladder of success fostered elite male sexual anxieties, while the equation of public prestige with inner moral worth in a culture of ritual display led both scholars and the state to project their ideals of virtue onto the emblematic Ming figure of the chaste woman.[39] Literary representations of the frustrated scholarly male or ardent chaste female were certainly commonplace in late Ming writing. But I want to avoid reading them as reflections of a cultural pathology repressing natural human drives. Medicine here is an alternative lens — better understood as constructing a culturally specific form of normality, shaping the experience of embodiment. In deploying ideal norms of sexual continence and psycho-physical self-mastery, Ming medicine owed much to Zhu

38. Under the category of miscellaneous disorders in women, Xue Ji included 102 cases, of which eighty-two name an underlying syndrome. Liver Fire accounts for eighteen of these, the most frequent diagnosis. Out of twenty-eight cases where a patient's emotional state is commented on, twenty-five women are identified as angry (*nu*).

39. Such women were more often widows than virgins, since chastity was understood basically as sexual "loyalty" of wives to their husbands, a virtue with profound political resonances in Ming China. For a psychoanalytic approach to the spread of the chaste widow cult in the Yuan and Ming, see T'ien 1988. Elvin 1984, Holmgren 1985, Carlitz 1991 and 1997, Mann 1997, and Birge 1995 develop anthropological, economic, and social perspectives.

Zhenheng's morally significant natural philosophy of the body as the site of the superior man's self-cultivation. If late Ming gentry women found themselves more restricted than their Song foremothers had been, confined spatially within sex-segregated walls and physically by their bound feet, these dispositions of their persons also marked their participation in a bodily culture of restraint and self-control emblematic of moral order.

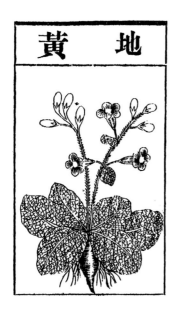

CHAPTER 5

To Benefit Yin

Fuke *and Late Ming*
Medical Culture

In the previous chapters I have written of the evolution
of *fuke* as a textual discourse but only tangentially of the lives of the
healers and patients who were the subjects of that discourse. As I turn
to the late sixteenth and seventeenth centuries, my task as a historian
changes. Textual traces no longer swim in and out of view, appearing
as flotsam on a vast unrecoverable stream of past life; rather, they crowd
the field of vision, churning up the surface images of a time of change —
of urbanization, of the spread of a money economy, of the loosening of
status boundaries, of cultural experiment and religious syncretism. The
documents that produce these historical riches are both a more accessible
record and in themselves evidence of the gradual Ming maturation of a
cultural nexus of power ordered around the printed word. Thus the *fuke*
of the late Ming can tell a story of medical authors knowable as individuals, whose lives were embedded in well-studied social networks of

politics, commerce and culture. These authors link to audiences as well—to readers both male and female—hinting of the social identities of patients as well as healers. Taking up the last segment of my survey of *fuke* as a textual tradition spanning Song through Ming, I locate it in a late sixteenth- and early seventeenth-century medical culture that forms the context for the remaining chapters of this book.

A good introduction to what "separate prescriptions" for women had come to mean by the end of the Ming dynasty is an enormously popular work produced in the early seventeenth century, *To Benefit Yin: A Comprehensive Guide (Ji yin gangmu)*. Here the legacy of Chen Ziming was doubly layered over, not only by Xue Ji's revisionism but also by the contributions of three important late Ming authorities who claimed to draw freely on all schools of medical thought: Wang Kentang (1549–1613), Wu Zhiwang (1552–1628), and Wang Qi (c. 1600–1668). Their summation of *fuke*, in contrast with that of the Southern Song four hundred years earlier, came out of a cultural context where not only the ideas of learned medicine but also the nature of textuality and the social configuration of communities of readers and writers had changed significantly.

By the late Ming the ideal of the literati physician had been well established for several hundred years. It now shaped the education, clinical strategies and cultural self-representation of most literate physicians, including many who came from hereditary lineages of family practitioners or who derived income from pharmacy shops. Such medical men were not dependent upon state office or patronage but were now part of a broader urban social stratum that included merchants, artists and scholars, with whom even the highest level of degree-holding officials might informally associate. On the one hand medicine had become well accepted as a respectable vocation for men who dropped off the ladder of official achievement, whether because of examination failure, financial need, or political alienation or disgrace. On the other hand, the commercial opportunities of a sophisticated national market in materia medica meant that doctoring was a economic step up for some, and a physician might become a wealthy man.[1] With the refining polish of literati culture extending down from

---

1. For Ming pharmacies run by famous physicians Wang Ji, Xu Chunfu, and Wang Yilong, among others, see Dong Guangdong and Liu Huiling 1995. The authors believe that in the Qing dynasty it gradually became more common for such shops to be owned by nonphysicians. Ximen Qing, protagonist of *Jin ping mei* (see

above and the emollient influence of commercial wealth spreading upward from below, learned physicians might be part of an elite in
which status boundaries were blurred by the influence of money, talent or celebrity.

Similarly, by the late Ming print had come to be the most prestigious
and powerful tool of cultural reproduction, overshadowing oral and
manuscript technologies. Commercially produced books outstripped
state-sponsored ones in volume, in diversity of genres, and levels of
audience addressed. Popular vernacular works democratized literati
knowledge downward, and also drew the folkways of the village world
onto their pages. In medicine the printed book as a source of authority
and guide to practice had become so ubiquitous that authors of prefaces
liked to complain that "ox carts are weighted down" by the volumes
available. They also complained of confusion, as medical classics and the
works elucidating Jin-Yuan lineages of learning acquired new layers of
exegesis, while the practice-based wisdom of clinicians produced hundreds of books of prescriptions, each bearing a healer's personal therapeutic signature.

Among these were case history collections, a Ming genre of medical
publishing increasingly available in the sixteenth century. It also became more common for successful local practitioners to seek the prestige of print for their hitherto "secret" family traditions. Philanthropic
impulses added to the flood, as private gentlemen seeking Buddhist
merit in charitable good works came forward to print the manuscript
whose lore had saved a stricken family member, or the old pharmacy
text just discovered in a local scholar's library. As literacy grew among
ordinary commoners, there was demand for printed household handbooks in an easy-to-consult format, or for sections on medicine in
comprehensive popular almanacs, side by side with information on
the calendar, ritual and husbandry. The newly expansive urban, com-
mercialized culture that supported such a knowledge industry did not
extend over the whole countryside but was identified with the trading
and administrative centers of core regions, particularly Jiangnan—the
lower Yangzi river system, where most of the Ming-era doctors I discuss lived. (See figure 10.) Yet the geographical reach of print communication was widespread enough that medical publishing as a charitable undertaking was sometimes justified because it offered assistance

---

chapter 8), is a famous late Ming fictional representation of a wealthy drug wholesaler
who was not a doctor. For Jiangnan "Confucian physicians," see Chao Yuanling 1995:
150–213.

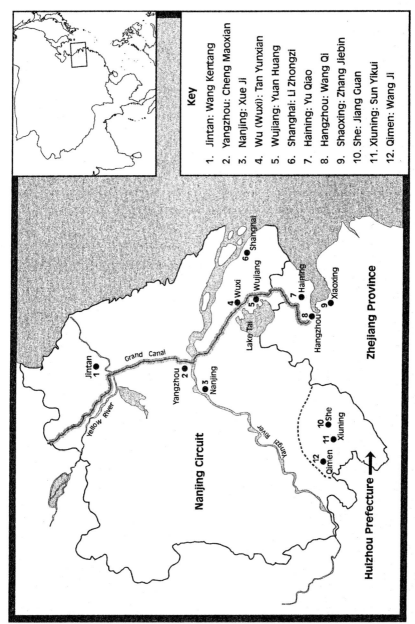

Key

1. Jintan: Wang Kentang
2. Yangzhou: Cheng Maoxian
3. Nanjing: Xue Ji
4. Wu (Wuxi): Tan Yunxian
5. Wujiang: Yuan Huang
6. Shanghai: Li Zhongzi
7. Haining: Yu Qiao
8. Hangzhou: Wang Qi
9. Shaoxing: Zhang Jiebin
10. She: Jiang Guan
11. Xiuning: Sun Yikui
12. Qimen: Wang Ji

Figure 10. Map of Ming Jiangnan, indicating native places of doctors discussed in text.

to remote hamlets and mountain villages that lacked skilled local doctors of their own.

The Making of *To Benefit Yin*

Unlike the earlier Song and Ming works I have surveyed, *To Benefit Yin* was a learned medical treatise published under the name of a gentleman of rank in the tiny elite of national office holders. It was also a commercial publishing venture aimed at a cultured reading public that extended to commoners and included women. The scholar-official who is considered the primary author was Wu Zhiwang, a *jinshi* degree holder and minor civil and military official from Shaanxi province who in the 1590s served as a magistrate in Jiangdu county around the Jiangnan city of Yangzhou.[2] In making his compilation Wu said he had relied heavily upon the *Guideline for the Treatment of Female Disorders* by Wang Kentang, a more famous classmate in the *jinshi* examinations of 1589 and a man who abandoned national office for medicine.[3] But the work gained wide readership because of its popular second edition, which appeared thirty-five years after Wu's death, edited and rearranged by the well-known Hangzhou literatus and publisher Wang Qi.[4]

If Wu Zhiwang and Wang Kentang were among a small number Ming-era officials who also sought a public role as medical authorities, Wang Qi was a Huizhou merchant[5] — part of the free-spirited world of Jiangnan artists, entrepreneurs and bon vivants whose lives embraced both the pleasures of the late Ming urban "floating world" and the turbulence of the Ming-Qing dynastic transition in the 1640s and 1650s. His family book business, the Huanduzhai ("Returning to Reading

2. Wu Zhiwang 1620, 1621, *Ji yin gangmu*, with preface by the author. These two early editions quickly became rare, though it is said that the work circulated in his home district in hand copies.

3. Wang Kentang 1608, *Nüke zheng zhi zhunsheng*. First published as part of Wang's 44-juan collected works. The two men may have been acquainted, not only because they passed the national exams in the same year but because both served in the military campaign in Korea in 1593.

4. Wu Zhiwang 1665, *Ji yin gangmu*, edited and with a preface by Wang Qi. Although Wu Zhiwang is named as the primary author of this revised edition in most bibliographies, I refer to it hereafter in my notes as the Wang Qi edition.

5. Huizhou prefecture, made up of six counties in southern Anhui roughly due west of Hangzhou, was famous for both its merchants and its physicians. The medical culture of the region is often referred to as Xin'an, after a famous local mountain. See Grant 1996: chapter 2.

Studio"), produced fiction, drama, travel guides for merchants, examination aids, medical works, model letters and other how-to books for daily living. Wang Qi brought to the enterprise wide social connections among prominent literati as well as the marketing network for which Huizhou merchants were famous. Ellen Widmer has shown how the Huanduzhai's publishing list reflected the personal interests and talents of Wang and his circle, and how the studio attached to his book shop was a social and intellectual center for literati in and out of officialdom. All this helped the Huanduzhai tailor its products to a well-defined reading community. It also reached out to what Widmer calls "weaker readers" in the commoner class, and to "female talent" — by printing writings by and for women.[6]

Wu Zhiwang, Wang Kentang and Wang Qi moved comfortably in interlocking official, literary and medical circles. The first two were well known as national-level officials, but they also collected medical disciples and recorded their clinical experiences in case histories; medical authorship is what gained them fame. Medicine was less central to Wang Qi, who wrote novels, managed his family's publishing business, and called himself a serious follower of Daoism. Practicing doctors were only one of several groups among his network of kin and associates, which included ranking scholars, unemployed literati and Ming loyalists, and a number of women poets. His medical persona was explained this way by Cha Wang, a doctor friend who helped edit *To Benefit Yin:* "[He] is a student of the Dao who uses medicine to explore the Dao, which does not exhaust the Dao. He uses the Dao to broaden medicine without busying himself with [the details of] medicine. . . . As for me, I only know about disease [*bing*]." Though he may have relied on Cha Wang as a consultant, Wang Qi promoted himself successfully as a medically learned commentator on the text of *To Benefit Yin.*[7]

In this world, the distinction between literati physician (*ru yi*) and physician by family inheritance or vocation (*shi yi*) need mean very little.

---

6. Widmer 1989 and 1996. See also Hanson 1995.

7. Cha Wang said he studied medicine for twenty years and aspired to write his own work of *fuke*. The 1665 edition lists Wu Zhiwang as author, Wang Qi as critical commentator (*jianshi*), and Cha Wang as consultant (*canyue*). See Cha Wang's preface to the 1665 edition held in the Cabinet Library, Tokyo. My thanks to Ellen Widmer for making the prefaces to this version available to me. They do not appear in the 1665 edition held in the rare book library of the Zhongyi Yanjiuyuan in Beijing. But woodblock books could add or discard pages even within a single "edition." Widmer 1996 has other examples of such variations in the surviving products of the Huanduzhai.

Here scholars who did not claim to be doctors and physicians recognized as literati mingled socially and shared knowledge. How members of such a medical and cultural elite related to humbler working practitioners is another question. There is the curious fact that Wang Qi included in his 1665 edition of *To Benefit Yin* a preface by one Min Sheng, a man who claimed that the text was based on the family traditions of a hereditary physician from Zhejiang who had been an intimate of Min's father. Wu, he said, had discovered and published it.[8] The implication — that *To Benefit Yin* owed more to a lineage of obscure "hereditary doctors" than to the high official who appropriated their work — shows how the ideal of the literati physician continued to be contested, and how "secret" family traditions outside the sphere of print culture remained a jealously guarded alternative source of medical authority.

Min Sheng's story also shows that conflicting claims to authentic medical authorship were now part of the cultural scene. When Wang Qi omitted Wu Zhiwang's original preface from his edition, and also excised Wu's personal case histories, he appeared to be subtly seconding Min. Nonetheless, in spite of these moves, the result did not construct individual authorship as we understand it today. *To Benefit Yin,* like its predecessors, was a composite product, a bricolage rather than a tract, its components to be taken up, modified and abandoned as successive users saw fit. Wu Zhiwang himself, in that discarded preface to the 1620 edition, placed the work in a line of descent from the earlier eminent medical masters who were liberally quoted in its pages. These intellectual antecedents ran from the *Inner Canon* through Chen Ziming, the Jin-Yuan masters and Xue Ji, up to Wang Kentang. Then, just as Wu Zhiwang claimed the special authority of Wang Kentang, his more famous contemporary, for his text, so a few decades later Wang Qi pronounced (disingenuously, it seems) that he was publishing this now rare "cinnabar classic" unaltered.

In sum, the text that gained such wide popularity after 1665 (there were thirty-four known reprintings before the end of the imperial era)[9] was an eclectic work within which multiple authorial "voices" jostled together. All three major compilers followed the basic topical outline of Chen Ziming's work, preserving Song and Ming views from many

8. See 1665 edition held in Tokyo Cabinet Library, preface by Min Sheng. Min claimed that this physician, Jin Hanfeng, had been intimate with his family. Jin is mentioned briefly in He Shixi 1991, 2:50 as a late Ming physician from Wuxing, near Lake Tai.

9. See Yu Ying'ao preface to Chen Ziming. See also Xue Qinglu 1991: 431–32.

sources side by side, leaving interpretation open. Nonetheless, the 1665 text permits a reading, emphasized by Wu Zhiwang's adaptations of Wang Kentang and Wang Qi's further critical commentary, of a characteristic late Ming approach, distinguished from earlier texts in both format and viewpoint. In the succession of prefaces, the three compilers made claims that showed where clinical fashion had changed since the Southern Song or even since Xue Ji's day eighty years earlier.[10]

They rejected Chen Ziming's diagnostic categories as "based on little more than Wind and Cold," leading to an overemphasis on expelling pathogens with fiercely "heating" remedies. They complained that his prescriptions failed to balance the five flavors properly, addressing discrete symptoms rather than underlying patterns. If many of Chen Ziming's prescriptions were now dismissed as uncouth, his nosological categories, passed along by Xue Ji, were thought overelaborate, redundant and confusing, without clear guidelines for the user. The late Ming compilers also criticized the Jin-Yuan revisionism of Zhu Zhenheng and Xue Ji. Although Zhu's pharmaceutical repertory was known to be flexible in practice, his signature strategy of "nourish yin and make Fire descend" was one-sided, too fearful of Ministerial Fire and too slow to boost yang with warming ingredients in cases of depleted generative vitalities.[11]

10. My discussion is based on a comparison of the three texts: Wang Kentang's *Nüke,* Wu Zhiwang's 1620 *Ji yin gangmu* in 5 juan, and Wang Qi's 1665 edition in 14 juan. The Wu Zhiwang text drew on Wang Kentang most heavily for its outline of topics, a number of discussions, and the many case histories from famous Yuan and Ming physicians. Wu eliminated Wang's references to pre-Song classics, including the *Zhen jiu jiayi jing,* a classic of acupuncture, and dropped most of the Song nosology of miscellaneous disorders inherited from Chen Ziming. He expanded the sections on genital disorders, lactation and sexuality. Wang Qi, in addition to providing a running commentary in his "eyebrow" notes, excised most of Wu Zhiwang's own case histories and a number of his discussions, adding a substantial number of prescriptions as well as putting other prescriptions under new headings. He substituted his own preface for Wu's original. Wang Kentang emerges as a more conservative historical scholar of medicine, while Wu Zhiwang included brief notes on birth ritual therapies that the two Wangs dismissed as superstition. Wu's strong views on diet and health represent another personal note. See also Jiang and Li 1988, and Cao Bingzhang 1936, *Tiyao,* juan 9, 10–11.

11. The influential mid-Ming Huizhou physician Wang Ji had attacked Zhu for overemphasizing "bitter and cooling" as against "warming and replenishing" therapeutic strategies. Wang Ji wanted to promote the use of ginseng in combination with astragalus root (*huangqi*) for yin depletion disorders like *xulao* consumptions as well as for Cold Damage fevers. He complained that Zhu's influence encouraged clients to fear heating ingredients whenever their symptoms involved the loss of blood or other fluids. See Grant 1996, chapter 2. In chapter seven, I discuss the practice of a seventeenth-century doctor who espoused "warming and replenishing" methods.

Xue Ji, on the other hand, had been an overly opinionated partisan of Spleen-stomach therapies, and in his zeal to revise Song pharmacy had rejected many useful old formulas along with the outmoded ones.

Accordingly, *To Benefit Yin* was designed to be both catholic and selective. It included case histories from the Jin-Yuan masters Li Gao and Zhu Zhenheng, and from Xue Ji, but added many from Wang Ji as well. The compilers tempered their appreciation of famous old Song and pre-Song classical formulas with warnings against ignorant appropriation of ill-understood prescriptions from the ancients. A majority of the formulas actually cited came neither from Song or Jin-Yuan masters but from the more eclectic writings of mid- and late Ming popular experts, like Wan Quan, Li Yan and Gong Tingxian.[12]

A selling point of *To Benefit Yin* was clear, practical organization: "Not only doctors but . . . ordinary gentlemen can put a copy on the shelf for household use," promised the cover page of the 1665 edition. Topics were introduced by syndrome clusters, emphasizing symptoms; discussion minimized historical exegesis, facilitating bedside use by the sick and their families. Visual features of graphic design supported a subtle intertextuality. Wang Qi's own voluminous "eyebrow notes" along the top of the page, supplemented by an appendix to the 1665 edition under his name, concluded the chain of commentary and criticism with a decidedly personal voice. The voice of this latter-day "gentleman admirer of medicine" is heard throughout, by turns cautionary and admiring, now educating the reader about symptom relief, now dissecting distinct herbal strands in the symphonic whole of a prescription formula, now explaining the cosmological relationships that constituted its deeper meaning.

In Wang Qi's eyebrow notes, late Ming readers heard an enthusiastic literatus explain the refinements of the art of prescription so that they could become, like himself, a connoisseur of its language of the concrete. Each materia medica has its own invariable nature, like an instrument in an orchestra. It is not that angelica loses its own intrinsic qualities in combination with other ingredients, he said, but that its nature can either be reinforced and enhanced or counterbalanced and attenuated.

---

12. Wan Quan (1488–1578) was the most famous member of a Hubei medical lineage. Texts based on his family tradition circulated widely in central and south China in the late Ming. Li Yan was the author of *Yixue ru men*, 1575, and Gong Tingxian's *Wan bing hui chun*, 1587, was also reprinted by the Huanduzhai. According to Jiang and Li 1988, in the Wang Qi edition of *Ji yin gangmu* sixty-five percent of the prescriptions were from these sources rather than from earlier authorities like Xue Ji or Zhu Zhenheng.

A traditional system of classification ordered the proportions and functions of each herb in a formula according to a hierarchy, designating one drug as ruler (*jun*), with minister (*chen*), assistant (*zuo*) and envoy (*shi*) in supporting positions.[13] Wang Qi showed how each prescription should also embody yin and yang qualities in order to produce an formula of balanced ingredients counteracting the imbalance of the sickness. Thus the materia medica in a prescription should combine a hierarchical order of ingredients and also an appropriate balance of complementary opposites.

Take, for example, his analysis of a Five Ingredients Replenishing pill recommended for amenorrhea. This prescription assumes that the sufferer will need first to boost Blood and second to clear away any pathological Fire that may have attacked fluids. It also assumes that for effective drug action Blood will be dependent on *qi*. The relationship of the five ingredients involves both a hierarchy of drug actions and a balance between yin and yang:

	Yin		Yang
(1)	dried *dihuang* (to replenish Blood)		ginseng (to replenish *qi*)
(2)	poria fungus (to stimulate fluids)		Lycium bark (to clear heat)
(3)		ox-knee (*niuxi*) acts as envoy to lead menstrual flow down and out of body	

Here the prescription orchestrates the herbs to produce three effects in descending order: they increase the production of body fluids, reduce body heat and stimulate menstrual discharge. But Wang Qi explained the deep structure of the formula in terms of a larger pattern: "Dried *dihuang* replenishes Heavenly Water; ginseng grows Heavenly *qi*. It is said that Water is produced from *qi*; thus if *qi* does not descend [from Heaven] Water cannot be produced. So we use white poria fungus [*baifuling*] to make Heavenly *qi* descend [as water] and Lycium bark [*digupi*] to clean *qi* of its excess Fire; ox-knee [*niuxi*] leads the ingredients below.

13. This standard classification followed the *Su wen*. For its place in the *bencao* tradition, and alternative meanings of these categories, see Unschuld 1986: 116, and Farquhar 1994: 181–82.

This is underlying theme of the prescription."[14] In this prescription the formula aims for an overall yin yang balance of the first two ingredients, while at the next level the "yin within yang" powers of poria fungus allow *qi* to lead, encompassing Blood yet reinforcing that the main task at hand is to engender earthly Water so that fluid becomes menses and finds its proper descending path. Ox-knee was often prescribed to expel menstrual or even gestational Blood (as an abortifacient), but when Wang Qi placed it last, in the subsidiary "envoy" position, he was showing that the deep structure of the formula was not about symptom relief. The yin yang pattern was similar to those at work in religious and ritual practice and enshrined in metaphysics and philosophy.

As in this example of ox-knee to stimulate uterine bleeding, Wang Qi's comments on pharmacy often called attention to drug properties for symptom relief—how they produced sweat, purged bowels or eased pain. He also took for granted that efficacy was sometimes bound up in a logic of concrete natural symbols of a familiar kind: gall for courage, deer horn for potency, cinnabar for longevity. But these empirical and magical aspects were less central to his late Ming art of pharmacy than the power of the prescription to materialize in exquisite balance the hidden natural relationships at work in the body as in the world. Such medicine offered a sufferer balm through bodily incorporation of a specific microcosmic energy system configuring dynamic relationships of yin and yang. Still, the prescription was by no means purely symbolic: the healer managed the material world of symptoms, and did not just ritually manipulate herbs understood primarily as signifiers of cosmic relationships. Efficacy pertained to both. Wang Qi's commentaries on formulas and materia medica formed an accessible guide through these multiple layers of interpretation, and helped make *To Benefit Yin* abidingly popular with readers.

Female Ailment and Cure in *To Benefit Yin*

Eyebrow notes, prefaces and other commentary made readers of *To Benefit Yin* well aware that when medicine rejected Chen

---

14. Wang Qi ed., eyebrow note, 51. See *Zhong yao da cidian* 1:820, 1597–98, for *fuling* and *digupi*. While indicating his general belief that *qi* should lead in *fuke* formulas, Wang Qi did not list exact quantities, presumably leaving that to be adjusted to individual circumstances. Five Ingredients Replenishing pill was originally a formula of the Song state medical bureau. See Zhu Bangxian 1991: 360.

Ziming's "leadership of Blood," the nature of bodily gender itself was at stake. The medical consultant on the work, Cha Wang, reported how his friend Wang Qi asked directly, "Are there differences between medicine for males and for females?" Cha Wang replied:

> Male and female are cured in the same way. Yin and yang are based on one principle, and there is no basis for difference. Where one may differentiate is in accordance with the Classic's saying, "Disorders of the two yang [tracts] act on the Heart and Spleen systems, and so sometimes [males are] impotent and females don't menstruate."[15] The ancients said that miscellaneous disorders are alike in women and men, except for those in pregnancy and postpartum. The *Encyclopedia of Sagely Benefaction*[16] includes within its thirteen disciplines [*ke*] a segment [*men*] on women's miscellaneous disorders, but the discourse is abstruse and not worth reading.[17]

Their own goal, he said, should be to produce a work that eliminated the vague and confusing categories of the ancients, concentrating on those disorders which are verifiably special to women alone. Following Cha Wang, the case for the primacy of the human body over the gendered one can be teased out of *To Benefit Yin*'s critique of "miscellaneous disorders" in *fuke* and its suggestions that the root of fertility problems in both sexes may more often be found in the metabolic function of digestion.

First of all, the compilers performed major surgery on the category of "miscellaneous disorders" of women. Wang Qi's notes argued that Wind was never an internal factor in etiology. This meant its direct links to action on Blood were illusory. So Wind-stroke (*zhongfeng*), both apathetic (*dian*) and agitated (*kuang*) types of madness, Heart pain, and Cold Damage fevers were dropped. Blood Wind, which in the Song imagination had taken such a variety of forms, was reclassified as an aspect of a streamlined nosology of "depletion exhaustion," and linked to menstrual dysfunction in wasting disorders. Foot *qi* (*jiaoqi*), which in older *fuke* had been treated with drugs to drive out Wind, was moved

15. I read Cha Wang as interpreting the *Su wen* to argue that fertility problems are likely to be rooted in malfunctioning Heart and Spleen systems. For a similar seventeenth-century view, see Zhang Jiebin 1624: 119–20.

16. The *Sheng ji zonglu* was a twelfth-century collection on pharmacy, compiled under the emperor Huizong's sponsorship as a companion to his *Sheng ji jing*. Published by the medical bureau of the Jin dynasty, it represented the Song learned tradition in the north in the Jin-Yuan, but lost currency thereafter.

17. Wang Qi ed., preface by Cha Wang.

to the postpartum section.[18] Pharmacologically, the old repertory of medicines acting on the body's Wind system was rejected as too powerfully acrid and heating for today's weaker constitutions, and healers were advised to consider alternative diagnoses based on a root problem of Liver function.[19]

If many old "miscellaneous disorders" in women were discarded, others lost relevance due to a more compartmentalized understanding of the body's interior. Here medical authorities were making more distinctions between reproductive, excretory and other functions. Piles, constipation, anal prolapse and urinary retention were dropped, while other abnormal urinary discharges were reclassified with genital problems (*qian yin*). Some syndromes based on visible blood, as in nosebleeds or bloody sputum or vomit, were also eliminated from *fuke*, suggesting that they no longer obviously implicated the generative functions of Blood.

What remained of "miscellaneous disorders" of women were streamlined versions of the broad categories of "depletion exhaustion" (*xulao*) and "swellings and accumulations" (*jiju*). Concerning the latter, *To Benefit Yin* maintained traditional gender-specific categories of abdominal growths: *jia* in female and *shan* in males. The narrative also continued to link depletion exhaustion with Kidney and sexual function. But Wang Qi's eyebrow notes were skeptical. Males can have *jia*-type swellings and females can have *shan* types, he said. As for depletion exhaustion, although the root of the illness in males and females may be different, "the visible signs of depletion exhaustion are quite similar [in males and females]."[20]

As miscellaneous disorders receded in importance, the genital region (*qian yin, yin hu*) got more attention. *To Benefit Yin* showed how Ming

18. Wang Qi ed., 426–27. This shift would seem to be more in line with the modern identification of *jiaoqi* with beriberi, to which pregnant and nursing mothers are especially vulnerable. In the seventeenth-century context, debates reflected re-evaluations of *jiaoqi* associated with the ideas of Li Gao. Li had suggested that it had a "northern" form of internal etiology and a "southern" one of external etiology, where the agency was Heat and Damp. By the late Ming several traditions conflicted: the picture of *jiaoqi* as a internal disorder of Kidney function, implicating sexuality, was in conflict with newer environmental theories. While many medical authorities tried to harmonize these two approaches, the practical issue in *fuke*, as elsewhere, was the choice of a therapy: whether to treat the disorder with drugs to drive out Wind (the classical *fuke* strategy), or to focus on Heat and Damp, or to privilege postpartum formulas to circulate and replenish Blood.

19. See Jiang and Li 1988: 116. For Wang Qi's eyebrow notes on Wind, see 105, 122, 127.

20. Wang Qi ed., eyebrow notes, 122, 149, 157.

diagnostic categories of Damp Heat, phlegm, and Liver stasis (or Liver Fire) allowed for sophisticated therapeutic strategies that worked from within rather than at the body surface. Interpreting the *Inner Canon,* doctors theorized that the *zujueyin* tract governs the "creation and transformation of generative *qi* [*zu qi*]." Here holistic reproductive functions were linked to specific surface genitalia.[21] For various categories of genital sores, itching, swellings or infestations, Wu Zhiwang offered a repertory of infusions working through the Liver, Spleen or Kidney systems.[22] At the end of this section, the bound foot made a rare appearance in a medical text with a recipe for a pain-relieving salve. In this way, importantly, the woman's "lotus foot" was identified as a genital zone of the body.

To Benefit Yin also shows how discourse concerning medical interventions to curb fertility or to terminate pregnancy was more highly charged than it had been in the Song. Although Chinese medicine never spoke of fertility control in the twentieth-century idiom of contraception, Chen Ziming had offered prescriptions that promised to render barren those "nuns, prostitutes, or ailing wives" who might wish to "cut off birth [*duan chan*]." Similarly, Chen's text concluded its discussion of spontaneous miscarriage with a brief addendum: "When, due to other illness a woman's fetus cannot be tranquilized, it is permissible to abort [*ke xiazhe*]."[23] Then and later, medical authorities, ever situational in orientation, avoided an absolute stand: medicine had the resources and doctors had the judgment and skill to act responsibly. However precious descendants were to a family, there was no absolute right to fetal life overriding a mother's health, nor were women who were weary of repeated childbearing necessarily stigmatized.

But in *To Benefit Yin* Chen Ziming's old advice was hemmed around with new strictures, and with examples from cases that drove home the risks to women who resorted to such expedients. Most came from Xue Ji. Where Chen Ziming had warned against bitterly cooling materia medica—liquid mercury (*shuiyin*), gadflies (*mengchong*) or leeches (*shuizhi*)—to sterilize, he had offered alternatives that he said were safer.[24]

---

21. See Wang Kentang, *Nüke*, 1; Wang Qi ed., eyebrow note, 70.

22. Wang Qi ed., 213–33. See also Ren Yingqiu 1980: 326–28, praising Wu Zhiwang's synthesis of these issues.

23. Chen Ziming, juan 13, 384.

24. Chen Ziming, juan 13, 384–85. Materia medica recommended included ox-knee (*niuxi*), Tibetan crocus (*honghua*), various kinds of fermented wheat paste (*mianqu*), and silkworm paper (*canzhi*). This last was paper on which silkworms had

But, in Xue Ji's words, "Most methods that sterilize use strong violent [drugs] and many never recover." Xue's cautionary examples were two wives of men among his clients who "said themselves that their bodies had been debilitated both outwardly and inwardly, so that with the slightest fatigue they fall ill."[25] As for inducing an abortion, doctors "may discuss it, but should take great care." The example that followed told of a man who had failed to follow Xue's advice that his sick wife let nature take its course. The result was calamity: a female doctor (*nü yi*) resolved matters with massive doses of ox-knee (*niuxi*) and the unfortunate woman aborted, hemorrhaged and died. Other cases showed the doctor either saving the baby or cleaning up the complications of a woman's own botched job of it.[26] Drawing on Xue Ji, *To Benefit Yin* here represented medical strategies to limit female fertility as dangerous, and implied that orthodox male authority was there to protect women from the risks they ran in acting on their own. A terrain ridden with gender conflict was exposed, while the entry of such charged social issues into medical discourse also reflected heightened cultural self-consciousness about the body as a locus of individual responsibility involving moral praise or blame.

Finally, as the territory covered by *fuke* contracted to a more limited range of disorders "unique to women alone," menstruation assumed proportionally greater significance. Diagnostic possibilities multiplied as doctors emphasized that the circulation of Blood and *qi* themselves depended on the importance of the metabolic functions of Heart and Spleen and Liver, while on the level of primordial *qi*, managing pathological Fire and protecting Kidney Water were vital. *To Benefit Yin* offered rich examples of Ming refinement and elaboration of menstrual nosology. While Four Ingredients infusion remained a basic remedy, these further considerations shaped the narrative on variants. Fifty-three supplementary formulas were also included.[27]

Some were based on the idea that it was important to privilege drug action on *qi*. Wang Qi warned that without appropriate adjustments in the formula, Four Ingredients posed risks to *qi* Blood balance. *Dihuang*,

---

hatched, depositing husks and other detritus in the process. Like other silkworm byproducts, it was used to stop bleeding.

25. Wang Qi ed., quoting Xue Ji, 209.

26. Wang Qi ed., 333–37, quoting cases of Xue Ji. For a further late Ming warning about the danger of abortion and sterilization, see editor's comment in Jiang Guan, juan 11, 328.

27. See Wang Qi ed., 16–42.

for example, which increases Kidney Water, can stagnate *qi,* while angelica's mild, Blood-moving warmth may disperse *qi* upward. Or in cases of amenorrhea, "though strategies to reduce *qi* and boost Blood are standard in *nüke,* remember that Blood is mated with *qi;* when *qi* heats Blood heats [in response]. . . . When *qi* is disordered, regulate it; when *qi* is cold, warm it; when *qi* is depleted, replenish it. In both males and females, yang vigor naturally promotes yin growth."[28]

Still further, Wang Qi suggested that one regulate the menses to harmonize with latent seasonal influences. Materia medica could be adjusted to draw upon the seasonal affinities of herbs themselves, as Four Ingredients complete the full cycle of a year. The sweet, acrid, moist and warm spirit of angelica produces the harmonious warmth of spring; lovage's acrid, warming and dispersing action enacts the efflorescence of summer; peony root, sour and concentrated, incorporates autumnal gathering; and dried *dihuang*'s richness embodies the storage of winter. However, Wang Qi warned that as with seasonal change, materia medica will be properly dynamic only as one leading factor establishes a momentum: "Without a chief their qualities will not manifest."[29] By doubling proportions appropriate to the season, the body's interior climate might be strengthened to enhance the benefits of the environmental moment. Another method was to adjust the proportions in the herbs to stimulate an independent "seasonal" effect within the body, growing and burgeoning or preserving and keeping. In this way the skillful pharmacist might rely upon angelica and lovage alone to encourage menstrual flow, while peony root and *dihuang* could be turned to stop bleeding. Similarly, angelica itself could be imagined as internally differentiated: being a root, its "head" fostered upward motion, stopping bleeding, while its "tail" had an affinity for descent. With these strategies as a foundation, a full repertory of materia medica to act on *qi,* and to address specific organ-system functions might be added. Readings like these, seeing in prescriptions for menstrual regulation elegant embodiments of cosmological relationships and forces driving all phenomena, made pharmacy culturally resonant and sold books about *fuke.*[30]

28. Wang Qi ed., 49.
29. Wang Qi ed., 17.
30. Li Shizhen offered similar views about prescriptions and seasons, but explained them further in terms of *wu yun liu qi* doctrines. See *Bencao gangmu,* juan 1 in vol. 1:73–74. See Ma Dazheng 1991: 210–14, for further elaborations in Ming approaches to menstruation.

Finally, Wang Qi's approach to menstrual regulation incorporated the teachings of Zhu Zhenheng about the relationship of Fire, desires and generative vitalities. Ministerial Fire lodged in the Liver system is the source of sexual desires in both males and females, he said. This is further demonstrated by the cosmological affinities between Liver, the phase of Wood and the mating season of spring. To make Fire descend and nourish yin Blood is the strategy of choice when unsatisfied passion deranges the menses. Danxi's (i.e., Zhu Zhenheng's) methods are good for cases of depletion heat affecting Liver and Kidney yin. In cases of amenorrhea, look to the hidden feelings she can't express that have stirred Heart Fire and caused *qi* stasis, inhibiting appetite so that she grows thin and emaciated.[31] By means of comments like these, Wang Qi showed he understood Zhu Zhenheng's body of Ministerial Fire as linking sexual desires, emotions and body heat in a way directly relevant to female disorder.

My foregoing account has emphasized how far *To Benefit Yin* further revised the legacy of Chen Ziming and his Ming interpreter Xue Ji. Changes in styles of prescribing were explained in terms of the primacy of *qi* in the Blood-*qi* pair, the importance of Fire as both generative and pathological body heat, and by the location of the roots of disorders in Liver, Spleen-stomach and Heart system functioning. Nosological categories suggested a more bounded body, where functional vitalities were more closely harnessed to physiological structures. There was also more interest in how the body's interior might be compartmentalized, so that the medicine that is "unique to women alone" was directed toward discrete localized sites of sexual and gestational function.[32] The relationship of emotion and illness was conceptualized in terms of a dialectic of interaction between the Heart system and the Kidney and Liver systems, site of primordial *qi*, while the Spleen-stomach served as the material basis of metabolic "*qi* of grains" (*gu qi*), processed from food and drink. *To Benefit Yin* rejected the Song "leadership of Blood" and ignored the

---

31. Wang Qi ed., eyebrow notes, 3, 12, 31, 43, 49.

32. All of this might be glossed as a greater sensitivity to issues of anatomy than was apparent in the Song or Yuan. It is also true that medical drawings purporting to depict *zang* and *fu* organ systems came into fashion in the seventeenth century, while Ming learned physicians debated the morphology of the Kidney system and speculated about the influence of the womb's shape on the sex of offspring (see below, chapter six). However, this kind of interest in bodily structures was meant to answer questions about functions understood in the familiar idiom of yin yang and the Five Phases, not to reorient medicine toward anatomical observation for its own sake.

Song construction of female bodily gender around diffuse forms of "yin influence" associated with the inner and outer circulation of Wind and Cold. Instead the Liver system gained importance as the functioning center of the specifically female forms of generative vitality dependent upon Blood function, while Blood in general was more firmly subordinated to *qi* in the pairing of yin yang primary vitalities.

However, by stressing these features of *To Benefit Yin,* and in particular the voice of Wang Qi's eyebrow notes, my interpretation of innovation in late Ming medicine is overstated. That voice offered one cultured reading out of many possible ones. Above all, its point of view both complements and conflicts with the many-layered elements of an eclectic text. Readers could easily sift through passages harking back to a symptom-based approach, or to the strategies assuming the leadership of Blood destabilized by Wind and Cold that filtered down in passages from Chen Ziming. Elsewhere in the text one might find popular and well-established therapies for menstrual problems around the tropes of Cold, congested, dirty, or stagnant Blood, requiring drugs to cleanse, cool, and harmonize it or to move and break it up.

Concerning postpartum, also, even as *To Benefit Yin* recommended Zhu Zhenheng's replenishing approach, one finds the cultured man of medicine facing doubts based on older Song constructions of delivery and its aftermath. Warming and replenishing medicines generate heat; they produce bodily fullness, threatening retention and accompanying pain, or stagnation of circulation flow. So imagined, they were poor pain relievers, and in excess might overwhelm threatened yin fluids. In obstetrics particularly, they could seem risky when women feared difficult labor or faced the still common association of birth Blood with pollution, requiring postpartum cleansing of the "noxious dew" (*e lu*). Old formulas to repress overactive fetal *qi* in pregnancy or to break up and move bad Blood after parturition retained a place in the text.[33]

One leitmotif, then, was the repeated warnings (driven home by the examples from the cases of famous physicians) about the crudity of standard therapies based on a belief in the "leadership of Blood." Early onset, flooding, or dark purplish clotting of menses were not to be read as simple symptoms of Blood heat; menstrual stoppage was not always stagnation from Cold or "dry Blood"; nor was pain necessarily congested Blood, nor hemorrhage and discoloration bad or dirty Blood. In thinking about deep pattern, *To Benefit Yin* assumed that, in contrast

33. See Wang Qi ed., 361, 397, for examples.

with Song norms, in *fuke* it is generally safer to boost *qi* than to repress it. While harmonizing and vivifying Blood are generally beneficent activities protecting vulnerable yin fluids, ill-considered action to move and break up Blood not only threatened fertility but exacerbated risks to females from yin depletion. I think, then, that Wang Qi's finely theorized vision of the prescription art had to coexist alongside approaches to *fuke* therapy closer to old norms. In his recorded menstrual case histories, some repeated in *To Benefit Yin*, Xue Ji had criticized women patients who dosed themselves with formulas that acted directly on Blood to "move the menses" (*tong jing*) or that addressed pain with remedies to "clear heat" (*qing re*) or "drive out Wind" (*qu feng*).[34] Moreover, such modes of menstrual regulation could be construed as dangerous if a woman's amenorrhea was in fact a pregnancy. As the list of materia medica deemed liable to destabilize a fetus expanded, remedies that "moved Blood" (*tong xue*) or "attacked downward" (*gong xia*) to purge were ambiguously linked to abortifacients. When the literati doctor customized a *fuke* prescription to the individual case, he did more than show his therapeutic subtlety. He established his distance from conventional "standard formulas" that in irresponsible hands might inadvertently or deliberately threaten a woman's fecundity.[35]

However, clients did not always use such physicians. In late Ming cities, shops did a profitable business in ready-made compounds. Some offered up-to-date versions of "standard formulas"(*cheng fang*) in powder, tablet or pill form; others advertised their "secret" formulas. These

34. See Xue Ji's "Tiao jing men" section, in ZGYXDC 5:479–88. Of the forty-three cases in this section, a therapeutic strategy is named in thirty-two. Eighteen of these recommend to "replenish center and boost *qi*" (*bu zhong yi qi*). "Replenish spleen" formulas are recommended ten times.

35. Francesca Bray has analyzed the medical issue of abortion in late imperial China in terms of the social control of the reproductive technology of menstrual regulation. The male-dominated medical profession was concerned that the decisions about female reproduction be made by responsible (patriarchal) family superiors, but menstrual regulating medicines were available to women who wished to take these matters into their own hands. Bray argues that the issue of control did not always pit men against women, for husbands sometimes sought abortifacients for their sickly wives. Further, menstrual regulating medicines played a role in the power relations of women themselves in polygamous elite families, where senior women were in the position to monitor the fertility of daughters-in-law, maids and concubines of the household. For evidence of these issues in a seventeenth-century doctor's practice, see below, chapter seven. Even in today's TCM the boundary between many formulas that regulate the menses and abortifacients remains ambiguous, and in Singapore and Taipei clinics advertising "menstrual regulation" are known to be abortion mills. See Bray 1995: 244–49, and Bray 1997: 335–68.

shops also supplied ordinary itinerant healers with the contents of medicine bags to take on their rounds. Although many were associated with well-known medical names, some shops were accused of harboring abortionists.[36] The literati physicians' warnings against standard prescriptions suggest to me that people continued to seek old, easily available remedies that were familiar, and that they expected formulas to address their symptoms directly—moving Blood to move the menses, driving out Wind to stop pain, or leading *qi* to purge. Such formulas could be dangerous, or put to transgressive uses. They remained part of a popular repertory that persisted in tension with the sophisticated philosophical pharmacy of the literati expert.

Obstetrics on the Margins of Print Culture

The medical innovations of *To Benefit Yin* did not extend to its discussion of childbirth. In the sections on pregnancy and postpartum, Chen Ziming and Xue Ji—the latter both on his own account and as the editor of Chen Ziming—dominated discussion. Among the scattered other voices quoted from time to time, those from post-Song texts were few.[37] Advice on labor and delivery had changed little since the thirteenth century, except for the virtual erasure of ritual obstetrics.[38] Wu Zhiwang, interestingly, included in his 1620 edition of the text a list of avoidances for pregnancy and instructions for the orientation of the birth bed and placenta burial—but such techniques of "prayer and incantation" (*zhuyou fa*) had been left out of Wang Kentang's *Nüke,* while Wang Qi dismissed them in a curt eyebrow note.[39] As telling as rejection, perhaps, was indifference.

---

36. See Dong and Liu 1995. For complaints about shops in late Ming Hangzhou that "cut off the way of birth" for a living, see Yue Fujia, *Miaoyizhai yixue zhengyin zhongzi bian,* author's preface dated 1635.

37. In the chapters on pregnancy (juan 8 and 9), Chen Ziming is quoted twenty-seven times and Xue Ji twenty-two times, and there are only six identifiable citations from other post-Song texts. Compare the chapters on menstrual regulation and on menstrual blockage (juan 1 and 2): here Chen Ziming is quoted twelve times and Xue Ji fifteen, while there are thirty-three identifiable citations from Jin-Yuan masters and their Ming successors. (Throughout, Chen Ziming is quoted according to the wording in Xue Ji's version of his work.)

38. Ma Dazheng 1991: 225–26, notes how case histories narrating obstetrical emergencies became even rarer after the Song.

39. Wang Kentang, preface to *Nüke zheng zhi zhunsheng;* Wu Zhiwang 1620, juan 4, 10b–11a; Wang Qi ed., juan 10, 352.

A text attributed to Wan Quan, leader of a popular medical lineage of the mid-Ming centered in Honan, simply noted in passing that "those who are good at such things can do them, but if they are omitted, it doesn't matter."[40]

The search for late Ming textual traces of obstetrical knowledge leads past *To Benefit Yin* back to ephemeral publications linked to Song traditions and to the elusive world of handwritten and oral transmission. One compilation that had a limited print circulation in the late Ming was titled *One Hundred Question Birth Treasury* (*Chan bao baiwen*). Although Ming printers put the names of Zhu Zhenheng and Wang Kentang on a five-juan version that I have seen, that text is based on Qi Zhongfu's Song original, to which neither Zhu nor Wang added any discernable editorial voice of their own. But it includes an obstetrical juan titled *Birth Treasury Miscellany* (*Chan bao zalu*), which is attributed to Qi Zhongfu but is not part of today's standard edition of his classic.[41] It offers practical and ritual advice on childbirth along the line of Southern Song originals by Yu Chong and Li Shisheng. In other words, the medical manuscript tradition associated with Qi Zhongfu was a fluid one, freely appropriated and adapted by those claiming the authority of Song or later masters for obstetrical expertise.[42]

Further, manuscripts occasionally surface in today's archives bearing traces of the anonymous recordkeeping that supported the medical practice of obstetrics as a domestic art or a craft of humble local midwives and doctors. Consider, for example, the anonymous *Collection for Safeguarding the Blessed Event* (*Chanyu baoqing ji*), a title rich in echoes of the so-called oldest surviving text on birth, the Song *Childbirth Treasury Collection* by Guo Jizhong and Li Shisheng. This is a handbook, copied not more than one or two hundred years ago, in a

40. See Wan Quan 1667, *Wan shi furen ke,* 37. These texts were valued as glimpses of lineage practitioners' wisdom of a kind that did not usually get published. It was said that Wan Quan agreed to print his family's medical notebooks because none of his ten sons was both fit and able to succeed him.

41. Although the authorship of the *Chan bao baiwen* is as unclear as the text is variable, I have followed Ma Jixing in naming Qi Zhongfu as the author of the undated printed version held in the rare book library of the Zhongyi Yanjiuyuan. An obstetrical juan seems to have been included in the 1571 and 1640 editions of the *Nüke baiwen* itself. However, it was dropped from the 1737 edition, which is the basis for the best known modern reprints. Okanishi Tameto accepts the two-juan *Nüke baiwen* as authentic, and sees the obstetrical title as an early—perhaps Yuan—accretion to the original. See Ma Jixing 1990: 226, and Okanishi Tameto 1948: 523–24.

42. See Ma Jixing 1990: 226.

spidery and not-too-accurate calligraphy. It is based on Song textual traditions: Qi Zhongfu's *One Hundred Questions*, with an obstetrical supplement, and the "Ten Topics on Birth" of Yang Zijian. A fragmentary preface to this handbook claims to be from a man named Wang Qin of the Southern Song. It tells a familiar tale of a manuscript original found in a relative's cupboard, from which a unique prescription formula was used to save a life. Wang Qin wrote of hoping to find a publisher for his text, but nothing reveals that this happened, or that the late Qing copyist had any notion of the variant strands of transmission associated with Qi Zhongfu or Yang Zijian antecedent to his or her home notebook. Nonetheless, the manuscript is marked with red ink *dian* punctuation marks, showing it was once read carefully for use.[43]

Similar traces may be read into manuscripts held today in the library of the Academy of Traditional Chinese Medicine in Beijing. One, titled *True Protection of the Female Origin*, is also derivative of *One Hundred Questions* but traces its lineage to the Song *fuke* traditions of the Xue and Guo families. Again, a Qing-era copybook version starts with a preface for which Song dates are given, in which an ancestral Dr. Xue commits his family's medical secrets to his descendants. Later in the text, writers in the fourteenth and twenty-second generation, now surnamed Li, add comments.[44]

Interestingly, an appendix to the 1665 edition of *To Benefit Yin* shows that Wang Qi was aware of the inadequacy of the obstetrical advice in the main text and that he personally tried to correct it. Wang's preface

43. Manuscript held in the East Asian Collection of the Library of Congress.

44. *Kun yuan shi bao.* Undated handwritten text held in the rare book library of the Zhongyi Yanjiuyuan in Beijing. Based on the preface, the library identifies the author as Xue Xian (fl. 1265), but the physical text is probably early nineteenth century. The whole is "copied by Li." My reading suggests a composite text assembled by a later descendant, surnamed Li, who has succeeded to the hereditary tradition claiming Xue as founder. There is much evidence of oral transmission, including a *Wan jin fang* of one hundred prescriptions, coded by means of a medical poem of one hundred words, each one "labelling" a specific prescription. The poem is a mnemonic filing system, enabling the doctor to call up specific prescriptions from memory. The text includes an interesting defense of secrecy in medical practice: irresponsible students from the outside might transmit errors. It also warns against overreliance on pulse diagnosis with women patients and urges that the doctor force them to speak about their symptoms. Since I have no way of locating the text precisely in time or space, it can only stand here as a cautionary example of the limitations of the medical record enshrined in print culture. The library has two other, later handwritten texts which are variants of the same medical lineage tradition(s). In one, verses on the ten months of gestation have comments by a "Fifth Sister Liu."

to this appendix, "Trivia for Safeguarding Life" (*Bao sheng suishi*),[45] advertised it as filling a gap in the literature, noting that neither *fuke* nor pediatrics dealt with the critical transition of birth and neonatal life. Assuming the voice of an elderly recluse, Wang Qi sketched a self portrait: "Already advanced in years, my goal is to nourish long life; having put aside household responsibilities, I nurse my ailments in a mountain temple, while devoting myself to the printing of books on trivial matters [*suishi*] such as geography and travel routes."[46] The present work, another such "trivial matter," nonetheless might save women in difficult labors and protect newborns in their first perilous week of life. The brief text offered practical, homespun advice on both labor and neonatal care. It touched on the timing of labor (irregular contractions are false labor) and techniques of breast feeding (before you begin, extract the stale "night milk"; don't nurse when overheated). It included detailed instructions on cutting the newborn's umbilical cord: "Wait until the baby has been washed off before cutting the cord, to avoid illness from exposure to water. . . . Tie it with string four or five inches from the body. . . . Gnaw it with your teeth; don't use knife or scissors, to avoid damage from Cold *qi*."[47]

Such practical advice aimed to bridge the gap between learned discourse and the medical skills of women concerned with birth. It was culled mostly from respected ancient authorities in pediatrics, but also from an obscure source entitled *Essential Oral Instructions for Families in Childbirth* (*Chan jia yaojue*). It showed the mother and child as interrelated, both by a material bond that the event of birth only partially severed and also by their interdependent function in an overall moral economy devoted to ensuring family posterity. However, in keeping with the neglect of obstetrics in the printed record of Ming medicine, Wang Qi's "Trivia" disappeared from subsequent editions of his *fuke*. If it was ever printed separately, that work too has vanished.[48]

---

45. Wang Qi ed., 577–86. The modern (1958) reprint omits the original prefaces, together with the separate title page that suggests that the text may have been packaged and sold separately as a pamphlet.

46. Wang Qi ed., 577.

47. Wang Qi ed., obstetrical appendix, 580. The advice is identical with that in Sun Simiao's *Beiji qianjin yaofang* from the Tang dynasty.

48. Xue Qinglu 1991: 452, mentions a *Bao sheng suishi* printed in 1689 and attributed to Wang Qi, a copy of which is held in the library of the Shanghai Zhongyi Xueyuan. The claim that this 14-juan work is the same as Wang Qi's appendix to the 1665 edition of *Ji yin gangmu* is implausible. See also Cao Bingzhang 1936, *Tiyao,*

Medicine, Birth Pollution
and Pediatric Disease

By the end of the Ming, Song-style birth rituals had almost disappeared from the repertory of medical advice published in texts on *fuke*. Nonetheless, although the ritual dangers of birth were now medically de-emphasized, preoccupations previously visible in obstetrics shifted shape. Now medicalized, pollution beliefs resurfaced in pediatrics, particularly in the syndrome of fetal poison (*tai du*), where neonatal and childhood diseases were seen as the delayed consequence of gestational contamination. When this contamination was identified with the dread Ming childhood killer, smallpox, it contributed to learned Ming theorizing on epidemics and their etiology. When the origin of "fetal poison" was traced back to the sexual heat of intercourse at conception, the rhetoric of birth pollution colored the subtext of Ming moral discourse on eros and health. As specialties in learned medicine, pediatrics and *fuke* had evolved side by side, bound by their common importance to the survival of the family collective, and medical thought easily represented the bodies of parents and child as joined. Paradoxically, theories of fetal poison spread as Ming elite physicians who found themselves at the margins of the maternal sphere of birth increased their involvement with those mothers' infants by taking up the pediatrics of smallpox as an urgent new medical specialty.[49]

Wang Qi's obstetrical "Trivia" indirectly showed something of both older and more recent medical thinking on the relationship of fetal contamination and infant disease. Among his recommendations for newborns were two prescriptions to be taken in the first weeks of life. They were culled from the *Essential Oral Instructions for Families in Childbirth*. Classified as medicines for "reducing pox" (*xi dou*), the first was a paste made of roasted and dried umbilical cord: ingested by the child, this medicine evoked the generative power of the "root" of the child's own life. The other recipe had as its main ingredients cinnabar powder, *huanglian* and licorice — materia medica which for centuries had been

juan 9, 10–11. Cao thinks a pediatric supplement to *Ji yin gangmu* was later advertised but may never have been printed.

49. Xue Qinglu 1991: 496–526 surveys the voluminous specialty literature on poxes (*douzhen*) in children produced between the thirteenth century and the end of the imperial era. Measles and other childhood eruptive fevers were also part of the syndrome complex.

used in one form or another as cleansing and cooling tonics for newborns.[50] From Sun Simiao on down, experts had promoted such tonics to purify the child of the residues of gestation — not only birth blood but its fetal stool, fetal hair or clotted matter in the newborn's mouth — promising also that such remedies prevented skin disease later on.[51] In one way, then, Wang Qi's formulas followed an old established tradition of medicinal purification of the newborn. But when Wang Qi explained that his soft "reducing pox" (*xi dou*) pellets, smeared inside the child's mouth or on the nursing mother's nipple, would cause its "fetal poison to follow stool and urine passing away out of the body," he was responding to medical conditions of the more recent past. This medicine aimed not only to prevent infant eczemas and rashes but to ensure that the later inevitable case of smallpox would be a mild one. Its spread in China as an endemic childhood disease had produced a rereading of gestational contamination in a distinctively Ming idiom.

Wang Kentang was among many in the late Ming who talked about smallpox as a historical disease and theorized its etiology. Wang thought that the term "bean" (*dou*) for the distinctive smallpox pustules had appeared first in the annals of the Jianwu emperor of the Eastern Han (25 C.E.), associated with a pestilence brought by nomadic invaders; and he also noticed that association of smallpox with fetal poison was a matter of record only "since the Song and Yuan" dynasties. Another famous late Ming physician, Sun Yikui, had a similar analysis, pointing to early case histories of the famous twelfth- and thirteenth-century pediatricians Qian Yi and Chen Wenzhong.[52] It was only after smallpox had lost its epidemic character (no longer breaking out so infrequently that it found victims in adult populations) and had become established as an endemic disease striking in childhood that the term "fetal poison" could name its dread impact on child mortality. Wang Kentang and others deduced from the historical and regional epidemiology of smallpox that environmental influence had to be a vector of contamination. But then, seeing it strike Chinese universally in childhood and seeing that survivors were immune thereafter, they imagined an inborn toxic

50. Wang Qi ed., 585–86.

51. Sun Simiao, *Beiji qianjin yaofang*, juan 5, 76; Liu Fang 1150, *You you xin shu*, juan 4, 84–85.

52. Wang Kentang 1602, juan 1, 1–8; Sun Yikui 1584, juan 27, 1004–5. Marta Hanson 1997 argues that the story of the Eastern Han origins of smallpox was a mid-fifteenth-century invention to explain the presumed Southern homeland of the disease. For a Song overview see Liu Fang 1150, juan 18, 656–67.

heat latent in the child's body waiting for the appropriate environmental stimulus to be drawn out. "Only when internal contamination [*ran*] and external [epidemic] *qi* clash against one another does it develop."[53] Unlike ordinary skin eruptions, which were treated by medicines to disperse and evaporate, the purulent "bean" (*dou*) rash had to ripen and bloom for a successful expulsion of the poison. For children, smallpox became more than an illness — it was a bodily passage through the polluted stages of neonatal and infant disease to childhood health and the hope of living to grow up.

Sometime in the Song era, then, physicians had begun to distinguish the symptoms of smallpox from those of other fevers and rashes of childhood, and to write about smallpox as a separate medical discipline (*ke*).[54] In the same period a new term — "fetal poison" (*tai du*) — began to name a root of some neonatal and childhood illnesses marked by discharges via skin eruptions or feverish rashes. These were illnesses of internal, not external, origin, etiologically identified with the latent influence of gestational heat. Smallpox became one such illness. In the earlier Northern Song formulation of Qian Yi, fetal pollution was imagined as transmitted via the "dirty Blood" the child ate in utero, visible in the fetal stool and clotted matter in a newborn's mouth. Others pointed to a mother's spicy diet, or to the influence of heating medicines she consumed in pregnancy.[55]

However, where Song authorities saw the origins of fetal poison in the pollution of the mother's gestational Blood, Ming experts on small-

53. Wang Kentang 1602, juan 1, 2.

54. Earlier, more ambiguous records that some scholars have read as accounts of smallpox did not associate the syndrome with children. Even Qian Yi (1032–1113) and Pang Anshi (1042–1099), who are among the earliest cited authorities on the matter, did not systematically distinguish smallpox from Cold Damage fevers — which in children often were accompanied by different sorts of rashes (*zhen* or *chuang*). However, Pang Anshi and Zhu Zhenheng both described recognizable outbreaks, the first of many after the fourteenth century. See Chia-feng Chang 1996: 24–32. Northern Song understandings are summarized in Liu Fang 1150, juan 18, 656–63.

55. As a pediatric category, fetal poison was associated not only with smallpox but with a widening array of neonatal disorders. Zhu Zhenheng used the term to explain the internal, as opposed to external, origins of one infant's scalp and face eczema, and of another's fever with erratic rash. See Liu Fang 1150: 658, and Zhu Zhenheng, *Ge zhi yu lun,* in SKQS 746:645–46. The compilers of *Ming yi lei an* and its successor, *Xu ming yi lei an,* saw fetal poison at work in syndromes where foul matter was discharged through a child's skin, or via its urine or stool. See Jiang Guan, juan 12, 345–46, and Wei Zhixiu, juan 27, 378–79. Ming and Qing pediatric texts included under fetal poison neonatal disorders like "goose mouth" and "heavy tongue." Some added to the list "navel Wind," which biomedical experts today identify with neonatal tetanus. See Furth 1987: 19–21, 26–27.

pox looked to sexual heat. Wan Quan popularized Ming understandings of the pediatrics of smallpox as a disorder of internal Ministerial Fire deposited in the infant's body from the heat of sexual desire at the time of conception. Under the stimulus of external environmental Fire factors of seasonal *qi* — also called Ministerial Fire and Princely Fire in *wu yun liu qi* theory — this latent internal Fire would one day react just as a magnet attracts needles, agitating the child's Blood and producing the heat and foul skin rash of the disease. "Smallpox [*douzhen*] arises from the fetal poison of the father and mother stored at the [child's] Vital Gate [*ming men*]. The Vital Gate is the Ministerial Fire of the right Kidney, the foundation of human birth and transformation. This is why the poison is stored there. If a winter is mild, yang *qi* turbulence arises and human beings respond; their Ministerial Fire is aroused, and in the spring and summer when [Fire *qi*] has matured, its poison is released like a contagion."[56] Here fetal poison was read as an aspect of Zhu Zhenheng's body of Ministerial Fire, linked via *wu yun liu qi* reasoning to recurring environmental cycles of Fire influence. Stored at the Vital Gate yet released as disease, this Fire was at once generative and destructive, making smallpox a blight parents bestowed along with life itself as a byproduct of the necessary impurity of sexual congress.

Even though Ming authorities continued to warn women against improper diet or conduct during pregnancy, most elite physicians like Wang Kentang and Sun Yikui rejected the notion that mothers were the sole source of fetal poison. As a sexual disease smallpox was linked rhetorically with the androgynous body of Ministerial Fire, and so with male bodily powers and responsibilities.[57] If fathers and mothers as sexual partners shared responsibility for their children's fetal poison, smallpox was nonetheless also surrounded with popular rituals calling atten-

56. Wan Quan 1667: 152.

57. Chang Chia-feng discusses Ming learned medical debates over the exact mechanisms by which human desires produce fetal poison. Some suggested that the mother's yin poison produced smallpox, while the father's yang poison would only develop into measles. Others argued the opposite. Some blamed male use of aphrodisiacs or urged abstention from intercourse during pregnancy as an added precaution. While some continued to repeat the older Song theory that the child in utero eats dirty maternal blood, others argued that in fact the fetus is nourished safely via the umbilical cord. Chang's research corrects my earlier view (Furth 1987) that fetal poison was blamed on the mother alone — an interpretation I derived from seventeenth and eighteenth-century popular pediatric texts. Such misogynistic views focusing on the pregnant woman's emotions and desires did continue to circulate in both Ming and Qing popular writings. See Chia-feng Chang 1996: 54–66.

tion to its special relationship to the female gestational body. Menstrual blood and the blood of parturition had an affinity for the red, weeping inflammation of smallpox pustules. Parents were to abstain from intercourse during their child's illness, and menstruating women were to keep out of the sickroom. Evil smells—of sweat, of menses, of suppuration—were imagined as mutually reinforcing, requiring an antidote in fragrant incense burned at the bedside. Adolescents of both sexes were considered medically susceptible to severe cases; in boys sexual arousal and in girls menstruation were understood as intensifiers, and some physicians developed therapies adjusted for a postpubescent female's menstrual cycle in relationship to the malady.[58]

In sum, if by the late Ming the pollution of the mother's body was medically de-emphasized, the pollution of the child's body was exaggerated. Since Zhu Zhenheng, learned healers had frowned on therapies purging postpartum mothers of their "noxious dew." But they had developed new ways to name the newborn child as unclean. For late Ming mothers, if their gestational bodies were no longer seen as a major source of danger to themselves as well as to neonatal life, mother and child continued to be conjoined through infancy and lactation and beyond, until the inevitable crisis of smallpox had passed. Lessening the dangers of this crisis was directly linked to the regulation of parental desires. For mothers their responsibilities for their children's health had become more a matter of personal ethical conduct and less one of fate and ritual mediation. For fathers, these responsibilities were linked more intimately to the moral management of marital intercourse.

Continuity and Change in *Fuke:* Layered Knowledge

The past two chapters have traced shifts in learned medicine between the beginning of the Yuan dynasty in 1279 and the fall of the Ming in 1644—a period of about four hundred years. By twentieth-century standards the medical culture of Zhu Zhenheng and that of Wang Qi will not seem very far apart. One reason is that some change added layers more than it transformed foundations. Just as the rise of literati physicians as a medical elite pushed other kinds of practitioners to lower rungs of a more socially differentiated healer hierarchy, so med-

58. See Wan Quan, n.d.; Sun Yikui 1584, juan 28, 1048; Chia-feng Chang 1996: 93.

ical revisionism meant simply that many older therapies — like acupuncture, moxibustion and rituals — survived as part of popular medical culture. No clear narrative of progress can be imposed upon a medical world where possibilities multiplied without being sorted out according to the implicit standard of a hegemonic science. Tradition remained important to doctors, who on the one hand depended for their authority on history exemplified in textual canon and ancient masters, while on the other hand they had to satisfy clients who understood their afflictions in terms of a deeply conservative language of bodily experience. What does the historian's story of change in the Ming dynasty look like under these circumstances?

I have found a narrative of the expansion and the contraction of gynecology. As the paradigm of the "leadership of Blood" came to be partially eclipsed by the teachings of the Jin-Yuan masters and their successors, medical writers gradually limited the scope of "separate prescriptions" for women. They privileged therapies that took organ systems as a point of departure, as well as those said to act on *qi* to lead Blood. Female disorders were limited to a narrower range of gestational pathologies, and they were tied to a subtly more sexualized body with a measure of anatomical specificity as well as holistic qualities. At the same time, elite doctors moved from an accommodation to a criticism of ritual therapies in obstetrics, while the learned clinician turned away from strategies based on cleansing women's birth pollution of Blood, instead stressing postpartum yin and yang depletion. Pollution beliefs survived, however, in the disguised and medicalized form of "fetal poison," now associated with sexual heat in conception and gestation and with diseases that afflicted children.

From a broader historical perspective, however, these changes in *fuke* were limited ones. *Fuke* shifted with changing styles in practice, it did not drive them. Its broad social utility remained as before to help secure family descent lines by safeguarding women's fertility and fecundity. In the late Ming, as in the Song, the female subjects of medical discourse were seen primarily as childbearers. If fewer of their illnesses were judged relevant to reproductive health, this just brought out more clearly what medicine's primary agenda ought to be. It was to safeguard female primary vitalities and to make sure that other illnesses in fertile, pregnant and postpartum women were not prescribed for in a way that might damage their reproductive health.

Between the Song and the late Ming, therapeutic change in *fuke* added complexity more than it transformed foundations. The late Ming criticism of earlier styles of therapy was not so trenchant as to stifle alternatives or preclude user choice. Song gynecology survived as a variation within perennial ways of thinking that never really ceased to occupy the discursive high ground. At the most fundamental level the body of learned medical discourse remained androgynous, and Ming language of yin and yang reflected that emphasis upon process, transmutation and change over substance, structure and fixed essences. Fundamentally, also, the rhetoric of the medical body had always been masculine, and Ming language of the Blood and *qi* relationship reflected the belief in an immutable natural and human hierarchy that included gender. Finally, Ming medicine may have rejected childbirth rituals and obstetrical pharmaceutics that conveyed essentialized representations of the female body as unclean, but doctors continued to live with conflicting paradigms of a gestational body of female impurity and of an idealized androgynous body of generation.

Nonetheless, in spite of all of this, Ming medical rhetoric did speak about the body in a recognizably Ming idiom. A text like *To Benefit Yin* said something distinctive about the sexual powers of the body and about its relationship to the universe at large. Late Ming *fuke* did not return to Sun Simiao's unbounded female "gathering place of yin influences," or to the Song obstetrical body open to the influence of Wind and Cold, of sky spirits, directional *qi* and baleful ghosts. In the pages of *To Benefit Yin*, late Ming women readers did not find Sun's famous description of why the "the roots of their illnesses are deep and their cure is difficult."[59]

Both the hostility to ritual medicine and the shift to narrower definitions of disorder "specific to women alone" were part of a larger late Ming rereading of the relationship of body and cosmos. Medicine was changing in ways that support John Henderson's arguments, made about another ancient Chinese science, astronomy, that by the seventeenth century natural philosophers had turned away from correlative cosmology.[60] In medicine as elsewhere, late sixteenth- and seventeenth-

---

59. Sun Simiao, *Beiji qianjin yaofang*, juan 2, 16. In the Ming Sun Simiao's famous passage was paraphrased in the *fuke* sections of several versions of the *Danxi xinfa* attributed to Zhu Zhenheng. It circulated in Ming-Qing editions of *Nüke baiwen*. But it was drastically truncated in Xue Ji's rendition of Chen Ziming, and disappeared entirely from *Ji yin gangmu*.

60. Henderson 1984. Such an argument cannot really be derived from the evidence of *fuke* alone. If Henderson's analysis is applicable, one would expect to find literati doctors beginning to discard explanatory systems based on the formal, often numerological models of time and change of the *Yijing*, the divinatory cosmometry

century interpreters were taking note of anomaly and unpredictability in the human and natural world in ways that led to an emphasis upon the local and concrete over macrocosmic patterns. Certainly the late Ming medical body was not only less ritualized but also more bounded. In the discourse on the centrality of Spleen-stomach function, health was imagined as based on the material functions of assimilation of food and drink. In thinking about epidemic disease, physicians groped toward understanding the relationship of sick bodies to specific and localized environmental agencies of contamination. The discourse on fetal poison — analyzed here for its cultural construction of sex, gender and parent-child relationships — was also one manifestation of learned medicine's search for ways to understand more concretely how internal functions and external environment interact to produce such disease. The body of Ministerial Fire and Kidney Water derived from Zhu Zhenheng was imagined less in terms of the cosmic forces of time, season and change, and more in terms of a finite human life cycle and of a psychophysical moral economy of embodiment. Finally, in late Ming medicine one can see how the body's sexual powers were becoming more a focus of human management and control, and through this of moral responsibility. Following Foucault one can find in late Ming medicine and society a clash between libertinism and ideals of sexual sobriety, both attesting to a heightened significance accorded the sexual as a locus of personal meaning and social power.

Nonetheless the generative body in both women and men continued to be evoked with metaphors showing their participation in the creative powers of Heaven and Earth. This generative body continued to elude twentieth-century forms of rationalism or materialism. It may be that for reflective seventeenth-century minds, Heaven was being emptied of nameable qualities and contents while Earth was fuller than ever with the teeming multiplicity of things, even as patterns of change seemed to elude the formal order of numbers and fixed correspondences. But yin yang and the Five Phases remained metaphors for a deeper organic unity behind the flux of experience. Belief in the complementarity of macrocosm and microcosm remained a basic article of faith. Inhabiting a more bounded body, enjoined to ground human nature in ethical norms, Hu-

---

of Heavenly Stems and Branches, or the *wu yun liu qi* cycles of climatic change. This would mean a challenge to much in Song and Jin-Yuan views as well as to older Han versions of the cosmology of systematic correspondences. Marta Hanson's work on Qing approaches to epidemic disease (Hanson 1997) begins to address some of these issues.

manity, as the third in the perennial triad, would need to reshape that complementarity within the self. Perhaps much of what scholars have called the subjectivism and individualism of late Ming thought was about this. One way that inward turn took medical form is in a concern with internal alchemy (*nei dan*) — a discourse on the generative body, fertility and longevity particularly important for the construction of male bodily gender. This discourse, as shown in the network of readers and writers surrounding *To Benefit Yin*, is where my story turns next.

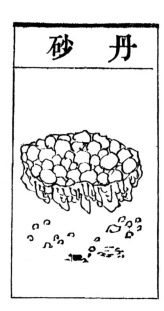

CHAPTER 6

"Nourishing Life"

*Ming Bodies of
Generation and Longevity*

Sixteenth- and seventeenth-century writers on medicine
may have neglected the gestational body of obstetrics, but they were
fascinated with the generative body of fertility. While a few printed texts
on obstetrics echoed Song themes, Ming publishers turned out dozens
of new works that addressed the intertwined topics of "multiplying descendants" (*guang si*) and attaining longevity by "nourishing life" (*yang
sheng, she sheng*).[1] The subject of fertility connected the bodies of men,
women and children, and Ming texts on begetting also undertook to
instruct men on female gestational functions—menstrual regulation as

1. A crude measure is the number of titles surviving in PRC libraries today, as
listed in Xue Qinglu 1991. The pattern is as follows: for the years between 1600 and
1800, twenty-one titles are classified as *chanke*, sixteen as *guang si*, and sixty-one as
yang sheng. See 452–53, 469–70, 608–12.

a guide to female fertility, but also on health in pregnancy. In addition, *fuke* and the discourse on "nourishing life" overlapped in their concern for the more mundane technologies of reproduction: age of marriage, matching of partners for health and bodily compatibility, and above all the techniques of intercourse for conception and the successful begetting of boys as opposed to girls. These were socially critical issues that had long attracted the attention of the medical world, and on which many authorities over the centuries had something to say. Finally, the discourse on *yang sheng* was linked historically with teachings about the sexual "art of the bed-chamber" (*fang shu*) that linked eros, fertility and health.[2] By incorporating materials from the Ming literature on nourishing life, *To Benefit Yin* brought together in a work of *fuke* discussion on matters bearing directly on male sexual life.

Further, for those who nourished life, the deeper structure of fertility was linked to longevity as an equally profound manifestation of the body's generative potential. Here I find the relationship of males and females to be an ambiguous one. The fruitful mating couple was imagined as a yin yang pair—homologous partners, not differentiated according to a gendered hierarchy. However, erotic scripts stressed male initiative and female compliance, while the generative ideal of longevity was a bodily achievement appropriate to patriarchs and sages. In these ways the discourse on nourishing life can be read as a master narrative for the construction of bodily identity for males. Still, when the topic of discussion was longevity, the gestational bodies of women reappeared disguised in metaphors figuring the process of the longevity-seeker's self-renewal and rebirth. In sum, I see the medical art of nourishing life as complementing *fuke* by constructing male gender identity. In so doing, it offers yet another perspective on the tensions between generation and gestation in the androgynous medical body.

If a central subject of *fuke* was a woman's gestational body—whose visible functions males did not share—thinking about conception, fertility and sexual differentiation in the womb all focused attention on their common endowment of generative vitality. This included sexual intercourse and its meaning as body function and erotic performance. Here medical authors had to consider issues that were also culturally charged for them as men: the production and management of sexual desire, the fulfillment of the Confucian family duty to produce heirs, and the attainment of the most venerated high cultural moral ideal—

2. For the medieval literature see Van Gulik 1974, Song Shugong 1991, Furth 1994.

the sage. The elite culture of the late Ming—thought to be decadent in politics, permissive in social mores, experimental and syncretic in philosophy and religion, and romantic in aesthetics and the arts—fostered open and eclectic discourse on the body of generativity as a masculine ideal. Through it upper class men worked out identities as lovers, fathers and men of wisdom.

A point of departure for discussing these issues is the chapter on "seeking descendants" in *To Benefit Yin*. Though intended to aid women, rhetorically *To Benefit Yin* was addressed primarily to men, whom convention deemed responsible for family management and who were the normal purchasers as well as producers of printed books. Breaking with earlier *fuke* narratives, the compilers developed their discussion of conception and fertility using excerpts from contemporary authors of the burgeoning *yang sheng* genre, making their work innovative in its sexual frankness while revealing its paternalistic voice with especial clarity. Wang Kentang and Wu Zhiwang appear to have shaped the text through their personal selection of *yang sheng* experts to cite. One was Chen Chuliang, known as the author of two short works on techniques for attaining long life published in 1588.[3] Another was Yu Qiao (1522–1566), a one-time imperial medical officer at Nanjing and author of the mid-sixteenth-century *Essential Words on Propagating Descendants*, which was drawn upon extensively by later medical experts.[4] Most important was the voice of Yuan Huang (Yuan Liaofan, 1533–1606), famous in his day as an official, a military man and one of the more original figures in late Ming syncretic religious thought. Since he earned a *jinshi* degree in 1586 and participated in the Korean military campaign of 1593, Yuan Huang may have known Wu Zhiwang or Wang Kentang personally. Finally, Wu Zhiwang in turn did not confine his advice on fertility and longevity to the pages of *To Benefit Yin* but expanded them for a male audience directly in a companion work titled *To Benefit Yang*, published in 1626 to capitalize on the popular success of his *fuke*.[5] The following

3. Chen Chuliang, "Immortal Prescriptions from the Family Tradition of Master Chen of Wulin" (*Wulin Chen shi jiazhuan xian fang*) and *Buddha's Way of Prescribing for Long Life and Immortality* (*Fo fa ling shou danfang*). Since I have been unable to see a copy of the original texts, my knowledge of his work comes entirely from *To Benefit Yin*.

4. Yu Qiao, *Guang si yaoyu*, 1544.

5. Wu Zhiwang, *Ji yang gangmu*, 1626. In spite of its title, this was a work of general medicine, taking the male body as the norm, and not a *nanke* in the modern sense of a treatise on male sexual disfunction. Juan 67 ("Zhong zi"), 68 ("Yang sheng"), and 69 ("Yang lao") deal with fertility and longevity, and parallel the *fuke* most closely. Unlike *Ji yin gangmu*, *To Benefit Yang* soon disappeared from circula-

analysis is based on the intertextual web linking these works with one another and with a circle of readers extending to Wang Qi's Huanduzhai in the middle seventeenth century.

Yuan Huang and Ming Inner Alchemy

In Yuan Huang the late Ming worlds of officialdom and of medicine were particularly intertwined. His family had practiced medicine for four generations in Wujiang, Jiangsu, after an eminent ancestor had been caught in the crossfire of the Yongle usurpation that deposed the second Ming emperor (1403 C.E.), suffering political disgrace as a result. As the descendant who succeeded in the national examinations and restored the lineage to official fame, Yuan Huang's life reflected the family's eclectic intellectual interests, extending beyond medicine to mathematics, hydraulics and military affairs. Further, his family's vicissitudes of fortune spurred Yuan Huang's lifelong philosophical preoccupation with the relation between moral responsibility and karmic retribution and reward. *To Benefit Yin* was heavily indebted to one of Yuan's two known essays on nourishing life, *Veracious Explanation of the Blessing of Heirs (Qi si zhenquan)*, published in 1591. This work was inspired by Yuan's personal quest for a son, born finally when he was forty-eight.[6] While the *Veracious Explanation* made a very personal Buddhist case for the power of a man's good deeds to transform his fate, its medical system was virtually identical with that in Yuan Huang's short Daoist tract *Three Essentials for Furthering Life*, published at the same time.[7]

Yuan Huang recommended a technology to ensure a fertile body

---

tion, its printing blocks destroyed in the Manchu invasion of 1644. It is known today on the basis of a nineteenth-century scholar's editorial reconstruction of a rare copy of the original first edition.

6. Yuan Huang, *Qi si zhenquan*, 1591. Yuan was close to scholars of the Taizhou school of neo-Confucianism, as well as being a disciple of a famous Buddhist monk, Fawei. He popularized a revival of the Buddhist practice of self-examination by means of daily "ledgers of merit and demerit"—reinterpreting karmic law as an internalist ethic of virtue for its own sake. A major study of Yuan Huang's life is Brokaw 1991. For the medical tradition in the Yuan family, see 64–75.

7. Yuan Huang, *She sheng san yao*, 1591. The word *she* is virtually untranslatable, carrying the image of a lodestone gathering filings or of blotting paper absorbing water. The passages on "nourishing Essence," "cultivating *qi*" and "focusing Psyche" in Yuan's *Veracious Explanation* are identical with those in this text, which was transmitted as Daoist and published in a modern supplement to the canonical Daoist encyclopedia, the *Daozang*.

subject to human control, disciplined by sexual and spiritual exercises as well as by diet and pharmacy. He understood fertility and longevity as linked because both depended theoretically on a common set of assumptions about the generative body that linked the powers and pleasures of sexual function with the possibilities of sagely transcendence and bodily immortality. The deep structure of such a body was based on "inner alchemy" (*nei dan*), a sprawling tradition of philosophy and body practice identified originally with the religious Daoism of medieval China, but also long associated with esoteric medical teachings. Sometime in the Song period, in the hands of medical authorities like Kou Congzhi and Liu Wansu, inner alchemy body practices for longevity were incorporated into the medical discourse on nourishing life. The medieval "external alchemy" (*wai dan*) of religious Daoism shaped inner alchemy's foundational metaphor of the body as a crucible (*ding*) and furnace (*lu*) where gross material may be refined and purified.

Inner alchemy was too visionary for ordinary language, and too secretive for common history. This makes it especially difficult to define or summarize.[8] The practitioner's most ambitious goal went beyond prolonging one's years to reversing the aging process altogether to attain immortality. Where ordinary medicine maintained health, the medicine of the internal alchemist was an elixir (*dan*) that an adept produced out of the resources of his own person. The realization of the body of immortality was an arduous process of lifelong self-cultivation — a higher discipline against which more standard medical regimens for health and longevity stood as a preliminary, lower stage. On one level the association of inner alchemy and medicine was based on metaphor. It did not mean that every doctor was also a practitioner and teacher of the immortalist's art. In the late Ming internal alchemy was a multidimensional aspect of upper class philosophical eclecticism and religious syncretism as well. However, Yuan Huang reveals how the language of inner alchemy had come to shape the way many Ming medical authors and audiences imagined the body of generation. Metaphors, then, ran both

8. For *nei dan*, see Needham 1983: 20–218; Robinet 1989; Baldrian-Hussein 1989–90. Defining *nei dan* is elusive, but Robinet argues that its four basic characteristics are: (1) emphasis upon training the mind as well as the body, (2) syncretism of the three teachings, Confucianism, Daoism and Buddhism; (3) use of the *Yijing* as cosmography; (4) the model of alchemy, that is, the transmutation of base metals into precious ones. See 299–302. Baldrian-Hussein argues that the term *nei dan* was not commonly used before the ninth century, and was first applied to a full range of longevity techniques in the Song. See 187.

ways, linking the medical body of reproduction and the utopian body of immortality seekers.

In Yuan Huang, readers were exposed to the teachings of a medical lineage that is known to have transmitted techniques of inner alchemy—including sexual hygiene, meditation, breath control and visualization of the body's inner landscape—as an unwritten esoteric aspect of medical learning and practice. Yuan Hao (1414–1494), Yuan Huang's great-grandfather and founder of the family's medical lineage, explained their importance in his "household instructions" to his sons on the principles of the medical arts:

> From of old, the Way of Medicine has extended to the Way of Immortals [*xian dao*]. Those who wish to study medicine must grasp the precepts concerning the Mysterious Gateway and the cultivation [of *qi*] and nour-ishment [of Essence]; they must attend carefully to the oral instructions concerning the Gate of the Mysterious Female, the Door of Birth, and holding the Center to nourish one's *qi*; and to the principles of visualizing the apertures and visualizing the marvels. Seek out an illustrious teacher and go personally to his home district and enter his dwelling. When you have understood fully, then the vicissitudes of disease and the processes of Creation will all be clear, and curing disorders cannot be anything but easy! Further, when a man's illnesses cannot be cured with materia med-ica, instruct him in these methods, and he who makes use of their merits will not fail to heal. . . . A day and a night of regulated breathing can [reverse] twenty years of chronic illness. One exposure to Heaven's yang *qi* and all things grow and bloom. One "return" of a man's primal *qi* makes his whole body harmonious.[9]

As doctors, the men of the Yuan lineage were here taught about a range of body practices. By managing seminal essence and breath, one developed an inner ability both to "guard the center" and to circulate one's primal *qi* as a countercurrent, reversing its natural tendency to dispersal. The paths of such movement up and down from the "Gate of the Mysterious Female" at the generative centers below the navel through the visceral trunk to the "bright hall" (*ming tang*) behind the eyes and the "ball of mud" (*niwan*) of the brain followed the pathways of the circulation channel system and its openings, so that one visualized *zang* and *fu* organ systems as terrain linked by pathways in a tapestried

9. Yuan Hao, "Yuan shi jiaxun" (Yuan Family Instructions) in the fifteenth-century *Yuan shi congshu* (Collected Writings of the Yuan Family). The quote is from the section "Min zhi pian" (On the place of a commoner), number six of ten precepts on medical practice. I am grateful to Cynthia Brokaw for providing me with a pho-tocopy of this text.

interior landscape. This is my crude approximation of the meditating body Yuan Hao instructed his sons to study and practice.

However, Yuan Huang's teachings on the family's traditions imagined the alchemical body as the functioning nexus of three primary vitalities: Essence (*jing*), *qi*, and Psyche (*shen*) — a theorization considered by scholars today as central to the body of internal alchemy. I read Yuan Huang's interpretation as having a particular Ming flavor, showing internal alchemy as an eclectic strand in medical thought, addressing questions about the boundaries of life and death that medical doctrines based on the cycles of yin yang and the Five Phases ignored.

Although Essence, *qi*, and Psyche or Spirit were always basic components of the Chinese medical body, the *Inner Canon* had not argued for a triangular relationship among these three vitalities as central to a vigorous long life, or to its version of sagehood.[10] In the Yellow Emperor's body psychic activity was not the subject of any distinct analysis. On the other hand, in the mature inner alchemy of the Song dynasty, as described by Isabelle Robinet, the work of self-cultivation that began with the refinement of Essence moved in a three-stage process to the purification of *qi* and finally to the self-transcendence of Psyche reverting to the original Emptiness — a mystical extinction of consciousness not unlike Buddhist Nirvana.[11]

Yuan Huang's body of inner alchemy was achieved through meditation disciplines focusing the practitioner on mastering the complex interdependence of the three. (See figures 11 and 12.) The inner alchemist located himself in relation to the critical boundaries of birth and death in time; his ideal was conservationist, his model of bodily health one of apertures well defended and of a center able to dominate peripheries, marshalling finite energies against the erosions of time. The relationship of primordial *qi*, the generative vitality of Essence, and the embodied consciousness of Psyche marked out a human being's passage from birth to death. If Heavenly *qi* from outside the domain of time

10. The *Inner Canon*'s core teaching on longevity is found in chapter one of the *Su wen*, where the emperor is advised to cultivate tranquility, detachment and nonstriving in order to "guard one's Essence and Spirit within." It also spoke enigmatically of avoiding the "seven damages" (*qi sun*) and cultivating the "eight benefits" (*ba yi*). See *Su wen* 1:7–9 and 5:22. See also Song Shugong 1991: 125–28. However, as the "three treasures," *jing*, *qi*, and *shen* played an important role in medieval religious Daoist thought on bodily immortality. In the context of this trinity *shen* has spiritualist connotations indicated in my translation by a capitalized Psyche.

11. Robinet 1989: 318–20.

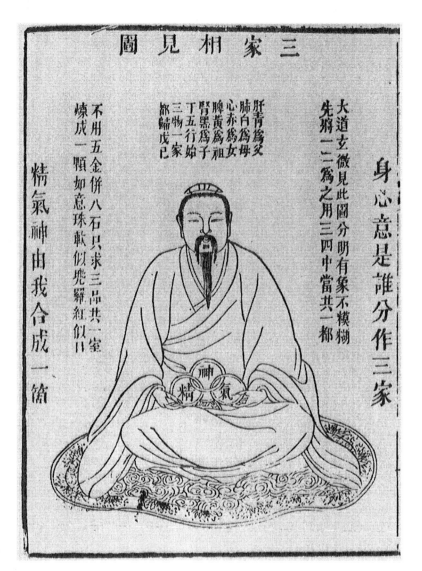

Figure 11. The Ming alchemical body: the unity of Essence, *qi,* and Psyche. From Yin Zhenren, *Xingming gui zhi* (Leading to the Core of Life), first published in 1615. Reproduced from woodblock edition held in the Needham Research Institute, Cambridge, England.

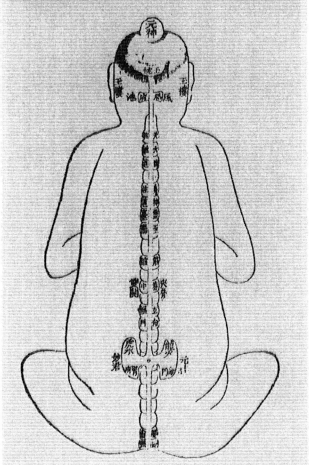

Figure 12. The Ming alchemical body: cultivating the immortal embryo. The vital Essence moves upward along the
Superintendent channel to the crown of the head. The drawing identifies medical apertures along the path of the spine;
the caption lists more fanciful spots in the Daoist interior
landscape. From Yin Zhenren, *Xingming gui zhi* (Leading to
the Core of Life), first published in 1615. Reproduced from
woodblock edition held in the Needham Research Institute,
Cambridge, England.

(*xiantian*) enters the embryonic human form at conception and underlies all primary vitalities as the primordial *qi*, in the course of temporal existence (*houtian*) *qi* gradually assumes the decayed form of material breath sustained by the function of the lungs. If consciousness—Psyche—is "ready" at the end of the ten months of gestation, as the child is born, it sustains the conscious human experience (unless disturbed in delirium or the "soul loss" of spirit possession) until dissipated at death. As a primal vitality Psyche is purest in those moments of unselfconscious awareness that precede deliberate thought or effort. But in the course of mundane life, Psyche takes the decayed form of ordinary mental activity with all of its restlessness, worries and longings (*shen silü*).

Of the three vitalities, Essence, the vitality that presides over bodily renewal, is the one directly associated with generativity in the sexual sense. This vitality is dispersed in yin Blood in childhood and develops with growth, attaining its purest and most concentrated form in the adolescent virgin youth. But with the beginning of sexual activity "his true body already lacks something and his true form has already been punctured." Essence as its materialization is latent in the body until the Ministerial Fire of sexual arousal agitates the underlying true yin Blood. Distilled from this aroused Blood as it flows through the Vital Gate, Essence has assumed its grosser form as seminal ejaculate and is available for use. Hereafter the Essence that is produced from food and drink must make up for what has been expended, but "what can be produced this way is limited and what can be expended is boundless." In this body of finite resources, a man's ability to nourish life in mature years may depend upon whether in youth he slept alone.[12] Furthermore, "Essence is developed from Blood, and it's not just in the bed-chamber that it can be overconsumed," said Yuan Huang. Within the larger scheme of the generative body and its vitalities, seminal essence depends upon Blood as the yin aspect of the Blood-*qi* pair. In this larger sense, generative Blood is here imagined as depleted through sensory stimuli—the overactivity of the seeing eyes, the listening ears, the tasting mouth—as well as through the disorders of anger or lust inciting Ministerial Fire.

Thus, in the body of Ming inner alchemy, sexual vitality is only one aspect of a triad that must be understood and managed in its complex interdependence. As Yuan Huang put it, "True Essence in the body is like the sap in wood; Psyche relies on it like a fish in water, *qi* relies on

---

12. Yuan Huang, *She sheng san yao*, 1a/b; similar wording in Yu Qiao, *Guang si yaoyu*, 29.

it like mist gathering in the valley."[13] If nourishing Essence is a matter of regulating sexual energy, nourishing *qi* is a matter of regulating breath. While the *qi* that suffuses every bone and sinew of the body is maintained through the function of respiration, the sage manages his breath so that activity and rest are balanced, no motion is sudden and no transition forced. He manages his life so that anger and worry can not derange him within, and so that stormy inclement weather cannot buffet him without. Quietistic breathing is like the imperceptible breath of a young fish in spring water, or of hibernating insects in winter. Finally, primordial *qi* is nourished through "fetal eating" and "fetal breathing." Here the practitioner swallows the *qi* that is concentrated in the saliva spring below the tongue, and he "breathes" from the navel, drawing on the *qi* of Heaven and Earth, bypassing ordinary respiration as a fetus relies on the *qi* of its mother during uterine life.

Finally, if "gathering Essence depends on nourishing *qi*, nourishing *qi* depends upon focusing one's Psyche [*cun shen*]."[14] Focusing Psyche may have been the most complex of all inner alchemy disciplines for Yuan Huang, involving as it did the paradox of unknowing knowledge and unwilled thought. On the one hand, Yuan explained that we intuit Psyche spontaneously in the fleeting impulses preceding intentional thought, in the mental life of children, in dreams or in trances. On the other hand, Psyche is focused through disciplined meditation on an internal bodily geography differentiated according to apertures along the Conception and Superintendent channels, pathways for the "return" of primal *qi*. Such meditation starts as mentally arduous concentration on specific locales within the self, where success means illumination and rejuvenation, while failure — incorrect "focusing" — may produce sensory disorientation and even disease:

> There is a focus point between the eyebrows; it is called "true man who has no place," since he goes in and out of the doors of the face. Focus and you may gather there a round globe of light; miss and your Fire floats about and you get red in the face. There is a focus point at the roof of the mouth; it is called "teeth piercing the primal pearl," and the three passes meet there. Focus and you can pass across the magpie

13. Yuan Huang, *Qi si zhenquan*, 11.

14. *Cun shen* goes back to old Daoist classics like the *Yellow Court Classic* (*Huang ting jing*), where *shen* are literally "spirits" animating the various parts of the interior body. In that interpretation "focusing the Psyche" would mean visualizing the body's spiritual denizens. Yuan Huang, however, rejected the "visualizing the apertures and visualizing the marvels" of his great-grandfather. See *She sheng san yao*, 3a/b.

bridge, flying along the Conception and Superintendent channels; miss and your Essence will not return to the source. There is a focus point at the center of the Heart, for it is said that [the body's] hundred bones and myriad apertures connect with one another in the Heart. Focus there and you can nourish your Psyche and gather your thoughts, and your beard and hair will stay forever black. Miss and it will make you bent over, not upright and at ease. . . . There is a focus point below the Heart and above the navel; it is called the "true site of the Spleen palace"; the four emblems follow there. Focus and your center will be replete and in contact with Principle; miss and it will make you overeat and yet be constantly hungry. There is a focus point at the navel, where it is said that the stem of fate is tied, circulating breath. Focus and you can nourish your primal spirit, strengthen your bowels and open your passageways. Miss and your *qi* will sink and stagnate. There is a focus point in the lower cinnabar field, as it is said that "*qi* returns to the primal sea" and that "medicine is found in Kun village" [female principle, point of origin for primal Water]. Focus and drums can arouse primal yang, returning Essence to the eyes; miss and your phallus will rise up quickly and ejaculate carelessly. There is a focus point at the genitals, linking sight and the affairs of yang [sex], as it is said that in the exchange between Heart and Kidney the furthermost point lies in the eyes. Focus to take Kan to fill Li; miss and your seminal fluids will wander without a goal.[15]

In Yuan Huang's body of generation, then, focusing Psyche is the most complex of the interlocking self-cultivation techniques of the inner alchemist, whose unstated goal is a kind of self-transcendence through the body. The language of inner alchemy strikes an outsider as that of a fanciful and poetically imagined cosmic body populated with spirits and animals, buildings and roads, streams, peaks and valleys, in a topographical landscape of the interior traveller's voyage into a fantastical realm. However, Yuan Huang shows how the alchemical body was mapped precisely onto the medical one of circulation channels and *zang* and *fu* organ systems (see especially figures 2m and 2n) and how the poetical inner journeys were correlated with body states imagined in concrete somatic terms. On one level the inner alchemical journey directly strengthened the physical and sexual powers of the body. But it

15. Yuan Huang, *She sheng san yao*, 3b; *Qi si zhenquan*, 15–16. The names are names of apertures along the Conception tract. The "magpie bridge" in many inner alchemy systems of visualization links the upper and lower halves of the trunk. The "four emblems" may refer to four magical animals identified with the first four hexagrams of the *Yijing*, and therefore with cosmogenesis and primal differentiation. *Kan* and *li*, hexagrams twenty-nine and thirty in the *Yijing*, in alchemical symbolism stand for the marital couple, the earthly counterparts to *qian* and *kun* in Heaven.

also was imagined as a process of rejuvenation and rebirth for which the most profound metaphor was gestation and the most realized body that of an infant in the womb. Here the alchemical *dan* was not medicine but embryo.

Sex, Self-Cultivation and Male Fertility

"Refining the elixir" (*lian dan*) or "returning the elixir" (*huan dan*) involves far more than control of Essence as a sexual vitality; begetting heirs, according to Yuan Huang, requires only a rudimentary command of practice. The larger process, however, is one whereby circulated vitalities assume ever more concentrated and ethereal form. At the same time, the concreteness of inner alchemy as body experience gives some clues as to how those influenced by it might have experienced what moderns think of as the sexual body, defined by erotic experience. Like Zhu Zhenheng in his earlier reading of the *Inner Canon*, Yuan Huang emphasized that "Heart and Kidney are tied together" in an exchange of Fire and Water. For the inner alchemist this evokes Psyche's tendency to initiate erotic arousal through the workings of thought, and arousal's manifestation in a flow of fluids. Moreover, these two centers found their outermost peripheries in the external genitals below and the eyes above—calling attention to the role of sight in the production of desire. Therefore, the full repertory of the self-cultivation practices of nourishing *qi* and focusing Psyche was to play a role in the management of sexual arousal to attain the detachment and control that made it possible to "lessen desire" through the calculated diminishment of external sensory stimulus.

If the generative body of inner alchemy controlled desire by setting boundaries to sensory excitation without, the techniques of gathering Essence referred to the sexual body's contribution to generativity within. On the material level what was to be gathered was semen, using basic techniques of reserving semen in intercourse known since early times. "Returning Essence to nourish the brain" was not explicitly part of the Yellow Emperor's teachings on longevity but had its locus classicus in medieval "bed-chamber arts" taught by Sun Simiao and many others. Joseph Needham has described this technique as "coitus reservatus," whereby manual pressure on the base of the scrotum at the moment of ejaculation diverts semen into the urethra and bladder. But I think that Yuan Huang and his contemporaries believed that all kinds of movements of Ministerial Fire—experienced as heightened sexual tension without climax — could, if managed properly, advance the project of "nourishing Essence."

If a man's seminal Essence is depleted in a variety of moralized ways, it can be positively nourished by meditation exercises that stimulate and direct generative heat in keeping with the body's natural rhythms of arousal. In the early hours of the morning, taking advantage of ascending yang influences, seated in loose garments, he begins with regulated breathing, concentrating his Psyche thereby. The nourishment of Essence is accomplished through ritual self-massage, linking external genital stimulation to the nourishment of the deeper centers of Kidney function behind the navel.[16] The Essence so reserved initially as semen is imagined as transformable into a precious elixir rising and falling imperceptibly in the body along the Conception and Superintendent channels, nourishing the brain and gathering as the sweet dew of saliva before returning to the generative root in the lower cinnabar field. Such circulation, accomplished in harmony with the rhythms of day, month and year, would accomplish what Needham has called a "redemptive hygiene" — prolonging a youthful appearance, extending life and placing immortality itself within reach.

In medieval China the project of nourishing Essence had been associated with the amorous arts of the bed-chamber, recommended in manuals addressed to aristocratic males. Here the goal had been imagined as achieved through the erotic manipulation of multiple females, provoking one's partners' orgasms while withholding one's own. The question of whether this in fact was either a desirable or natural sexual script for a man was controversial, and erotically explicit "bed-chamber manuals" teaching that female orgasm can nourish the male disappeared from public circulation early in the Song dynasty, condemned by moralists as an excuse for licentiousness. The famous scholar-official Su Shi was an influential early critic. The old teachings continued to circulate underground or in some Daoist circles as esoteric practices, now branded by mainstream society as transgressive and pornographic.[17] As illicit temptation, bed-chamber arts did not cease to fascinate, as shown

16. Yuan Huang, *Qi si zhenquan*, 13.
17. For the decline of "bed-chamber arts" see Song Shugong, 1991: 289–90; Wile 1992: 146–92; and Furth 1994. The underground Ming-Qing transmission of these traditions was associated with the Daoist immortal Zhang Sanfeng, a shadowy figure variously said to have lived in the Song, Yuan or early Ming who was rhetorically identified with the "sexual school" of Daoism from the Ming forward. Wile translates three elliptically worded treatises on sexual alchemy attributed to Zhang. See 146–48. A hagiographic biography of Zhang is discussed in Anna Sidel 1970.

in the tropes of Ming erotic fiction and when occasionally they surfaced in stories about the imperial court. The Jiajing emperor (1522–1566) was accused of practicing "Daoist rites" with young girls, some of whom died, prompting, it was said, an attempt on the emperor's life by several palace women. In the early seventeenth century, the untimely death of the young heir to the Wanli emperor was attributed by some to his overindulgence with eight beauties presented as presents.[18]

In spite of scandals like these, Ming medical authorities could turn to a more respected source of teachings on the bed-chamber arts — Sun Simiao, whose writings continued to be honored as medical classics. Already in the seventh century Sun had criticized not the exploitation of females implicit in the art of the bed-chamber but the male fantasies of power that lured reckless youth to play with fire this way. In Sun Simiao, pursuit of longevity through multiple sexual partners had been recommended as appropriate in men over forty, whose passions had moderated enough to allow them to approach the process with the necessary detachment. Moreover, Sun had shifted emphasis from the manipulation of female arousal to male self-control through focused visualization techniques similar to those in internal alchemy, and his commonsense solution to the problem of male loss of vitality through sexual expenditure was neither abstinence nor boudoir athletics but moderation. In a famous metaphor that doctors echoed down the centuries, Sun warned that qi is finite, like a lamp's supply of oil, which may either flare up and burn out or, through careful conservation and use, last a full span of years.[19]

When Ming-era physicians criticized the bed-chamber arts, they took off from Zhu Zhenheng's comments on Sun Simiao. Zhu considered the matter from the point of view of the vulnerable masculinity of the body of yang surplus and yin deficiency. Suggesting that Sun's advice had been directed at middle-aged men who needed to make up for a dissipated youth, Zhu pointed to the superiority of prevention over cure and called for a sexual script in which the male "stops" rather than "steals."[20] In bodies where the yang of Ministerial Fire is always in

18. The scandal concerning the Jiajing emperor was reported in Shen Defu, *Wanli yehhuo bian*, juan 3. The mysterious death of the Wanli emperor's heir rocked the court in 1620. Some attributed it to a mysterious "red pill"—a monk's medicine containing "red lead," a yang replenisher made up of sublimed menstrual blood mixed with arsenic. See Peterson 1979: 134–37. For "red lead" as medicine see below, 216.

19. Sun Simiao, "Fang zhong bu yi" (Replenishing Benefits of the Bed-chamber), in *Beiji qianjin yaofang*, juan 27, 488–91.

20. Zhu Zhenheng, *Ge zhi yu lun*, in SKQS 746:671–72.

surplus and the yin of generative Water is always deficient, sexual restraint was not based on a puritanical distrust of the "natural" body but
on an ethic of prudence advocated in the name of harmony with nature's
deeper truth. It was in support of such constructions of the natural that
Yuan Huang, like Wan Quan and other Ming medical authorities, condemned the bed-chamber arts of "plucking *qi*" or "stealing Essence"
from women as transgressive sexual practices dangerous to health. *To
Benefit Yin* quoted these words:

> Master Yuan Liaofan says, "The Way of gathering Essence is: one, reduce
> desire; two, avoid overexertion; three, restrain anger; four, abstain from
> wine; five, moderate diet. Nowadays those who talk of 'nourishing life'
> often speak of 'gathering yin to replenish yang,' and of prolonged [sexual]
> combat without emission. This is a great mistake. The Kidneys are the
> storehouse of Essence, and when males and females engage in the sex act
> they must disturb Kidney function. When Kidneys are activated, Essence
> and Blood follow and flow out. Even if one emits nothing externally,
> Essence has already left the palace. Before one has managed to curb it,
> even as one's member softens a few drops of true Essence may leak out.
> This is [a common] experience. When the fire is blazing, who can restore
> the firewood?"[21]

Caught between the snares of enchantment awaiting the would-be
boudoir athlete and the introspective nights of solitary exercise practiced
by the longevity seeker, the ordinary sensual male seeking medical advice
could turn to numbers. Guidelines concerning coital frequency, adjusted
for age and constitution, had been supplied by doctors from Sun Simiao
on down to Yu Qiao, Yuan Huang and Wu Zhiwang. Suggestions for
young men varied: every four days? every five days? twice a month?
Should males over sixty abstain entirely, or try it once a month? The
exact numbers were less important than their cautionary rhetoric calling
attention to generative vitality as a finite and measurable resource.[22]
They reinforced criticisms of the old bed-chamber arts as what Foucault

---

21. Wang Qi ed., 180–81. See also Yuan Huang, *Qi si zhenquan*, 12–13.

22. The numbers in Sun Simiao: for a man at twenty, every four days; at thirty,
every eight days; at forty, every sixteen days; at fifty, every twenty days; and at sixty,
once a month or not at all. See "Fang shu bu yi," 489. Yu Qiao's text included the
following: at twenty, when "one cannot help it," once every five days; at thirty once
every ten days; at forty once a month. See *Guang si yaoyu*, "Lun tong zhuang" (On
youth and maturity), 29. Wu Zhiwang claimed to follow the *Baopuzi*, allowing males
under twenty-one ejaculation every two days, males under thirty every three days,
under forty every ten days, over forty once a month, and over fifty once every three
months, while those in their sixties should "shut the door." See Wu Zhiwang 1626,
juan 69, 4a.

might call a discourse of incitement. Not everyone took the stricter view: the essayist Xie Zhaozhe (1567–1624) said that worry and anxiety could do more damage than sexual intercourse, while the irreverent playwright Li Yu lampooned midnight meditation to "nourish life": it just interferes with a good night's sleep, he said.[23] But even libertines like Li Yu (1611–1680) embraced the ideal of moderation, while the experience of the respected scholar Gu Yanwu (1618–1682) showed the risks believed to follow from the wrong medical advice. Left without a living heir at sixty, he was persuaded by the eminent physician and poet Fu Shan that he could take a concubine; two years later, claiming exhaustion, Gu dismissed her, and Fu Shan was criticized roundly by the scholar's friends.

Bed-chamber arts and inner alchemy, then, while presenting males with conflicting models of what kind of performance was sexually natural and desirable, nonetheless were opposites sharing a common set of assumptions—that is, a shared habitus. This included an underlying view of primary vitalities as embodied in material, quantifiable amounts of stuff whose deployment in the temporal world (*houtian*) guided the human life cycle along a path from growth and generativity to decline and death. Still, these vitalities linked the human body to sources of creativity and transcendent power outside of time (*xiantian*), and these were unquantifiable and infinite. This mysticism of the body encouraged a detachment of the sexual from the social realm. While the medieval bed-chamber arts have been rightly criticized inside and outside of China for their manipulative exploitation of women, the Ming self-cultivation ideal of inner alchemy also enlisted the sexual drive for inward-turning personal goals of sagehood. Both bed-chamber arts and inner alchemy were comparatively indifferent to the social dimensions of erotic experience as a human interaction. They neither defined the "sexual" in a modernist mode around privately shared bodily pleasures nor romanticized an art of love imbued with sentiment and passion. Rather they encouraged in males a detached sort of desireless desire, or even indifference toward women.[24]

This picture will be modified, however, if we see Ming discourse on the generative body of internal alchemy as positioning the erotic at the

23. Xie Zhaozhe, n.d. [1977], juan 5, 120; Li Yu 1671, juan 15, 17b–21a; juan 16, 17a–26b. Li Yu, who came from a medical family, larded his "Casual Expressions" with satirical riffs on the medical classics, such as his list of the "seven medicines for the mind" of the hedonist, a takeoff on the *Inner Canon*'s "seven harms."

24. Judith Zeitlin notes that in Ming fiction sexual intercourse with multiple partners is presented as far less dangerous than falling in love. (Personal communication.)

fulcrum of body experiences, implicating human longevity and even immortality on one hand and generativity ensuring the social reproduction of the family on the other. In *Veracious Explanation* Yuan Huang relied on the inner alchemical self-cultivation of Essence, *qi*, and Psyche to produce the foundation of a fertile male body of "flourishing Essence" (*jing wang*). For mature men lacking heirs, the procreative duty of a head of household took unquestioned priority over the body's other uses and aspirations. All the prescribed alchemical disciplines of the senses, the monitoring of Ministerial Fire and Princely Fire, the control of anger and drunkenness, the attention to diet and to meditation exercise — all were properly directed at the goal of reproduction.

When the generative body worked to serve the family, eros was properly enlisted. Here *To Benefit Yin* supplemented the advice of Yuan Huang with the more mundane guide to sexual intercourse in Yu Qiao. Both emphasized that a fruitful coupling was a joyous one and that neither "solitary yang" nor "solitary yin" could conceive a child. In order to instruct bridegrooms, Wan Quan's popular text on begetting had even drawn upon the language of the old bed-chamber manuals about the signs of female arousal and the proper male conduct of intercourse.[25] Yu Qiao had advice for males with unruly phalluses, whether suffering from the limpness of "weak yang," the excessive rigidity of Ministerial Fire, or the premature emissions of "yin depletion." As for women, "with their tranquil yin natures, many experience bitter couplings [*ku jiao*] and do not conceive," he said.[26] Although his recommendations that materia medica could assist coital happiness would seem to imply aphrodisiacs, in fact his Beginning of Joy pill contained standard *fuke* ingredients to nourish a wife's *qi* and Blood, while the male Thinking of Immortals formula combined ingredients to cool and tranquilize Heart on the one hand and to "roughen" and consolidate Essence on the other.[27] Her medicines aided a latent fertility, his fostered sexual control. Yuan Huang added considerations of the role of sentiment in

25. The reference to mutual orgasm is clear as explained by Wan Quan: "If yang Essence arrives first and yin does not respond, it is a case of 'solitary yang' . . . [and vice versa]." See *Wan shi jia chuan guang si jiyao*, juan 5, 25–29. See also Yu Qiao, 1.

26. Yu Qiao, 3.

27. Yu Qiao, 3. For the pharmaceutical formulas, see 7, 8. The Beginning of Joy pill of sixteen ingredients led with ginseng, *baishu*, licorice, and angelica. Thinking of Immortals formula featured buds of lotus flower (*lianhua*) and snake brambleseed (*shilianzi*) for cooling and tranquilizing, and Cherokee rose hips (*jinyingzi*), a very sour fruit whose tartness would assist the body in "gathering" and consolidating fluids.

fruitful marriages, noting that "when wives are happy and harmonious, then children come," just as the burgeoning of spring is the result of the harmony of Heaven and Earth. *Veracious Explanation* addressed male responsibility for domestic harmony in polygamous households. A man should temper authority with mildness and fairness, recalling the poet's words that "the realm of passion [*qingyu*] is not ruled by easygoing manners; the secrets of the boudoir do not show in one's deportment."[28]

By contrast with the rhetorical emphasis upon technique induced by much in advice literature on fertility and longevity, Yuan Huang's final admonitions appealed to sentiment in harmony with the late Ming cult of love (*qing*)[29] and to Daoist-inspired natural philosophy. It is when coitus is spontaneous, performed "without knowledge or thought," that conceptions occur, Heavenly *qi* descends, and Essence effects the transmission of life from one body to another in a generational continuum. Continence as a way of life for males was not based on abstinence but on appropriate reverence for reproductive powers vested in the body by nature. It was not imagined as repression of the sexual drive but as the ideal form of its expression. Where the dissipation of the rake bespeaks his folly and lack of self-control, the strong man enjoys a bodily wholeness and vitality marked by secure borders and a serene center. With this foundation, a man may proceed to the nuptial couch at the proper time. His ability either to release and get an heir, or to "reverse course" and increase his own longevity, is not a matter of heedless lust or laborious control but a reenactment of nature's creative spontaneity.

Here the male generative body was also an alchemical one. Male sexual powers were identified both with the reproductive function, which accomplishes the social mission of the family, and with generative vitality, which can replicate and extend the creative work of the cosmos at large. Such a patriarch's body is also that of a natural man, whom Ming gentlemen might have recognized in the seventeenth-century sketches I have reproduced in chapter one to illustrate the fourteen cardinal channels (figures 2a–2n). Ideal masculinity does not lodge in youth

28. Yuan Huang, *Qi si zhenquan*, 18. The term I have translated as "boudoir" (*yan si*, literally "swallow's privacy") alludes to a famous piece of advice on conjugal harmony offered the philosopher Mencius by his mother: "When you go into the *yan si* [i.e., women's chamber] make a noise to announce your presence in advance; to fail in this is unmannerly." See *Zhongwen da cidian* 20:457.

29. Ko 1994: 69–99, discusses the extraordinary popularity of late Ming plays, poems and short stories on romantic themes, and the importance of female as well as male readers in making them fashionable.

but in maturity; not in a muscular surface but in a vitality of inner circulation, and in bodily postures evoking both relaxed and easy motion and stability of center. A man's deeper generativity may be hinted at by an appearance that hides his years—the strong teeth, abundant black hair, and fresh complexion associated with ample Kidney function. But our drawings tell us these are not essential. A more powerful marker is the inner calm of a mature man's focused Psyche, one not prey to the wearisome buffeting of emotions and thought, but able instead to channel these as appropriate according to nature and ritual. In all these ways, medicine of internal alchemy in the Ming dynasty taught that the ideal of the sage was also the achievement of a realized masculinity.

Sexual Generation and the Female: Conception and the Sex of the Offspring

The role of each partner in the conception of an infant has been a potent question for science and society in many medical traditions. The mechanisms of conception lie concealed within, and the outcome of visible acts of coitus is unpredictable. In the face of explanatory appeals to fate and karma, medical experts in China, as elsewhere, looked for knowable patterns that could unlock the mystery of female fertility. In so doing, they reinforced the assumption that infertile unions were primarily a female problem, an influential view that in Ming China was upheld by the authority of Zhu Zhenheng. Beyond the mystery of conception itself is the fact that the act of begetting defines the family. Thinking of Aristotle's views on the matter, Thomas Laqueur has pointed out that "the biology of conception was at the same time a model of filiation."[30] In China's medical history, doctors do not seem to have been called upon to "name the Father" for the patriarchal family by privileging yang over yin in the procreative act itself. As embodiments of cosmic processes, the mating couple transmitted to their offspring the pattern of the species, and science did not concern itself with the inheritance of individual traits. When genealogists, following the philosopher Zhu Xi's theories of lineage, spoke of the *qi* transmitted from ancestors to descendants, they were talking about the agnatic descent

30. Laqueur 1990: 49.

line that made ancestral sacrifices efficacious, not the bodily *qi* and Blood that made both male and female babies.[31]

But filiation was at stake when every important medical account of conception was immediately followed by a consideration of the factors determining the sex of the fetus. For a Chinese man, after all, paternity meant the begetting of sons. Accordingly, in the discourse on sexual generation in medical literature, questions about the female bodily dispositions promoting or inhibiting conception were rhetorically linked to the issue of the sexual differentiation of the fetus, which in Ming times was assumed to occur at the same time.

Where conception created new life though the union of yin and yang, bestowing the unitary *qi* of Heaven, the subsequent division of yin and yang into male or female was the most fundamental endowment of the *qi* of Earth. *To Benefit Yin,* introducing its chapter on seeking descendants, glossed the matter with a syncretic twist: "What is it that congeals at the time of sexual union to make the fetus? Though it is none other than Essence and Blood, made up of the material dregs that exist in the temporal world [*houtian*], a tiny bit of perfected spirit *qi* from outside the realm of time [*xiantian zhen yi zhi ling qi*], moved to germinate by the feelings of desire [*qingyu*], miraculously is part of it."[32] Here Buddhist images named the gulf between the mundane world of material "dregs" and a numinous (*ling*) atemporal realm, while the facilitating role of sexual desire was added to the standard older medical account of male and female powers completing the work of Heaven as a yin yang pair embodying Earth.[33]

Here as elsewhere in Chinese cosmology, issues of timeliness and timing mattered greatly. The medical consensus that a woman's fertile period occurs as her menstrual flow ends and "new Blood begins to grow" had not changed over the centuries, nor had the belief that external phenomena might affect the decisive moment. Chen Ziming had pointed to a vast lore concerning auspicious and inauspicious stars, days, natural anomalies, spirits and demons capable of affecting the outcome of the sexual act. In the final analysis Chen Ziming had appealed to these as dimensions of an overarching fate: "The reasons for lacking an heir

---

31. For Zhu Xi the important question was to explain the efficacy of prayers to the ancestors, including the prayers of wives, who were not biologically related to husbands' forebearers. See Zhu Xi, *Zhuzi xingli yulei,* juan 3, "Gui shen," 26–44. My thanks to David Bello for pointing these passages out to me. See also Waltner 1990: 28–37.

32. Wang Qi ed., 179.

33. For comparison with early modern European views see Furth 1995.

are three: ancestral altars [bad karma], incompatible horoscopes [of the couple], illness in husband or wife." He had concluded that in obtaining sons, medicine might be less effective than the blessings of the Buddhist gods.[34] As a devout if syncretic Buddhist, on some level Yuan Huang would have agreed here with Chen Ziming, but *To Benefit Yin* not only neglected issues of supernatural influences but also emphasized aspects of the work of Yuan Huang and others that focused upon the internal workings of the human body and the ability of human actors to control it. This shift to an emphasis on internal agency not only marked the embodied self as more sharply bounded and centered, it also gave greater weight and seriousness to the issue of male or female responsibility for reproductive failure.

Keeping to the spirit of correspondence theory, *To Benefit Yin* called attention to the timeliness of yin yang influences in the diurnal and lunar cycles, according to which male cycles are daily and female ones are monthly. The male voices in *To Benefit Yin* spoke of their experience of a period of natural yang ascendancy in the hours of the early morning, between midnight and dawn. Reaching for a construction of the female body as analogous with their own, they discussed menstruation in the context of a female body discipline to enhance fertility. Where males nourished Essence, females were advised to regulate their menses, extending if necessary to a regimen of replenishing drugs in the morning to warm below and cooling doses before bedtime to cleanse above.[35] Even more strenuous was "driving the menses" (*gan jing*) with drugs to advance or retard the flow every month until a woman's cycle coincided with the lunar one. Here an ideal menstrual cycle was constructed as if, on analogy with male seminal Essence, it could be controlled to benefit from its natural affinity with yin yang rhythms of the seasonal calendar.[36]

Concerning the timing of intercourse itself, most people learned in medicine in the seventeenth century accepted the old theory that a woman was fertile during the first few days of a new menstrual cycle. Yu Qiao had imagined the couple's bodies as vessel and contents respectively. He advised males to cultivate their own "fullness" (*shi* = repletion) and to look for signs to "cast into the vacancy" (*xu* = deple-

---

34. Chen Ziming, juan 9, 287, 301.
35. Wang Qi ed., 179, quoting Chen Chuliang.
36. Wang Qi ed., 186–87, quoting an unknown *Qiu si quanshu* (Complete Book on Seeking Heirs).

tion) that occurred at the beginning of the woman's new cycle. Although no yin yang pair should get too far out of balance with one another, still Essence was best when replete, while Blood's generative power was greatest when most incipient. As her month advanced, the increasing abundance and repletion of Blood would move the coital couple out of balance; when replete cast into replete, no fruit would result.[37] The search for signs of such minute transitions deep in the female body produced ever more refined readings — of menstrual red turning to gold, as dirty old Blood is dispelled and precious new Blood begins to grow. A well-known doggerel verse, "Thirty [Chinese] hours, or two-and-one-half days; at [hour] twenty-eight or twenty-nine, the gentleman knows," was one guide to calculating the best moment for intercourse. Another — more recherché — method was to track diurnal cycles in the rhythms of the couple's pulses, in order to identify excesses in advance and correct them with medicines.

To Benefit Yin reported on these strategies, but it gave more space to Yuan Huang's method of determining female fertility by the most intimate of a woman's internal signs — her desire:

> Yuan Liaofan [Yuan Huang] says, "Living creatures all have a mating season. . . . The classics of inner alchemy [*dan jing*] teach that each month there is one hour of one day, in keeping with the rhythm of the menstrual cycle, when a woman will have a fertile period. In that hour, her *qi* will be steaming and hot. When she is swooning and longing, unable to control her desire, the moment is at hand. At this time one may reverse course and hold [semen] to make an immortal embryo, or let flow and release it to make a fetus. . . . When her desire is intense, within the womb something like a budding lotus flower . . . protrudes into the vagina. A wife will feel it when she washes herself below, but, ashamed, she is unwilling to speak. If the man can privately advise her beforehand, and have her speak of it herself, he will straightaway hit the mark."[38]

Here we see an amorous relationship based on spousal intimacy, but also one naturalizing feminine shame. The sexual script for a wife enjoined indirection and reserve. The desiring woman was figured in veiled metaphors: "The leaden cauldron [*ding*] is warming within; light shines through the curtains."[39] Thus eroticized, she was more a figure caught

---

37. Yu Qiao, 3–6.
38. Wang Qi ed., 182, quoting Yuan Huang, *Qi si zhenquan*, 18–19.
39. Wang Qi ed., 182, quoting Yuan Huang.

between modesty and instinct than a partner equal to her mate in continent self-mastery and sexual control. Although erotic arousal in both males and females was imagined to follow natural rhythms of timeliness, eros in women was an instinct more intimately tied to fertility. It was deployed to serve reproduction rather than a woman's own longevity as well. The fertile erotic encounter was imagined as an event guided and directed by the male partner.

In medieval China, the bodily processes by which a child was conceived and those which produced either a male or female could be imagined as separated in time. Sun Simiao had transmitted teachings concerning "fetal education" in the first three months, a period of indeterminacy where "the inner responds to the outer," making female responsibility for the outcome a matter of her conduct. In the Song and after, medical authorities assumed that the child's sex was fixed at the time of conception itself. Accordingly, teaching that the newly pregnant woman actually might change her baby's sex, like other pieces of the ritual *fuke* repertory, gradually disappeared from learned medical discourse, relegated to the domain of folk medical practices.

This fusion of conception and sexual differentiation intensified the significance of the sexual script according to which married couples engaged in intercourse. A perennial theory, which in the Ming dynasty was identified with the Daoist scriptures, taught that the child's sex is determined by whether coitus takes place on days one, three, or five (yang numbers) or days two, four, or six (yin numbers) of a woman's new menstrual cycle. Chen Ziming and his successors had offered an alternative popular view attributed to Chu Cheng, which focused upon the inner dialectic of the yin yang relationship working through the bodies of the mating couple in a way that translated biological chance into a process subject to human control. In *To Benefit Yin* Chu Cheng was quoted portraying sexual differentiation as the result of a drama of combat as Essence met Blood in intercourse: "When man and woman unite, the Essences of both are joyful. If yin Blood arrives first and yang Essence then dashes against it, the Blood opens to wrap around the Essence; Essence enters, making bone, and a male is formed. If yang *qi* enters first and yin Blood later joins it, the Essence opens to surround Blood; Blood enters to make the foundation and a female is formed."[40]

40. See Chen Ziming, juan 10, 308; Wang Qi ed., 183–84; Wu Zhiwang 1626, juan 67, 7a; and many others. For the original, see Chu Cheng, in SKQS 734:543, "Shou xing" (Receiving Form).

Drawing on the perennial Chinese topos of sexual intercourse as combat, the timing of orgasm is the decisive factor in determining the sex of the child. It is set by the partner who proves "victor" in the sexual contest. In Chu Cheng, then, procreative sexual scripts subtly replicated the model of sexual vitalities of the old bed-chamber arts—showing males and females as possessing equivalent and matching yin yang powers, possibly taking an adversarial turn: "Water can extinguish Fire." The combat of erotic adversaries was also a familiar Ming trope in popular fiction, lending further credence to Chu Cheng's biologizing of the battle of the sexes.

However, *To Benefit Yin* also showed how some late Ming medical authorities had come to raise serious questions about Chu Cheng, as well as about other perennial theories of sexual differentiation using yin and yang cosmology. At issue was the validity of external cosmological versus internal bodily explanations of the gendered powers of yin and yang. But also at stake were the powers and responsibilities of male and female partners for procreative success or failure. The Jin and Yuan masters had begun to raise these doubts, appealing to reason and experience. Following them, a spirit of curiosity and inquiry informed late Ming approaches. Questions of natural philosophy—science, if you will—combined with preoccupations shaped by gender ideology.

To Benefit Yin offered its readers a competent summary of a scholarly debate reported on in other late Ming sources as well, Li Shizhen and Xie Zhaozhe among others.[41] Among the Jin-Yuan masters, doubts about Chu Cheng's model of sexual differentiation had been voiced. Li Gao had rejected the old Daoist view of the influence of odd and even numbered days in the woman's personal monthly calendar, opining simply that boys were conceived on the first two days after the end of menses during the time of greatest "vacancy." Zhu Zhenheng thought that yin and yang had affinities for the right and left sides of the womb—possibly based upon his observation of a prolapsed uterus with its two "branches" (fallopian tubes). Accordingly, he suggested that odd and even numbered days exercised an external force of attraction on this internal anatomy.[42] However, observation of twins complicated this last picture, as did reports from men who claimed to have timed intercourse carefully

41. See Li Shizhen, juan 52, 4:2970–71; Xie Zhaozhe, juan 5, 118. The immediate sources for *Ji yin gangmu* were Yuan Huang and Wang Kentang.

42. Wang Qi ed., 184. For Zhu's observation of uterine prolapse see Ma Dazheng 1991: 192. The case is recorded in Jiang Guan, juan 11, 337.

or to have attained "victory" in erotic combat without the predicted results. As for those who suggested that the result was determined by whether yin or yang was relatively strong or weak in the encounter, Yuan Huang noted, "There are scrawny husbands and timorous wives who produce child after child without being able to stop; and there are also those of robust *qi* and Blood and unusual prowess who remain heirless." Zhu Zhenheng had blamed fruitless unions solely on the female's menstrual problems, but, Yuan pointed out, some women who were barren in one marriage proved fertile in a subsequent union.[43]

· After considering all these possibilities, *To Benefit Yin,* quoting Yuan Huang, linked conception, sexual pleasure and male dominance in the production of heirs as follows:

> To speak of the male leading is not about [his] youth or age, strength or weakness, health or sickness, or whether ejaculation is easy or difficult. If at the time of amorous arousal "the hundred pulses arrive in unison" [*bai mai qi dao*] . . . one can conceive a child. . . . The woman's Blood is able to complete and consolidate it because her "hundred pulses gather together" [*bai mai heju*]. Compared with the male's Essence [Blood] is necessarily less strong. Confucius said that *qian*'s ability to initiate is called great; and *kun*'s ability to grow is called extensive. Isn't this its meaning? As for the sex of the child, it's not a matter of whether Essence or Blood arrives first, or of the day of the woman's cycle, or of whether intercourse is before or after midnight, nor is it a matter of a strong woman mating with a weaker man, or vice versa. Only the difference between their two climaxes can determine victory or defeat. Thus if Essence in attaining climax has the wherewithal to defeat Blood, the child will be male; if Blood in attaining climax has the wherewithal to defeat Essence, the child will be female.[44]

43. Wang Qi ed., 185–86, quoting Yuan Huang, *Qi si zhenquan,* 19–20. Yuan cites a man named Zheng Wujian, whom I have not been able to identify. Other authorities, such as Wan Quan, denied that Zhu Zhenheng ignored male infertility.

44. Yuan Huang, *Qi si zhenquan,* 20; Wang Qi ed., 186; Wu Zhiwang 1626: juan 67, 8a/b. Yuan Huang, 21, further explained "the hundred pulses arrive in unison" (*bai mai qi dao*) as follows: "When a young man 'rides' a woman, in the beginning he feels an intensity and thirst for his goal; after ejaculation his whole body is joyful and at ease. This is what is called 'one hundred pulses arrive in unison' to conceive a child." In *Ji yang gangmu,* Wu Zhiwang argued that fully complete orgasm (involving every one of the hundred pulses) was necessary for success. He rejected the possibility that a defective ("irregular") orgasm might produce an offspring with physical defects. Here the quality of the orgasm seems to act as a template for the formation of a whole human being. The term may allude to hexagram 63 of the *Yijing,* named *jiji,* "completion." This hexagram joins *kan* and *li,* which figure the archetypical male and female on Earth, counterparts of *qian* and *kun* in Heaven. See Van Gulik 1974: 36–39.

In this Ming revision of Chu Cheng, pleasure more than control ruled the coital encounter, and orgasm ("the hundred pulses arrive together") on the part of both partners was deemed essential to successful conception. Such a construction of sexuality and fertility called for a marriage relationship involving intimate communication between husband and wife, a goal Yuan Huang championed elsewhere. Wifely pleasure was naturalized as less intense, in keeping with her role of compliance, while males were enjoined to be considerate.

On the one hand, this debate on the mechanisms underlying sexual differentiation reflected Ming learned medicine's concern to reason from experience. On the other hand, the internalist model of conception, fusing fertility and erotic intimacy itself, was less a triumph of empirical observation than an ideologically driven valorization of romance in gentry marriage. *To Benefit Yin* followed Yuan Huang in honoring sentiment, being protective of women and drawing paternalist morals from its science. "So isn't it an error . . . to blame mothers alone for miscarriages, or to attribute child mortality to the child?"[45] Ironically, in considering sexual intercourse and fertility, *To Benefit Yin*'s detachment from theories of cosmological correspondences based on yin yang and the Five Phases opened the door to paternalist gender ideology. While celebrating romance in marriage, joining eros and fertility, that ideology also inscribed female compliance and passivity on the virtuously procreative couple, while implying that males were responsible for controlling bodily outcomes.

Did Wu Zhiwang's narrative on fertility and longevity for males in *To Benefit Yang* offer the same interpretation of these issues as that found in *To Benefit Yin*? By and large, yes, but their differences are more interesting, because they suggest something of how male doctors negotiated gender boundaries in addressing sexual issues. While also indebted to Yuan Huang on the importance of mutual orgasm to fertility, *To Benefit Yang* emphasized male performance, linking its problems specifically to Zhu Zhenheng's body of yin deficiency threatened by uncontrolled Ministerial Fire. Quoting Zhu, Wu linked the aphorism "yang is always in surplus; yin is always deficient" directly to problems of male and female generative vitality.[46] His pharmaceutical strategy followed accordingly. Concerned with protecting vulnerable generative Water, Wu was vehement against misuse of hot, drying, acrid materia

45. Wang Qi ed., 186; Yuan Huang, *Qi si zhenquan*, 21.
46. Wu Zhiwang 1626, juan 67, 4b–5b.

medica for enhancement of vitality. Impotence, skin lesions, and infants prone to boils and fits and worse awaited those who indulged in the current medical fad for "potent" (*du*) and "fiercely strong" replenishing medicines, he said. Instead, males should use the mildly warming and nourishing staples of *fuke:* Four Ingredients formula to aid Blood, and Four Gentlemen infusion to support Spleen-stomach. These were "the Way of Kings in medicine." Females should take fragrant nutgrass (*xiangfu*) formulas, a *fuke* favorite that moved *qi,* opening stasis and permitting Blood to follow.[47] Emphasizing the replenishment of Blood in males and the stimulation of *qi* in females, Wu's strategy for the fertile couple was to bring each back toward a common balanced center.

Wu's warnings about the heating properties of northern foods—heavy meat stews, leeks and scallions, pickled condiments, sorghum liquor—pointed to a similar moral. Many materia medica on Wu's hit list of dangerous drugs, like aconite (*fuzi*), immature deer horn (*lurong*), rabbit silk (*tusi*), eucommia bark (*duzhong*) and bastard cardamom (*sharen*), were also identified as strongly heating replenishers acting on yang. In a work addressed to males, Zhu Zhenheng's pharmacology of "replenishing yin" emerges as more controversial, specific to a delicate, Southern literati body. The therapeutic properties of cooling versus heating, moistening versus drying, overlapped ambiguously in the language of pharmacy, acquiring different connotations depending upon the body in question.[48]

Wu Zhiwang's fertility remedies sought to promote balance in Zhu Zhenheng's androgynous body of yin deficiency, but his sexual scripts favored yang. He repeated Zhu Zhenheng's warnings concerning Sun Simiao's art of the bed-chamber, while at the same time revealing his admiration for "the mature man strong in substance who can see the enemy and not be moved." After all, "lustful women produce girls."[49] Thinking of the sexual battleground, he offered men medical assistance to better control the timing of sexual climax to ensure "victory," including materia medica to "lengthen or shorten the [orgasmic]

47. Wu Zhiwang 1626, juan 67, 1b–2a, 13a. Four Gentlemen infusion was Xue Ji's preferred formula for addressing menstrual and other problems of Blood storage through Spleen-stomach function.

48. In fact, in the late Ming, Zhu Zhenheng's pharmacy was being challenged by medical partisans of "warming and replenishing" strategies. One such physician is discussed below, in chapter seven.

49. Wu Zhiwang 1626, juan 67, 2b.

pulse, to slow up the speedy and speed up the slow, to activate the flaccid and repress the slippery."[50] A technique derived from Yu Qiao advocated timing intercourse to cast into "the vacancy" that would occur two-and-one-half days after the *beginning* of a woman's menstrual cycle, at the exact midpoint when newest Blood—the menstrual "gold"—offers maximal advantage to yang.[51] To beget a son, a bold man might ignore the standard advice that contact with menstrual blood was polluting for males. Such advice, proffered by Wu himself in other contexts, also flouted long-standing *fuke* wisdom that intercourse during the menses was unhealthy for women. (Yuan Huang, in fact, had rejected it.)

Such advice exposes the double-edged image of menstrual blood, both generative and polluting. The subject of materia medica for fertility led male medical authority to embrace further contradictory representations of the gestational body. *To Benefit Yang* offered its readers a number of prescriptions based on the pharmaceutical principle of "using man to replenish man" (*yi ren bu ren*). Some byproducts of gestation like human milk had long been esteemed as nourishment for the aged. Zhu Zhenheng had popularized "purple river cart" (*ziheche*)—human placenta—as a remedy to nourish yin in cases of wasting disorders. It was the lead ingredient in Great Creation pill (*Dazao wan*), a formula for serious yin depletions sometimes given barren women.[52] Like umbilical cord, "purple river cart" was a remedy whose polluting power could not be separated from its generative significance. Though this repelled some and made it controversial, Wu Zhiwang was not unusual in promoting these substances as boosters of primordial *qi*. But he went further, offering his male clients the fashionable late Ming esoteric medicines known as "autumn stone" (*qiushi*) and "red lead" (*hongqian*)—chemical distillates of human urine (imagined as surplus Essence) and of menstrual blood, respectively. In his day these were believed to be potent alchemical aids to "nourishing life." These medicines, unknown in antiquity, were based on the generative fluids of the human body itself, carefully collected from pubescent adolescents approaching their natural apogee of growth. Autumn stone was esoteric chemistry, based on techniques associated with the traditions of

50. Wu Zhiwang 1626, juan 67, 9b.
51. Wu Zhiwang 1626, juan 67, 11a–12a. Others traced this technique back to Li Gao. See Wang Qi ed., 185.
52. See Zhang Songgeng 1957; Li Shizhen, juan 52, 4:2965.

medieval alchemists (*fang shi*).[53] Red lead—ideally from a girl's first menses—was possibly black magic, said to be a formula of "foreign" origin, suspected of the murder of an emperor and transmitted by only a few doctors.[54]

In sum, *To Benefit Yang* showed that in spite of medicine's suspicion of bed-chamber arts and its skepticism concerning Chu Cheng's theories, sexual scripts for males did not easily break with the model of a contest between yin and yang in intercourse. In spite of his rhetoric against drug abuse, Wu continued to teach that both fertility and longevity were manipulable by pharmaceutical means, stimulating the consumption he also deplored. In red lead and autumn stone, pharmacy even found a substitute for sexual Essence as elixir: dangerous yet generative body substances exchangeable between persons as medicinal extracts. In all these ways, *To Benefit Yang* concerned itself with male vulnerabilities: it imagined an underlying body economy of homologous yin and yang vitalities but offered medical strategies for male advantage in the performance on which the propagation of male descendants depended. On the other hand, as a narrative on the sexual functions of women, *To Benefit Yin* incorporated Yuan Huang's version of a natural hierarchy of gendered generative powers, facilitating paternalistic consideration for female weakness while implying male responsibility for controlling the outcome.

Generation and Gestation in the Body of Immortality

Gestation had complex resonances in the late Ming discourse of "nourishing life." As a creative process it completed the work of Heavenly *qi*, endowing even its material byproducts with life-giving medicinal value. Texts on nourishing life included advice on pregnancy and postpartum in recognition of the interdependence of the bodies of men, women and infants in the project of propagating descendants. But the power of pollution, with all its taboos and avoidances, also clung to

53. Wu Zhiwang 1626, juan 68, 9a–12b. See also Wan Quan 1645: 42; and Needham 1982: 313–37. Needham argues for the empirical efficacy of urinary sublimates based on their ability to concentrate urinary steroids.

54. Wu Zhiwang 1626, juan 68, 9a. See also Miyasita 1982. For further late Ming views, see Li Shizhen, juan 52, 4:2946–47, 2952–54, 2963–66.

the blood of human fertility—attaching in different degrees to milk, menses, umbilicus or placental afterbirth. It was the alchemist, as distinct from the ordinary pharmacist, who taught how to manipulate it as symbol and surround it with ritual so as to tap its efficacy. For the practitioners of inner alchemy, such products of gestation were known to be potent because their own self-cultivation was a pregnancy of sorts. They had long appropriated the gestational female cauldron (*ding*) as a way of imagining the body at work fashioning its victory over decay and its immortal transformation.

In religious myth this gestational body was figured most richly in Daoist legends of the birth of Laozi. Any Ming reader could have found a version of the story in Laozi's biography in Sima Qian's famous work of ancient history, the *Shiji*. But Kristofer Schipper says the myth was not narrated fully in the textual tradition, being "both scandalous tale and initiation lesson" for liturgical Daoists. As Schipper conveys modern versions of the myth taught in Taiwanese Daoist cloisters, the sage's cosmogonic body has the protean powers of the hermaphrodite—combining male and female to give birth to a being identical to itself. The immortal embryo nourished within grows and rises in the body over the years, until, as the myth of Laozi's "old child" told it, the sage as mother gives birth to the male child that is his own renewed self. In this way the body of immortality is achieved, all energies nourished and recycled, bypassing the continuum of human birth and death. If the sage is gestating mother here, he is also child in utero, in "fetal breathing" depending upon the *qi* of Heaven and Earth as on a mother; when born with white hair and a beard as Laozi was, he is also simultaneously infant and mature, already the fully Realized One.[55]

The Ming medical discourse of nourishing life usually focused more modestly on human health and longevity, distinguishable from the utopian quest of immortality seekers and would-be transcendents. But it led to a body imagined in the language of poetry, its performances conjured up by means of a luxuriant repertory of images, allegory and metaphysical innuendo. Far from reflecting the metaphors of everyday life, alchemy transformed language in transforming the self, enabling polyvalent interpretations that were obviously savored as such. "When Kidney Water ascends and Heart Fire descends, *kan* [hexagram for yang] and *li* [hexagram for yin] mate spontaneously and my body's boys and

55. Schipper 1993: 113–29 ("Lao Tzu: The Body of the Tao"). This miraculous birth was said to be through the mother's side or armpit, recalling myths of the birth of Buddha.

girls unite and its boys and girls within are formed," said Wu Zhiwang, refusing to choose between cosmographic and bodily geography, or between the mundane and immortal modes of generation.[56] Readers of this, like Ming templegoers encountering the commonplace icons of pregnant holy men — lohans — displaying babies in their bellies, might be inspired to consider alchemical transformations as exceptions to the norm but were unlikely to imagine them as violations of nature itself.[57] Popularized as a moralization of health in the syncretic atmosphere of late Ming cultural life, inner alchemy appropriated the female gestational body to manifest the more mysterious dimensions of the universe's creativity. In Yuan Huang's syncretic adaptation, the cultivation of an immortal embryo was understood as related to Confucian teachings on "rectifying the mind" as well as Daoist teachings on the "obscure and formless outside of Time" (*xiantian huanghuang huhu*) and the Buddhist ideal of nirvana.[58]

Utopian Bodies and the Feminine

The texts on *fuke* and nourishing life looked at here do not tell us whether women could also seek to cultivate their bodies of Essence, *qi* and Psyche to nourish their generative vitality within and seek long life or immortality. In *To Benefit Yin* as in the literature on nourishing life itself, passages on internal alchemy took the androgynous body of generation as the norm, and they instructed men and women as yin yang couples to nourish Essence and Blood so as to approach a complementary homology of matched generative powers. But their conventional wisdom that men conserve Essence and women regulate menses did not easily show how menstrual regulation might mimic seminal conservation and recirculation, nor was the erotic woman supposed to be empowered on a par with males. Nonetheless, the late Ming annals

56. Wu Zhiwang 1626, juan 67, 16b–17a.

57. Ming narratives of pregnant males were often bawdy but rarely skeptical. A pregnant monk, with belly flesh peeled back to reveal the infant, was a standard icon among statues of the "five hundred lohans" in Buddhist temples, many still visited today. See photographs in Needham 1983. See also Furth 1988.

58. Yuan Huang, *She sheng san yao,* 2a. Also see Liu Ts'un-yan 1970 for an argument that Ming neo-Confucianism, particularly the thought of Wang Yangming, is permeated with Daoist approaches to self-cultivation. Liu quotes Wang Yangming on the relationship of Essence, *qi* and Psyche, and notes that Yuan Huang was quite influenced by Wang Yangming's thought.

of female religious devotion and practice are rich, and include some famous mystics who were daughters of elite families. The family of Ye Shaoyuan, Yuan Huang's adopted son, as recorded by Dorothy Ko, included women who practiced Chan Buddhist meditation and who sought inspiration from a famous female spirit-writing medium of Su-zhou. Ye Xiaoluan, a pious and sickly daughter who died young, was revered as a family "immortal."[59] Did any women like these ever construct their devotional discipline around the bodily practices of internal alchemy?

We probably will never know exactly. However, some seventeenth-century adepts and healers apparently did teach women a specifically female version of inner alchemy, "female golden cinnabar" (*nü jin dan*). This teaching established gender boundaries and negotiated female difference just as "separate prescriptions" did. At its core was an esoteric self-cultivation technique whereby menses as materialized primary vitality were to be suppressed, "beheading the red dragon" (*zhan chi long*). One account of this is attributed to Fu Shan (1607–1684), a mid-seventeenth-century doctor and poet from Shanxi famous for his *fuke*. Drawing the parallel between seminal Essence and menstrual Blood, Fu Shan's instructions called attention to the original pure *qi* hidden within these dross sediments, making their dispersal also a loss of Heavenly *qi* from the body. Choosing the midnight hour of the day before her period was due, a woman should loosen her clothing and sit cross-legged with the heel of her left foot pressed against her vagina. Concentrating her spirit, she should regulate her thoughts and breath while massaging her breasts to circulate and nourish her yin Essence, causing her menstrual Blood gradually to transform from red to yellow to white. Over the months her periods should decrease and diminish altogether, "beheading the red dragon" to enhance her primordial *qi*.[60] Other similar versions of inner alchemy for women were based on traditions in "ten precepts" attributed to Sun Buer (1119–1182), the Jin-Yuan dynasty nun famous as the only woman among the founders of the northern Quan-zhen school of religious Daoism.

Beheading the red dragon, however, emerges ambivalently as both purification and conservation. Though a girl's first menses were most

59. See Ko 1994: 195–202.
60. "Duan hong long." This text attributed to Fu Shan is based on an undated manuscript transmitted to Taiwan and published as an appendix to a Daoist anthology compiled by Xiao Tianshi in 1965. See 124–28.

precious, and the cessation of menstruation in middle age was a sign of the exhaustion of vitality, ordinary menstruating women were not clean. For her body to return to a primal state, an older woman had first to restore her menstrual cycle and then to travel further back to prepubescent wholeness. The purest generative fluid in the female body was the yin Blood flowing within her breasts as milk, not the contents of her womb, while her realized body was sometimes portrayed as that of a child and sometimes as that of a man. Whereas semen were nourished, menses were "beheaded," implying rejection. The ideal female practitioner was represented as chaste, not as a mother; she became immortal by reverting to infant integrity rather than by herself gestating an immortal embryo.[61]

In sum, such techniques did not belong in marital bedrooms, nor were they offered as an empowering construction of menopause. The linkage between inner alchemy, reproduction and the erotic was supported in late Ming medical discussion of the generative body, but inner alchemical modes of mystical gestation and birth were about the transformations of transcendence, not about the passages of parturition. In the art of nourishing life, fertility, not longevity, was the bodily aspiration assigned to women, and in the language of *fuke* cessation of menses was simply a sign of sickness or of old age. Internal alchemy for women was not adapted into medical discourse as an ideal of bodily health but remained an esoteric and explicitly religious practice.

In sum, late Ming medicine on nourishing life encouraged men to think about their sexual functions as powers of a body of generation. Sexual functions were more than erotic pleasures; they extended to inner sensations that had meaning as somatic markers of primal energy flows—pathological excitation of Fire, or regenerative amplification of harmonious and nourishing Essence and *qi*. Sexual energy could flow out of the body, or reversing course flow within, linking up with other primary vitalities to produce new or renewed life. The cultural construction of a fusion of sex and reproduction fits modern stereotypes of es-

---

61. See Sun Buer, "Xi Wang Mu nüxiu zhengtu shi ze" (Queen Mother of the West's Ten Precepts on the Correct Path of Women's Practice), translated in Wile 1992: 192–201. This work is believed to have been transmitted by the late-eighteenth-century scholar Shen Yibin (fl. 1795). See also Needham 1983: 237–40. Despeux 1990 discusses the earliest strands of the traditions around Sun Buer. Like most Daoist works, these texts can't be dated precisely, but Wile says that the earliest surviving *nü jin dan* texts are from the seventeenth century and that many practices were developed in Buddhist convents. See 193.

sentialist biological thinking about the female body. But the Ming body of generation here was neither: neither reductionistically material nor transcendently spiritual, it was nonetheless utopian in its claims that procreative human coupling mimics cosmogenesis and allows human beings to participate in the work of creation, extending and prolonging the chain of universal life. The creative powers of such a body might even overcome the withering of age, reversing time's arrow to exceed the natural limits of mortality. The alchemical gestating body bridges the human life cycle, placing the cultivator in touch with the past child he once was and the future new self he may yet become. Structured around the immortal embryo, the generative body aspired to an active androgyny, becoming both male and female, combining generation with gestation to figure the highest form of creative renewal.

In inner alchemy, the female body's gestational functions were adopted by male self-cultivators claiming an androgynous body for the sage. One obvious way to look at the meaning of this is as metaphor, a way in which "the body is good to think with," as the anthropologist Margaret Lock puts it.[62] Students of Daoism have often commented upon the importance of images of the feminine used to figure the Daoist Way, with its rejection of hierarchy, embrace of obscurity, and withdrawal from society—all the things that mark this religious path as yin. We have thought less about possible social meanings the gestating alchemical body may have had for men in their roles as Confucian patriarchs. However, as men of authority it was important for patriarchs to aspire to the Confucian virtue of "benevolence." What better way to portray power tempered by kindness and altruism than for a man to strive to embody the nurturing functions of the mother? Though extremely uncommon as a symbol of Confucian virtue, lactating men were occasionally offered as representations of family devotion. This was the moral of an unusual story of a man whose breasts miraculously gave milk after he was left with a suddenly orphaned newborn, child of his dead brother and sister-in-law. The tale illustrated the virtue of filial and brotherly feeling for the highly orthodox "Sacred Edict" of the Kangxi emperor in the late seventeenth century. (See figure 13.)

But if the utopian body of inner alchemy eluded most people, it posed special problems for women. Just as Daoist metaphors of creation and the feminine say little about the actual social or religious powers available to women believers, the place of women in the inner alchemical

62. Scheper-Hughes and Lock, 1989.

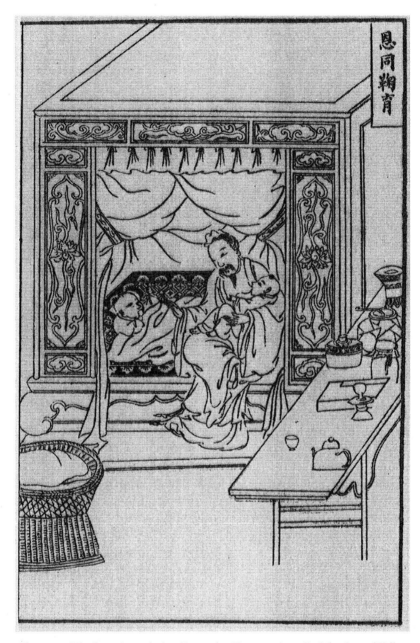

Figure 13. The lactating scholar. From the *Shengyu xiang jie* (The Sacred Edict, Illustrated and Explained).

enterprise remained ambiguous. Fertility, not longevity, was the bodily achievement expected of them by society, as texts on nourishing life made clear, while *fuke* continued to represent gestation as a bodily function involving depletion for mothers — loss rather than gain in the bodily exchange economy of measurable, materialized body vitalities. Nor did medicalization of pollution beliefs completely erase the negative constructions of menstruation and parturition as unclean. At the very least, for women to engage in alchemical cultivation would involve a breach of their mundane reproductive functions rather than an extension of them. To achieve immortality through the body was not just to tap an inner reservoir of creative potential but also to overcome something in the self that was both unclean and weak. Therefore, for women such self-cultivation may even have signified a socially transgressive rejection of both sex and procreation and an ascetic denial of the body rather than a project of self-transcendence through it.

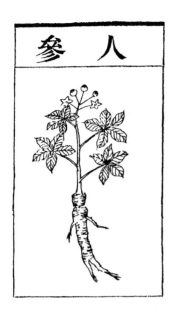

CHAPTER 7

A Doctor's Practice

*Narratives of the Clinical
Encounter in Late Ming
Yangzhou*

In the preceding chapters, medical classics and other prescriptive texts provided me with readings of modes of embodiment fostered by Chinese medical traditions. I have argued that the medical body here is a cultural construct because public, social knowledge of it is dependent on language. I have tried to show how the Yellow Emperor's language of symbolic correlations had to be linked to a language of symptoms and disease classification, integrated by means of metaphor and ultimately dependent upon the voicing of a phenomenology of experience. Thus I have claimed that the cultural production of such a body has necessarily been a dialogical process in which both sick people and physicians participated, within the context of clinical practice.

Clinical practice involves both words and actions in a dense social field of relationships that texts only partially trace. I have pointed to some of these practices — the rituals surrounding a Song parturition, the bodily self-cultivation of a Ming longevity seeker, the art of prescription itself as the central ritual of the doctor-patient encounter. I have also said that in Song to Ming China both illness and healing took place primarily at home, and that the social relations of medicine, including issues of power and knowledge, authority and gender, must take this context into account.

However, so far I have talked about no one individual's sick body in particular. In this chapter I turn to medical case histories to bring the patient into the story, and with her the domestic setting with its family relationships that are at the center of the clinical encounter. Here class and gender hierarchies surround and incorporate the doctor into a system of power, and a multiplicity of different voices combine and sometimes contend to define the meaning of the illness experience. But I am not turning away from discourse as culture in order to reveal to my readers a more concrete and truthful domain of social practice at the bedside. My major source, a seventeenth-century doctor's written record of some of his medical cases, is a text like the others. It constructs a representation, a textual "subject"; it is selective and interpretive, and as such is a part of the larger Ming medical discourse. It adds a new dimension because case histories construct experience as stories. Stories have a dramatic structure that shapes our understanding of the temporality of events, just as descriptive language gives meaning to inner bodily experience. Stories are cultural constructions not because of their resemblance to fiction but because storytelling — narrative fragments of biography — is a fundamental way for human beings to make the fact that we live in the dimension of time intelligible. Case histories add this essential diachronic dimension of illness, and reveal how the cultural meanings of medical embodiment cannot be disentangled from the system of signs we call social relations.

Although case histories were scattered through Chinese medical writings of all earlier periods, the individually authored and published case history collection was a Ming innovation. In part, the impulse behind such writing was a social effect of the late Ming publishing explosion, in light of the cultural ideal of the literati doctor (ru yi). Medical authorship confirmed that a physician was a man of learning, and in the absence of other markers of professional accomplishment or guild status it validated the reputations of his successors and disciples as well. Often the latter were involved in the compilation of case history collections, while lineage members, grateful clients and scholarly patrons contributed funds for publication.

But when literate healers chose the case history as a genre over others available—books of prescriptions or advice manuals, for example—they were saying something about textuality and the sources of medical authority itself. Case histories turned attention away from inherited canon and ancient masters, locating medical authority in the individual. The case called attention to the theoretical premise that illness is deeply mutable, both historically and environmentally, so that no two illness events are exactly alike, and healing becomes the practitioner's skillful response to a sufferer's many changes in condition. Using narrative techniques of plot—human predicament, suspense and their resolution—the case history could capture this fleeting process and reveal the logic behind the reasoning that produced a diagnosis, and the combination of drugs that effected a cure. In a typical case history narrative, the climax to the story was the doctor's itemization of one or more artfully crafted prescriptions, usually tied to an empirically successful outcome. Ming doctors used the case history format didactically, to advocate their own preferred pharmaceutical strategies and to give instruction on fine points of diagnosis and the clinical encounter. Some, like the doctor I will be talking about here, used it also as a vehicle for literary expression, displaying a persona as a man of letters as well as a physician. The late Ming was the golden age of case history writing in China, reflecting a medical culture that had become extremely decentralized, its sources of authority diffuse, its classical roots subject to question, requiring the successful physician to stand as an individual on his medical opinion and to look for social support from whatever literati or lineage identity his circumstances permitted.[1]

Cheng Congzhou (Cheng Maoxian, 1581–?) was such a doctor, a man who lived and practiced in Yangzhou in the 1610s and 1620s. According to his friends, Cheng was "a literati physician practicing in obscurity." Obscurity enshrouded his sole literary legacy, a small collection of ninety-three cases, together with some prefaces, which was apparently published in 1644—the year the Manchu invaders savagely sacked his

---

1. Farquhar 1994 and Hanson 1997 discuss the medical case history as a marker of the epistemological emphasis upon changing conditions of practice. Hanson explores the historical tensions between text and practice in the Ming-Qing discourse on epidemic fevers. For the Ming decline of a state role in medicine see Leung 1987.

home town of Yangzhou and brought the Ming dynasty to an end. Only one known copy of this text has survived. But obscurity is serendipity for the historian of the everyday. In a way that integrates literary and clinical storytelling, Cheng Maoxian's casebook is a vivid narrative of a doctor's practice and a demonstration of the richness of the case history genre.[2]

The case histories here open up my discussion of medical bodies in various ways. First, stories make it possible to see more closely how the abstract language of medical theory — the yin/yang, Blood/*qi*, depletion/repletion dyads of pattern analysis — was used in the context of an actual disorder. They also reveal indirectly the dialogues that explored the symptoms of illness, and they use metaphors that link bodily experience and the social world. It becomes easier to locate the various levels of medical discourse at work when medical language constructs body processes as abstract formal relationships; when it is phenomenological, naming experienced feelings; and when it operates as metaphor. While these levels are hardly independent of one another, they become analytically separable as traces of the account of a single illness. Second, the case history allows me to follow the clinical encounter from the doctor's point of view as a process whereby illness is named in a way that translates it into a known quantity — a disease — pointing to a technology of intervention and cure. Third, the case history is a story of the social relations of healing — involving not only a sufferer and a doctor, but family and community as well. It forms a matrix wherein relationships of gender, class and kinship are deployed. And finally, through these interactions as reported by the doctor, something of patient and family points of view are hinted at, suggesting popular understandings of the body and tensions between expert healers and their clients. Case histories, better than any other medical genre, show how medicine is in fact embedded in the social relations of daily life, and how the experience of illness is rendered intelligible by recourse to a cultural syntax requiring hermeneutical analysis.[3] Gender relations and gender ideology are an integral part of this story, but they are best seen in the context of Cheng's practice as a whole.

---

2. *Cheng Maoxian yi'an*, 2 juan. The author's preface is dated 1633, but Xue Qinglu 1991: 629, says the original was printed in 1644. The fashion for case histories was spread by Jiang Guan's anthology *Ming yi lei an* (1552), and more famous Ming masters of the genre included Wang Ji, Sun Yikui and Yu Chang.

3. My account of the case history and narrative theory is indebted to Good 1994: 135–65.

Cheng Maoxian: A Literati Physician

The following narrative tells the story of a woman's illness and recovery as recalled by Cheng Maoxian sometime in the early seventeenth century. Like her doctor, this lady lived in the prosperous commercial city of Yangzhou, center of the vital salt trade and entrepôt for the intersection of the Grand Canal and the lower Yangzi delta:

Fang Shunian's mother, the scholar's Honored Lady,[4] was sixty-three years old. Her constitution was naturally weak and emaciated. Her *qi* and Blood were both depleted. Normally all her six pulses were extremely "subtle" and "fine"; even when she caught cold they did not become very "big" or "pounding."

In the first fortnight of the sixth month of this year she happened to eat some melons and peaches. The night afterwards she suffered an attack of acute bowel uproar [*huoluan*] with repeated vomiting and diarrhea and pain in her belly.

So one dose of amplified Six Harmony infusion[5] was taken; the vomiting abated, but then she suffered from "stagnation downward" with many episodes of red and white discharge day and night. She felt nauseated and dry of mouth; her condition was grave; the pulses of both wrists were "flooding" and "large," particularly on the right arm.

From this I knew that it was a case [requiring] moving stagnation; medicines for dry vomiting syndromes were not suitable; even more, for one naturally depleted in both *qi* and Blood, there were further impediments. Moreover in cases of dysentery [*li*], "flooding" and "large" pulses were to be feared. For this reason I went ahead and used ingredients to "regulate the stomach" and "transform stagnation." After one or two days her mouth symptoms abated. Then I gave one dose of Transform Stagnation pill with costus [*muxiang*]. Her belly growled and she passed two dry turds, but the pain still did not abate.

Gradually she grew dispirited and ceased to eat or drink. On the eighth day she thought to sip some tea, but the tea leaves would not pass down her throat; lotus seed broth was too thick to go down. Everyone thought it was a case of "crooked mouth" [verge of death]. The attending

---

4. Honored Lady (*ru ren*) was a title awarded wives and mothers of civil officials. This and other forms of respectful address help identify the social position of patients and their families. In interpreting case histories I assume that persons named without an honorific, or identified by surname only, are of lower status relative to the doctor.

5. Six Harmony infusion (*Liu he tang*) was a well-known formula for summer dysenteries and "bowel uproar" disorders. It featured equal amounts of *banxia*, *baishu*, peach kernel (*taoren*) and ginseng with a pinch of cinnabar and other supporting ingredients. See *Jianming Zhongyi cidian*, 201.

maids all had swelling and suppuration on their hands, revealing the poisonous *qi* of the disease. The lady grasped her son's hand and said, "I am so weak and my illness has reached such a pass that I certainly will not live. You must prepare for my end, and avoid [my body] coming to grief in the summer weather." Shunian choked back his tears, and could not bear to reply.

I then used doses to "nourish the stomach" and "harmonize the center." After one or two days of regulation, the accumulated stagnation still was not entirely gone. Moreover, [I] estimated that it was time for "descending" action. So I used three qian of rhubarb [*dahuang*] in wine together with costus, betelnut [*binlang*], hawthorne [*shancha*], *ling-lian* [formula featuring golden-thread (*huanglian*) and skullcap (*huangqin*)] and such like. After one dose she evacuated a certain amount of accumulated filth and her pain lessened a little. In the course of a day and a night there were several tens [of evacuations].

Her chest still was not free, so next I used ginseng-*baishu* combination, *ling-lian* [formula], betelnut, costus, *gui-shao* [formula featuring angelica (*danggui*) and peony (*baishao*)], poria [*fuling*], hyacinth bean [*biandou*], licorice [*gancao*], et cetera, appropriately adjusted. The lady knew that I was using ginseng and feared that her chest would not ease but be stopped up from [excessive] supporting action. For this reason, over several days I added one-and-one-half qian of ginseng without letting her know. After these doses her chest was opened, and her stagnation downward abated.

One day the lady said to her son Shunian, "In the last few days my gullet has felt open; don't use ginseng any more." Shunian murmured assent but together with my unworthy self he secretly added ginseng without ill effects for several days.

At this time the eldest young gentleman, Wuqi, and the fourth young gentleman, Xiangheng, were both guests in Wu. They ordered a servant to proceed home [for news]. When the servant returned Wuqi interviewed him, asking who was in charge of the medicines. The servant said it was my unworthy self. Wuqi said, "Then there is nothing to worry about."

Indeed, the sufferer did recover, and after three months of convalescence was entirely well. Though the disorder was grave, she was restored to life. Half the merit was Shunian's, for the two reasons that he was a filial and friendly gentleman. First, he did not spare the ginseng; and second, he gave [me] complete charge. Had he looked for overnight success, or feared to use ginseng and astragalus root [*huangqi*], or, taking alarm, changed from Dr. Li to Dr. Chang, the lady his mother could scarcely have preserved her life [*yuan qi*].[6]

6. Cheng Congzhou, juan 1, 1a–2b. Li and Chang are common surnames, like Smith or Jones in English.

This was the case that Cheng Maoxian chose to place at the beginning of his collection. It shows medical practice as it ought to be, from the doctor's point of view. The physician is the trusted advisor of an elite family. Moreover, he is part of the pious moral enterprise of helping a filial son care for the health of his aged mother. The case is difficult, but there is no hint of expert disagreement or mercenary considerations, and the doctor is able to follow the sufferer through a course of successive pathological crises or "changes," adjusting his pharmacopoeia to each stage in the evolution of disorder until recovery is secured. The case shows both the art of prescription and the social relations of healing in an optimal light. The gender relationship valorized here is the conventional Confucian tie of filiality and affection between mother and son, but the story also hints of a woman's reservations about the paternalist control of her care.

The biographical information gleaned from Cheng's narrative of this and ninety-two other cases is slight. The Cheng family ancestral home was said to be in Xin'an, Anhui (Huizhou prefecture), and a branch of the lineage was resident in Chenzhou, just across the Yangzi from Yangzhou. But although Cheng spoke of himself as an outsider in Guangling (Yangzhou), he had lived there for twenty years, and most of the clients he wrote about belonged to local Yangzhou families. The picture sketched by the prefaces to his work suggest a gentleman amateur, a man whose father "entertained himself with lute and books" rather than practicing medicine.[7] As perhaps fit the son of a cultured dilettante, Cheng circulated the draft of his case history collection to his poetry club rather than to professional disciples. To club members, he was a bon vivant: as one put it, he saved the dying during the time not taken up with wine and versifying. They also were impressed by his somewhat abrupt, aloof manner, sustaining a reputation for profundity. This image was crafted by the admiring friends and kinsmen who wrote prefaces to his book, and was echoed in a more prestigious prefatory tribute from a visiting official who met him when passing through town in 1628.

However, this portrait of a cultivated eccentric did not tell the whole story. She county, Cheng's ancestral home, was at the heart of Huizhou prefecture and its rich medical culture. He mentioned a maternal grandfather, one Wu Muxi, said to be the author of his own medical casebook.[8] Cheng had "travelled in search of teachers" in Zhejiang and

7. Preface by Wu Kongjia.
8. Cheng Congzhou, juan 2, 14b. I have not been able to identify Wu Muxi or his work.

Jiangsu — a standard mode of medical apprenticeship. Finally, he had been known for healing in Yangzhou for twenty years, and his son aspired to carry on the paternal practice and become a doctor himself. Concerning this desire, the father had cautionary words:

> You, my son Deng, have urged me to gather [these cases] together, wishing to stock up a medicine bag [of your own]. My words to you are: these represent my aspiration to save lives and my insights at particular moments. You cannot see them as a made-to-order method. . . . If one wants to grasp the profound and attain comprehensive and penetrating [knowledge], one doesn't make a zither with glue and lacquer alone. One can't grasp a stallion galloping on the basis of its picture. Ascend slowly to the hall and enter the chamber in stages. If you do this, these cases may not be entirely useless to you. Consider these words. Don't boast that you have studied and mastered your father's books and then become a son of Ma Fu."[9]

Embroidering his parental admonitions in literary allusions, Cheng presented himself as both physician and gentleman, urbane yet serious about his vocation as healer. He was well read in medicine, even though he cited only a few medical masters and those infrequently.[10] He wrote in the cultured prose of a scholar, but his preface questioned his own written narrative from the perspective of one who located medical knowledge in practice. Not only his son but we as readers today are told to understand his writings as imperfect approximations of essentially transitory bodily events.

If Cheng expressed a philosophical Daoist's distrust of words, my modernist reading sees in the words of his stories how pain enters language and becomes cultural experience of the body. In the doctor's telling the sick person speaks his or her distress. The voices of family members and other intimates also intervene, explaining what has happened and recounting the events preceding the doctor's arrival, while the doctor's duty as expert is to recraft the narrative to reveal a deeper level of intelligibility, renaming it in a way that points toward a technology of intervention promising cure. Thus, the case history as a narrative begins

9. Author's preface. Ma Fu was a famous general of the Warring States era whose son was given a command and then disastrously lost an important battle.

10. He cited the *Inner Canon* and the *Canon of the Pulse* occasionally. He mentioned Zhang Zhongjing, author of the *Treatise on Cold Damage Disorders* (*Shanghan lun*); Tao Hua, the early Ming expert on Cold Damage; and Zhu Zhenheng. He quoted Kou Zongshi on female seclusion, critically evaluated the theories of several Jin-Yuan masters on Wind-stroke (*zhongfeng*), and commented on the Ming debate on conception and sexual differentiation discussed in the previous chapter.

by engaging in the paradoxical task of bringing words to bodily experience, words that may never grasp the unnameable essence of pain but which are the vehicle by which a phenomenology of its experience is made a shareable public property.[11] As Dr. Cheng crafted his tales, we can hear his patients' voices along with his own in a common language of symptoms and events. In the comments of sufferers and family members, now questioning or objecting, now reporting the story of their descent into illness, we can pick up something of their everyday interpretations of the body, and of the repertory of practices they turned to for help. In sum, while the case history works rhetorically as the doctor's tale, making him protagonist and hero, it is a record of a dialogic interaction involving multiple voices.

Patient Voices: Illness as Experience

As stories, cases begin with falling ill, an experience that occurred before the doctor arrived on the scene and which must be told and retrospectively reinterpreted. Many of the illnesses described by Dr. Cheng, like other medical writers, were febrile sicknesses—that array of acute attacks grouped as Cold Damage disorders, or named for a specific variety of seasonal *qi*.[12] Lady Fang's bowel uproar (*huoluan*) was one variant of such a disorder (biomedicine identifies it with cholera). In thinking about why one falls sick, these illness narratives grappled with its mystery by appealing to the sufferer's innate constitution, or to influences of external environment or vagaries of personal circumstances. To begin with, everyone has a natural constitution, like "the weakness and emaciation" of Fang Shunian's mother. Cheng was trained to recognize his clients' natural conditions of sturdy "repletion" or frail "depletion," or their tendency toward bodily heat or cold. A Hot and Dry nature predisposed a woman to menstrual irregularity. One "fat and white" was probably depleted in *qi* and susceptible to phlegm. A generalized sickliness might be a weakness of primordial *qi*.

Beyond the body that fate dealt a person lay the happenstance of outside influences identified with weather and unseasonable thermo-

11. Scarry 1985 argues that pain, because it eludes language, being unnameable, in effect "unmakes the world" of the sufferer.

12. Names in medical literature varied: Spring Warm (*chun wen*), Summer Heat (*shu re*) and Autumn Dry (*qiu zao*) were among the common terms.

dynamic conditions, the classic agents of disease doctors associated with seasonal *qi*. A sixth month "summer epidemic" gave Chang Weikang headache and fever; though his body ached he didn't sweat and his mouth was dry—a sign of pathogenic Cold influences producing heat. Fan Ziyan's sixth month summer fever produced a body "sunken and heavy, dry mouth and hot dry tongue, blocked bowels for six days." In her extreme heat the wife of Wang Mingde was delirious (*kuang*), with hot dry mouth, thirst, incoherent speech, stifled Heart and red face. Doctors and patients alike understood these febrile attacks to be linked to season in a complex way: commonest in hot weather, they still could be triggered by Cold influences latent in the body and environment. An ever-present potential agent of Cold was Wind—palpable as draft, night air, or unseasonable breezes, against which one was advised to close off curtains, rooms, doors and windows. Or food might be responsible: an accumulation from a diet overly rich in meat could lead to stopped bowels, torpor and Hot and Cold spells, as happened to the salt merchant Liu Yaozhou one windy autumn; or one might be damaged by foods Cold in nature consumed in hot weather, as happened to Shunian's mother.

Sometimes a significant moment when emotion destabilized psyche marked the turning point leading to malady. One day in the second month, as Madame Cheng was eating a bowl of rice, something happened to displease her; the rice stagnated within and her stomach ached. Angry with her maidservant but unable to punish her, Wu Junyun's wife went to bed filled with congestion and distress. Frightened one night when she overheard something her parents-in-law said about her behavior, Wu Jingko's wife, young Lady Wu, suffered a Wind-Cold attack (*fenghan*) the next morning. A fifty-year-old widow who worked with her son as an itinerant petty trader, due to a violent fit of anger suffered a sudden deathlike reverse movement of *qi*, rendering her insensible and incontinent for three days and nights. As for the man who drank wine and ate cold crabs in a season of ascending Cold (late autumn) and then engaged in sex, he was courting disaster. It came in the form of a fright in the night as he was awakened by the city fire patrol and saw that he had fallen asleep without his shirt. The next day he was prostrated with stomach pains complicated by yin Cold (*yin han*).

For males, falling ill might involve stories of travel and its stresses or temptations. One merchant went all day and evening at market without eating, working on his accounts; another, after eating hot beef, crossed the river to go down to the salt fields and suffered a Wind-Cold attack.

Another man returned home and fell ill, having visited a brothel in the city. Returning to his home in Hangzhou from the spring exams at the capital, a young scholar suffered respiratory distress and halted his journey at Yangzhou. Even a woman occasionally came to grief from going abroad, like the pregnant wife who was returning home in a sedan chair from visiting her natal relatives when overcome with vomiting from a Wind-Cold attack. Any sign of sexual function out of control might be the significant destabilizing factor: a youth secretly fretted about his wet dreams; a middle-aged man had a "little concubine" and suffered from "bed-chamber fatigue"; a husband worried that his wife's collapse was provoked by their intimacies the night before; a young man was embarrassed to confess that he visited a brothel.

In all of the above ways, one's natural constitution, the environmental vagaries of seasons and weather, or the exigencies of one's own conduct might retrospectively give meaning and pattern to falling ill. But sometimes the doctor was summoned because there had been a unexpected, inexplicable and sudden collapse: a baby refused to nurse and its belly swelled around the navel in a case of dangerous navel Wind (*qi feng*). A widow lady was unable to pass urine for three days, until her lower belly was distended and aching. Another time, one morning in the ninth month as she went to relieve herself at the latrine, a good wife of forty suddenly fell prostrate, and when she was propped up on the bed, "She turned her face to the wall, legs curled up under her. Her speech was slurred, she was unbearably faint, her body [felt] light as a feather." Such misfortune frightened because it struck without warning. All the narratives of falling ill tell of attempts to counterbalance thoughts of chance and fatality with recollections of personal lapses and misadventures. Such thoughts might blame the sufferer for her illness, but they also restored the possibility of control, shaping a medical culture of health care and illness prevention structured around morality and personal discipline.

Once ill, the sufferer struggled for words to name his or her distress in the phenomenological language of symptoms. There were many ways to experience illness's heat. "Fearing Cold, she feels hot and dry"—a set of sensations manifest on the skin. Constipation is hot, drying out the bowels' water. Internal heat is more insidious, as in the matron whose "static congestion" (*yujie*) and internal heat made her crave cold water, which she drank excessively. Each time her chest and gullet would clear somewhat; without cold water fiery Heat blazed within, hottest at night and cooler during the day. Heat could come in tidelike waves, now hot, now cold; it could concentrate on sensitive spots like the palms of the hand and the soles of the feet. If not all heat was the elevated temperature of fever, a fever at its worst, as in the sweating body of a child with a fever-rash (*zhen*), could be a sign of unexpelled Hot poisons within the belly.

Cold symptoms were less frequently mentioned, and they were also slower, more likely to be chronic. The wife of Wu Tounan was always cold, her hands and feet especially, and her vaginal discharge (*daixia*) was heavy, so even in early autumn she covered herself with blankets and required a brazier. There was also a widow whose feet and legs gradually grew cold and numb, spreading up past the knees, growing painful bit by bit until she could scarcely move about. Cold crept inward from the extremities toward vital body centers, a trajectory that resembled the creeping cold in the dying.

Others experienced distress as phlegm (*tan*), thought to be a specialty of the damp south. Scholar Lu Rongxi's honored aunt took to her bed with a cough that could only be eased by bringing up phlegm. But phlegm concentrated in the chest area could affect the Heart and cloud psyche, producing fainting or even bouts of madness, as in the attack of apoplexy that felled Jiang Zhongren after a quarrel over a chess game, which was cured when he was made to vomit several bowls. While phlegm usually was imagined as a viscosity clogging the body's central systems of function, it could appear below, in the form of vaginal discharge in women.

The symptom of distress most closely connected with negative emotion was stasis (*yu*), constricting the chest with a dry, full, suffocating sensation, thick like a bramble patch in a meadow. Stasis afflicted a retiring scholar who never showed his anger, and a man embroiled in a lawsuit suffered static congestion from anger. In women, stasis troubled the overburdened housewife whose breast burned with inner static heat and the new mother whose baby died. Dr. Cheng reported on the stasis that came with his own hangovers and the stasis accompanying the melancholy of alcoholism in one of his [poetry] "society friends."

One suffered illness at home. If illness narratives show people's faith in the power of the classical pharmacopoeia, as well as some knowledge of its resources, they also show people accustomed to choosing medicines for themselves. Family seniors dosed the junior members dependent on their care, sometimes including servants. Adult males turned to friends and associates at work as well as to kin. Young wives were in the charge of their husbands or his female relations; mothers and grandmothers saw to their children, sometimes including adult sons and married daughters. Occasionally fathers took charge as well, particularly when their young sons suffered the dangerous childhood disease of smallpox. Therapy, then, began with self and family care, and Cheng's narratives included reports on what he found out about this. So strategies followed by Dr. Cheng's patients before he appeared on the scene are clues to people's understanding of medicine and their own body processes, and to the structure of household relationships that surrounded illness.

If fevers from Cold Damage and related environmental pathogens were especially commonplace afflictions, sufferers generally first hoped that medicines that induced sweating and gently stimulated the bowels would bring relief, according to tried and true strategies associated with the classic *Treatise on Cold Damage Disorders*. They worried about intake and outflow: about food and drink, and about blocked bowels or their opposite. If struck by Wind, it was inadvisable to try to eat very much; in protracted cases sufferers were not opposed to driving out pathogens with the descending action (*xia*) of purgatives. A little diarrhea, like that in Yang Jingchuan's nine-year-old boy, might be harmless, but prolonged purulent stagnation downward (*zhixia*) was serious. When Hong Weizhi suffered a stomachache with loose bowels, fear of a full-blown dysentery provoked him to overdose himself on purgatives. When the wife of Wang Mingde caught cold (*ganmao*) they tried medicines to clear heat (*qing re*) and to transform stagnation, and when these failed they turned to costus and betelnut to move *qi* with descending action. When Fang Jisuo's daughter suffered feverishness and headache they tried a similar strategy: doses to sweat—release to the exterior (*fa biao*)—followed by formulas to move and ease bowels. Those in charge of Dr. Cheng's infant grandson tried the mildly cooling and purging tonic golden-thread (*huanglian*) for the child's case of diarrhea with fever. Though some feared strong purgatives like rhubarb (*dahuang*), others tried these freely when they came down with dysentery. One man got purgatives from "a friend", and another took "move diarrhea" (*tong li*) formulas until, the doctor later said, his stomach *qi* was badly damaged. In all these ways sufferers reacted to fevers and dysenteries as invasions, and with more or less vehemence sought to drive the pathogens out of the body along with sweat or stool or urine. Other disorders conjured up similar of views of the body's enemies. Wang Mingde's servant woman used doses to "drive out Wind" for her rash. Like other servants, she may have gotten her medicines from her employer. Two families thought their family member's feverish chest swellings were suppurations (*nong*) and wanted the doctor to drain them by prescribing to cough up phlegm. In all these cases, sufferers marshalled to attack the invader.

People were readiest to dose themselves with warming and replenishing medicines to boost Blood and *qi* when they thought primary vitalities were threatened. One such circumstance was convalescence; another was when someone's generative capabilities appeared weakened. Wang Miaochu's teenage daughter was approaching marriage age, so when she suffered from a sore throat, she was first doctored with an infusion of balloon flower root (for coughs) and then with Four Ingredients infusion to nourish her yin. Another feverish parturient mother, thought to be naturally depleted in constitution, was treated by the "household head" with ginseng infusion to boost *qi*. Fearing a failure to beget heirs, a middle-aged man dosed himself with replenishing ingredients for potency. In convalescence, food might serve as replenishing medicine, as the bowl of soup offered a young man with a bellyache by his servant, or the hot meat broth a girl gulped down when she was recovering from an epidemic fever (*yi*). Home remedies could extend to complex prescription formulas, but many were standard ones (*cheng fang*). Plain medicines (*su fang*) of a single ingredient were also common. When Cheng, like other doctors, warned about both types, he underscored their popularity for self-care.

Cheng's clients, then, were ready with home remedies based on an understanding of the commoner forms of drug action in terms of palpable body processes. Formulas to "release to exterior" (*fa biao*) produced sweating, those that "transformed stagnation" (*hua zhi*) eased bowel movement, those that "attacked downward" (*gong xia*) purged; "clear heat" (*qing re*) ingredients cooled. Blood-moving and Blood-nourishing ingredients eased the congestive repletions that produced the pains of headaches or rheumatism or dysmenorrhea, while "replenishing" tonics speeded convalescence, improved one's ability to resist illness, and aided generative vitality—shown as menstrual regularity in women and sexual potency in men. The medical ideal of harmonious and free-flowing circulation of *qi* may have been a matter of a generalized wellness, but the ill often sought improvement in sensible alteration of body state.

A pedagogical goal of Cheng's collection was to advocate his own preferred therapeutic strategy of "warming and replenishing" prescriptions, particularly in cases of febrile disorders. His first case history, of

Fang Shunian's mother, illustrated this technical lesson as well. Here he was following a trend among mid- and late Ming doctors critical of Zhu Zhengheng's signature approach: "nourish yin and make Fire descend." Like these critics Cheng argued that cooling and bitter ingredients damaged digestion, and instead he promised success with the most famous of systemic yang boosters, ginseng, often in combination with astragalus root (*huangqi*).[13] However, his cases show him arguing against patients (and other doctors) whose understanding of body process made them apprehensive about such an approach. Lady Fang's reservations were shared by others. As a powerful stimulant of *qi*, ginseng acts to warm and replenish, not drain, fostering sensations of fullness and repletion. It would not clear heat. Doctors and patients alike believed that it should not be prescribed for a Cold Damage fever needing release of pathogens, or where there is phlegm or other painful congestive accumulation requiring evacuation. When Xia Wentai's wife felt increased swelling and fullness in her chest and gullet, her husband blamed the ginseng the doctor had given. Believing his young wife's collapse was due to Wind-Cold attack, another husband and family wanted to reject a ginseng prescription, pointing to her distended stomach and constipated bowels. Yang Jingchuan didn't want to give ginseng and astragalus root to his sick young son suffering from lung heat with phlegm. Another father of a child with fever-rash (*zhen*) felt the same way, as did the families worried about their sick members' chesty suppurations (*nong*).

Cheng's stories of ginseng showed that clients could be cautious of the dangers of strong medicines in a body out of balance, even as their doctor often represented them as eager, credulous consumers of powerful materia medica, ignorant of the dangers their preferred remedies posed. But the conflicts over ginseng often also exposed a gulf between one expert's readings of yin and yang, Blood and *qi*, in terms of circulating primary vitalities, and sufferers experiencing these in terms of a phenomenology of bodily fullness or emptiness, or sensations of heat and cold. Constructions of disease as internal depletion and functional inadequacy were sometimes at war with notions of it as external invasion and alien presence.

---

13. Grant 1996: chapter 3, shows that this therapeutic strategy and an accompanying critique of Zhu Zhengheng was articulated by Wang Ji (1463–1539) in his *Medical Cases from Stone Mountain (Shishan yi'an)*. Wang's argument that yang boosters can also replenish yin supported the view that Blood necessarily follows *qi*, reemphasizing that visible pathogenic blood is not always a sign of Blood disorder.

The Clinical Encounter

The doctor's intervention marked a new stage in the history of an illness. A successful clinical encounter involved both a doctor's technical evaluation, leading to therapy, and a social negotiation of his authority as an expert. Illness, as experienced and described by the sufferer in the language of symptoms, had to be renamed—converted through pattern analysis into "disease," a medical diagnosis that unlocked the key to a therapeutic strategy.[14] Cheng's case histories were designed to illustrate significant displays of technical skill. They also revealed social challenges to his authority from clients, client families and other doctors. Narratives showed sufferers who were in acute distress, where home remedies had been ineffective, and sometimes where other doctors previously on the scene had failed to cure. If people's helplessness in the face of crisis bolstered a healer's standing, the danger of failure was also greater.

A good example is Cheng's technical and social management of the case of Fang Tingxian, the fifty-two-year-old household head mentioned earlier as much occupied with a "little concubine." Fang came down with a fever and stomachache one midsummer:

He had already tried several elderly doctors, who all treated him for Summer Heat [*shu re*], either releasing and dispersing or clearing [heat] with things like aromatic madder and Heavenly Water.[15] He took in every kind of miscellaneous ingredient. . . . After the twelfth day . . . the sick man was too stupefied and dazed to know anything. Everybody [else] was ignorant of the nature of materia medica, but seeing the doctors as men of repute, they just agreed to their directions. Who was there to discuss matters of Hot and Cold with? So they gave him more nitre and rhubarb and waited in vain for his bowels to move. The next morning they called me in haste.

When I arrived I saw him stretched out sleeping in a chair, eyeballs white, sweat pouring like rain, his whole body cold like metal or stone.

14. Here I am applying the medical anthropologist's distinction between "illness" as a subjective experiential perspective and "disease" as an expert's explanatory model of a disorder. See Good 1994: 53.

15. For aromatic madder (*xiangru*), see *Zhong yao da cidian* 2:1680. Li Shizhen called it an important herb to release to the exterior in summer fevers or bowel uproar, dispersing fluid and harmonizing Spleen. He warned against use in people with depleted *qi*. Heavenly Water (*tian shui*) may refer to Heavenly Water infusion, a mixture of talc and licorice used to clear summer Damp Heat. Some variants added cinnabar, increasing its "cooling" effect. See *Jianming Zhongyi cidian*, 110, 738.

His six pulses were gone. A servant stood by with a cloth continually wiping the sweat. But the sick man's panting breath, now stopping now starting, showed there was only a thread of life there. The main event was already over; I forcefully declined the case as hopeless. When the household heard these words they stood around me in a circle weeping. Holding out a babe in arms [its mother] said, "The Fong surname has only this one heir; if he expires who will raise [this babe]? I can see, Sir, you have a compassionate heart. Use extraordinary skill! Try for a long shot! You may earn the merit of saving a life or at least avoid future regret." Having spoken, she resumed weeping.

I could not just callously walk out the door. So I used a Live Pulse infusion[16] and forced it down his throat. The medicine took hold somewhat, the panting abated somewhat, and the sweating gradually ceased, his hands and feet warmed. His right pulse was faintly discernible, like pearls on a string, and he could speak. He asked to be raised up on a rattan platform. Then I used five qian of ginseng, three qian of aconite [*fuzi*], three qian of astragalus root, three qian of *baishu,* two qian of black dry ginger [*heiganjiang*], one qian of cinnamon heart [*rougui*] and two qian of burnt licorice in a single dose. He breathed and slept normally.

Toward evening the previous doctor returned, took his pulse and said, "Today his pulses are improved, happily, due to our actions yesterday." Fang's affinal kinsman, Wang Xianchen, knew this was wrong and questioned him, saying, "It would seem one can use ginseng in cases of such great depletion, can't one?" The doctor replied, "In Cold Damage cases one never uses the method of replenishing, not even a single pinch [*fen*] of ginseng."

Xianchen challenged this: "One definitely can't use one pinch; today he took a more than a liang twice."[17]

That night I came back and found his left pulse was also faintly discernible. I put a lantern by the bed to see the sick man's face and he stretched toward me and showed his tongue, wanting me to look at it. Seeing this, those in attendance were overjoyed that he had revived. I said, "Not yet. We must watch for changes [*bian*] in his condition." I gave another dose of the previous infusion. The next day his faculties were clearer but his lower abdomen still ached, so [I] used moxibustion on his *guan yuan* aperture.

Fang's younger brother hastened from Chenzhou, and on arriving

16. Live Pulse infusion (*Sheng mai san*) was a formula consisting of ginseng, lily-turf (*maimendong*) and schisandra (*wuweizi*), which boosted *qi* by conserving and building fluids, especially in one depleted from sweating. See *Jianming Zhongyi cidian,* 262.

17. A qian equals approximately five grams and a liang equals about fifty grams. These are very large doses of ginseng.

heard of the alarms and confusion of the previous days. Seeing today's tranquility, he thanked me, saying, happily our elder brother has escaped death. I said, "Not yet. We must watch for changes in his condition. If there is no change, he will live. If there is a critical change [*bian*], there is nothing I can do." I gave another dose of the previous infusion. Toward evening his stomach growled; he evacuated several stools and his hands and feet cooled again and his pulse vanished. The next day he had a diarrhea of ten or more movements. His urine stained the clothing. Everything was yellow and his stool smelled of rhubarb. I said, "This is the crisis; we have labored in vain." Younger brother interrogated me, saying, "For several days he has taken your worthy's medicines; why is he now suffering from diarrhea?" I said, "This is the excess of the previous doctors, it is not the fault of your humble servant. Your respected brother's disorder belongs to the category of 'yin Cold,' but the doctors treated it with cold ingredients. This is like using cold water on ice; how can it melt? Earlier he was given rhubarb twice, and then your brother's stomach *qi* was ruined and his bowel function stopped. In the last few days, due to warming and replenishing doses of ginseng and astragalus root, his primordial *qi* revived a bit. The medicine reactivated [function], but it is as if he had taken poison; how could he hope to live?" [I.e., the restoration of function revived the power of a toxin to work.] All nodded in assent. I said, "I deeply regret that we met too late." Though the invalid indeed did not recover, I still gave him three days of life to prepare for his end. This was my humble accomplishment. Had I met with him a few days earlier, I certainly could have preserved him trouble free. However, I don't know if those other doctors on hearing of his last crisis felt any chagrin or not.[18]

Like the case of Fang Shunian's mother, this narrative made an expert's argument for a particular pharmaceutical strategy — the use of "warming and replenishing" formulas in the treatment of a seasonal fever, a common variant of a Cold Damage disorder. Fang Tingxian's case was an excellent illustration of just those principles of diagnosis that were at stake. Fang's case of Damage from Cold had not responded to medical treatment because others had reacted to it as a simple case of Summer Heat, rather than tracking the sickness to a root pattern of "yin Cold" factors. Instead they had continued to try and drive out heat with febrifuges and purgatives. Here is the explanation Cheng offered Wang Xianchen, the sympathetic brother-in-law, after the event:

18. Cheng Congzhou, juan 1, 10b–12b.

The most difficult aspect of Cold Damage syndromes is [recognizing] yin Cold. Everybody can see a natural true yin Cold, but if at the onset of illness one is suffering from a "double yin," excessive cold and cooling medicines can lead to "center Cold" and extreme yin dryness [loss of fluids], which will have an appearance of fierce yang [*shanghan*'s hot dry fever]. . . . Everyone knows the "center Cold" syndromes of winter, but they don't recognize that latent yin influences can be at work in the fevers of the other three seasons.[19]

Cheng appealed here first to classical theory enshrined in the *Treatise on Cold Damage Disorders*. An accurate reading of signs and symptoms can trace the progress of disorder from the initial phases governed by yang channels and dominated by hot dry external symptoms of skin surface and upper body, to the later, more dangerous path along the yin channels, deeper, lower and closer to vital centers. As energy channels, yang and yin locate the direction of change in a pathological process — moving either up and out to cure through release of pathogenic *qi*, or down and in to entrench it as a dangerous depletion where hot dry symptoms dynamically relate to yin weakness, not yang excess. Moreover, susceptibility to a yin form of the disorder may depend upon latent influences. Sometimes these are seasonal, but they operate more subtly than a direct influence of the seasonal *qi* of the moment. Here they may be identified as internal: double yin (*jian yin*) or a preexisting weakness of Kidney function — in Mr. Fang's case a reference to his preoccupation with his "little concubine."

Beyond the deep reading of inner and outer forces at work supplied by pattern diagnosis was the charged issue of iatrogenic illness — of rival healers who failed to see the patterns beneath surface symptoms, or to time their interventions accurately or to recognize the dangerous oversensitivity of weak bodies to strong medicines. Against the danger from the doctors, Cheng claimed for himself the authority of experience, bolstered by an admission that: "During my twenty years in Yangzhou, I personally have seen yin syndromes that were mistaken for yang ones and treated with cooling and cold formulas that ended lives."[20] Thus the authority he claimed for his deep reading of the case began with the model of disease process in the classical text and ended with his individual practice.

In case after case, Cheng showed himself at odds with both other physicians and with the expectations of his clients. Concerning the

19. Cheng Congzhou, juan 1, 13a–b.
20. Cheng Congzhou, juan 1, 13a.

former, Cheng hammered home the reformist pharmacology of the advocate of warming and replenishing against cooling and cleansing. "Doctors won't use warming methods and so their patients get sicker." They don't understand that "releasing sweat in the early stages of sickness is best followed up with replenishing formulas later."[21] "Northerners fear ginseng and astragalus root like snakes or scorpions. Common doctors without firm views or knowledge of repletion and depletion, seeing it used with bad results, use these to slander it and curry favor with household heads and patient families."[22]

As for clients, he deplored the latter's short-term focus—"they only praise the virtue of the latest doctor's dose." They fixated on the relief of external (*biao*) symptoms as sign of cure.[23] Here Cheng sounded like an expert warning against the popular oversimplifications of the untutored public. However, his expert's emphasis on deep pattern was not always best in practice, and Cheng's own successful cases showed this. He too often followed the medical maxim "In emergencies, treat external symptoms first, and attend to the root later"—never more dramatically than when he prescribed to restore a comatose individual to consciousness, as in the case of Fang Tingxian.

Moreover, his clients' views about ginseng and other formulas were based on understandings of body function for which there was ample classical precedent. The notion that febrile disorders were attacks from Wind, or were hot or cold depending upon the immediate season's influence, or that Cold Damage produces heat, or that replenishing ingredients encourage bodily repletions—all these represented well-established conventions, part of a common understanding that did not sharply divide professional healer from layperson. His use of pattern analysis to expose a dynamic disease process at a deeper level of intelligibility stood in contrast to many sufferers' perceptions of the best healing strategy for expelling an evil. Their perceptions overlapped with the doctor's clinical wisdom, providing an acceptable basis for self-care. But Dr. Cheng often judged them inadequate in the complex crises of his practice.

The world of shared medical knowledge was also one of divided authority. Having their own views, and believing them to be well

21. Cheng Congzhou, juan 2, 17b–18a; juan 1, 17b.
22. Cheng Congzhou, juan 1, 25b–26a.
23. Cheng Congzhou, juan 1, 17b.

informed, clients could be fickle, turning from one healer to another. Rather than collegial allies, healers were more often rivals. Such conflicts intensified the doctor's dependence upon the social authority of the ranking members of the families he visited. In the case of Fang Shunian's mother, the gentleman doctor enjoyed the full confidence of a gentleman in charge of the sufferer. However, the narrative of Fang Tingxian shows how easily lines of authority could become muddled when doctors disagreed, or when family seniors themselves were in serious or life-threatening predicaments. In Fang Tingxian's case the collapse of a mature head of household left the family rudderless. The narrative picture is of the sick man left surrounded by servants and weeping women, with their pathetic tales of orphan children and appeals to religious sentiment. It is also implied that the revolving-door succession of rival doctors gained ascendancy because of this vacuum of family leadership. It could not be filled by the only male in sight, an affinal kinsman shown as a wry observer. Not until the sick man's younger lineage brother arrived was social order restored by the presence of a figure of authority capable of cooperating with the doctor in the correct management of the case. We also see the doctor's dilemma when a patient appeared past cure. To withdraw was moral and professional abdication; to stay was to risk being blamed if the patient died.

In sum, as a service provider lacking the resources of an unchallengeable science, even the authority of a literati doctor depended heavily on his social relationships. Further, medical emergencies forced doctors to seek the support of class and patriarchal authority in the family in just those crises most likely to disrupt normal hierarchy. No wonder that in Cheng's casebook the men of a gentry patient's family were depicted as more farsighted and more reliable props to medical authority than Cheng's fellow physicians, whom he most often lampooned as self-important quacks.

As for the family's women, they were useless as allies. In Cheng's narratives they were nearly invisible as anonymous "household members" and "persons in attendance" in roles of service. In Fang Tingxian's case they intrude on the drama as a chorus, wringing their hands and lamenting. But some women could have informal power in a family, as elders, as mothers, or by default when their husbands were sick. When women themselves were sick, negotiating through senior males could run into obstacles set by the gender barriers encouraging separate spheres of inner and outer. Gender, then, added further dimensions to Cheng's problems of authority in his practice.

Women in the Clinical Encounter

How were issues of medical authority negotiated when Cheng Maoxian attended a sick woman? Cheng gave no sign that he had any special interest in *fuke,* but most seventeenth-century clinicians were generalists at the bedside. Cheng wrote about almost as many females as males (forty-one of his ninety-three cases), including children. While he treated women, like men, for fevers and miscellaneous disorders, he was most often consulted about their gestational problems of pregnancy or postpartum. He also recounted cases of *daixia* where menstrual anomaly was the leading factor.[24] Thus, his therapeutic considerations of the illnesses of women were dominated by narratives of the problems of reproductive function.

Socially, the treatment of sick women, like that of other family members, was expected to take place under the guidance of male authority, as we have seen in the cases of Fang Shunian's mother and of merchant Fang Tingxian. In his case narratives, Cheng always began by naming an adult male. A sick woman had an identity as such a man's kinswoman, and by implication as his dependent. Cheng usually implied there was a personal relationship between himself and this man in charge, while his use of polite or familiar forms of address showed whether one should consider him a person of culture and standing. In the doctor's narrative such adult males, particularly those marked as literati, are the people with whom the finer points of diagnosis and treatment are discussed. Other persons on the scene are identified by relationship (mother, son and so forth), or relegated to the anonymous category of family members (*jia ren*) or household (*ju jia*). Medicine appears as a learned calling, the province of elite males, to which others—both women and lower class people—have access through their relationships with these men, the former through kinship and the latter as neighbors, clients and servants.

When a woman fell ill, an appropriate adult man was presumed to have called the doctor and legitimized his presence. He was expected to be present at the examination, and it was through him that the visiting expert discussed the case. (See figures 14a–14d.) However, by contrast

24. Out of 93 cases, 52 were male and 41 female (55% versus 44%). Among the females the breakdown was: 5 menstruation, 9 pregnancy, 8 postpartum, 2 vaginal discharge, 4 pediatric and 13 other.

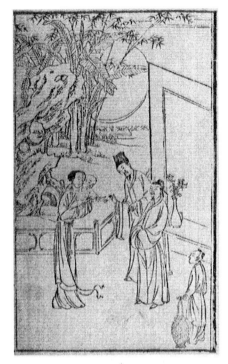 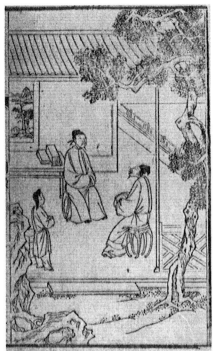

Figure 14a. Looking   Figure 14b. Asking

Figures 14a–14d. The doctor's visit and diagnosis. The physician enters the inner quarters to carry out his "four methods of diagnosis" on a boy with smallpox, escorted by the child's father. From Zhu Huiming, *Douzhen chuan xinlu* (Transmitted Essentials on Pox Disorders), first published in 1594. Reproduced from the 1786 edition held by the Gest Library, Princeton University.

with the ideal scenes illustrated here, it is clear that the sickrooms Cheng visited were often crowded places, even disorderly, and even when the sufferer was male, female kin and female servants were part of the bustle. More than once, Cheng's narrative took note of female tears. He laughed with Caihai's wife as her sick husband clamored for bowl after bowl of congee; he chided the mother and wife of Dongsi for bringing a painter of funeral portraits into the sickroom. Such tales called attention to humble families, and to the women who stepped in when a peasant householder sickened. But he also answered the questions of Cheng Yangchu's mother and sisters about Cheng's wife's threatened miscarriage, and argued with an "opinionated" grandmother about the

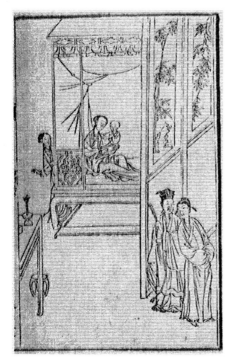

Figure 14c. Listening and smelling

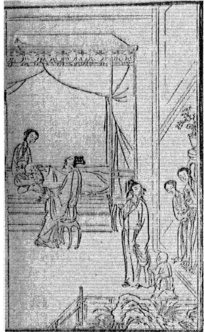

Figure 14d. Taking the pulse

proper prescription for her grandson's fever. In these two cases, women present showed they had opinions about proper pharmaceutical strategies based on some knowledge. This was also true of Lu Junxi's sister (or sister-in-law), who was in charge of preparing menstrual regulating prescriptions for her brother's new wife. Though often anonymous in the narrative, such family women could play an active role when the doctor came to call. The rules of modesty did not inhibit a social exchange between women who were in their proper place at home and an invited male visitor. In sum, the informality of gender boundaries at home served to confuse the gendered lines of authority that properly governed negotiations over medical treatment. The anonymous bystanders and household members represented in so many cases as now questioning or worrying, now skeptical or lamenting, included some of a family's women.

No matter who was sick, women, especially older women, could easily be in charge when no appropriate male family supervision existed.

Moreover, female sickness gave women authority, especially where pregnancy and birth or the illness of young children was involved. Where older matrons were involved, the formal authority accorded a male may have said rather little about the situation in the sickroom. Widow Liu, a fifty-year-old merchant trader, was the only woman Cheng named "in charge" of her own case as the head of her household—though she was in a coma from Wind-stroke most of the time and the doctor dealt with her son. In two cases the man named as in charge was a woman patient's nephew, a person unlikely to be authorized to supervise the illness of his senior kinswoman. Then there is the case of the wife of Cheng Yangchu who was hemorrhaging from a miscarriage. "Blood flowed out dripping, she was expiring over the commode, and the whole household surrounded her weeping. Yangchu's father, Zhengyu, reproved them, saying, 'What use are your tears? Call Mr. Cheng at once; maybe he can restore her.'" Here not only was the young husband named "in charge" not the household head, but the immediate caretakers were family women, to whom the sick woman's exasperated father-in-law addressed his order. Later, the sick person's kinswomen questioned the doctor.[25] In sum, since illness and healing both occurred at home, women were involved as family members, and the doctor's narrative shows him dealing with the informal as well as formal domestic hierarchies of which they were a part.

When a woman herself was sick, the ideals of patriarchal supervision often conflicted with the norms of female modesty. When Cheng instructed his readers on the importance of using all four standard methods of diagnosis—looking, asking, listening and smelling, and touching (pulse-taking)—the cases in question featured ill women. Touching was not a problem, since for Cheng as for others there was hardly any physical examination in the modern sense. The pulse provided the most important tactile evidence; he used it routinely with women, and even with male clients Cheng rarely went beyond it.[26] But as for "seeing" a sick

25. Cheng Congzhou, juan 1, 7a–8b.
26. Except for pulse-taking, Cheng rarely reported touching the sick. He applied moxibustion to Fang Tingxian in extremis; with another comatose sufferer he felt for pulses in the channels along the neck; with a desperately ill sick child left out to die, he lifted an eyelid to look at the pupil. But when one young man lay insensible and perhaps near death, he asked an attendant to feel if his feet were cold. He cared whether a swelling was painful or hard or moved under the skin, but I read his narratives as suggesting these were symptoms, reported verbally by the sufferer, rather than signs, independently arrived at by physical examination.

woman, Cheng quoted the famous complaint of the Song master of pharmacology, Kou Zongshi, about "curtains and screens" hiding her from view. He illustrated his point with an example from a case in which "pulse and symptom do not agree." Fearing that the delicate young gentry wife of Wu Jingke might be dying, he asked permission to see her face. It was granted.[27] This story bore out Kou's emphasis upon extremes of female modesty as a social marker of the upper class. Nonetheless, Cheng's telling of the tale showed the doctor surmounting the difficulty as confidant to an elite family, where protocol concerning "seeing" was matter of family honor in the hands of male authority.

Not all families were so fastidious. Cheng did not remark on the fact that a neighbor, Wang Mingde, called him into the sick chamber of his forty-five-year-old wife suffering from heat and delirium. After a ginseng infusion she recognized the doctor at her bedside and pointed, saying, "This is our neighbor Mr. Cheng."[28] Fang Jisuo even took his adolescent daughter to visit "doctors of the city gate" in town without results, after which he brought her personally to Cheng for questioning. In cases like these, the normative barriers to contact between sick women and a male outsider were negotiable when properly supervised.

The most serious gender barriers that Cheng faced were those imposed by his female clients themselves. Fang Jisuo's teenage daughter could not be diagnosed because she had been unwilling to speak about her vaginal discharge, and Cheng's triumph in the case was that after pulse and tongue examination he had ferreted out the truth by naming her symptoms directly. Of the four methods of diagnosis, "asking" was most difficult of all. Here modesty protected an intimate bodily space, suggesting a sexualized interpretation of it. Moreover, silence—the refusal to speak—was action that a woman herself controlled. Such silence struck at the key role of language in establishing illness symptoms. Whereas the authority of male householders and doctors over the management of a woman's illness is shown as subtly contested within the household, women as sufferers are shown supporting the conventions of modesty that safeguarded their honor. Although the etiquette concerning the separation of the sexes allowed authority to be adjusted according to issues of age, station and circumstances of the people involved, rituals of bodily decorum powerfully gendered the social relations of healing in Cheng's narratives of his female patients. Here female

27. Cheng Congzhou, juan 2, 54a–55a.
28. Cheng Congzhou, juan 2, 15b.

authority was understood as the more legitimate when it supported female modesty in the clinical encounter.

Female authority over the health of women in the home and female reticence in dealing with male doctors were especially noticeable when the diagnostic problem involved the core of Ming *fuke,* the sexual or gestational body. Cheng's narratives depict pregnancy as particularly troublesome. First, the facts of the matter were often shrouded in ambiguity. For women in the seventeenth century, a pregnancy as a known bodily experience emerged only gradually out of the liminality of menstrual irregularity, an uneasy digestion, and a sense of fullness, all of which could have many causes. For a doctor uncertainty was magnified by the challenges of diagnosis by pulse. The *Canon of the Pulse* defined pregnancy as a condition marked by symptoms of disorder in one whose pulse is normal, that is, it was a classic instance of the diagnostically challenging disjuncture where "pulse and symptom do not agree." Moreover, families called on Dr. Cheng not for symptom relief in cases of ordinary morning sickness, oedema, or urinary complaints, but where pregnancy itself was in doubt or in danger.

Sometime there was a conflict between a woman's belief about her condition and the doctor's diagnostic evidence using pulse. With the delicate, vegetarian wife of Kou Yufu, who at thirty-six was thought past childbearing, Cheng astounded her family with a textbook diagnosis of an early second-month pregnancy, based solely on her "floating, slippery, . . . and flowing" pulses. "When her belly gradually swelled and her fetus began to move, then they believed me." But he could also be mistaken. Lu Weiyuan's affinal kinswoman appeared to Cheng an unlikely candidate for pregnancy: she was in her forties, thin and overworked, and coughed a tiny amount of blood. He rejected her self-report that she was two months with child, but later she aborted, and he had to defend himself from the implication that his Spleen-restoring formula had caused the miscarriage.

A woman's silence about a suspected pregnancy made for an even more difficult case. Luo Hongyu's young concubine had missed her period for six months, and yet not only did she have no symptoms of distress but her pulses were "sunken, slow and . . . weak." Respectfully kowtowing, Cheng asked her if she felt fetal movement, but she would not speak to the doctor. Eventually the mystery was solved, not by diagnostic pulse or the "pregnancy detecting powder" he prescribed but when her husband privately elicited her history of menstrual irregularity. Finally, it seems that sometimes a woman's silence was a deliberate trap for the doctor. He reported the embarrassing instance when he found a doubtful "subtle, small and . . . sunken" pulse in Wu Duiyan's wife, who, it turned out, was eight months pregnant—a fact concealed from him behind her bed-curtains. For Cheng, these cases instructed the doctor to question the *Canon of the Pulse*'s reliability while leaving him with few diagnostic alternatives. They also show the social pressures supporting pulse diagnosis as the subtlest test of a physician's skills, and the problems it posed when used alone.

"Asking" a sick woman could signal to the family ignorance as well as impropriety in a doctor, even as Cheng, like other doctors, used his cases to warn medical men not to neglect it. Twice he reported how his correct diagnosis of a gestational illness turned on his willingness to "question closely": the pregnant wife of Mao-er had not told him about her improper diet of coarse buns while previously convalescent, and Wu Yanchao's young wife had concealed her "private thoughts" after childbirth.

Postpartum disorders were thought to be particularly tricky to diagnose, and Cheng emphasized their intricacies by specifically urging physicians to neglect none of the four methods of diagnosis in such situations. He also had to deal with the fact that postpartum recovery was normally managed by women themselves. Like many Ming physicians, he began with Zhu Zhenheng's famous aphorism that had revised Song dynasty norms of postpartum care: "After childbirth, give strong replenishers for *qi* and Blood, and treat other syndromes as secondary." He considered postpartum cleansing formulas to "break up Blood" and discharge afterbirth to be another example of an ill-advised remedy adopted by ignorant patients and their families. When Wu Yanchao's twenty-year-old wife, feeling pain in the bowels and an absence of postpartum flow, took doses to move Blood (*tong xue*) and ended up delirious, he criticized her caretakers for plying her with rich pork loin, chicken and eggs and overruled their objections to a formula to activate *qi* instead. When Bao Mingfu's wife damaged her Spleen from grief after losing her newborn to navel Wind, he scolded her caregivers similarly: "They use ingredients to drive out pathogens and break up Blood, piling depletion on depletion!"[29] Another young wife suffered complications because even though she was feverish and lacked strength, family members insisted that she rest propped upright on her couch (to assist postpartum discharge). Here the learned doctor saw himself at odds with

29. Cheng Congzhou, juan 2, 30b–31a.

family women who were taking care of a new mother in a medically traditional way. (See figures 15 and 16.)

On the other hand, sometimes families and doctors routinely treated postpartum illness as depletion. Following Zhu Zhenheng's strategy blindly, they failed to recognize indigestion from rich postpartum foods, or the "repletion heat" of a true Cold Damage fever. While he warned against remedies that could overwhelm frail constitutions, he added cases where his aggressive approach had been successful.[30] When after a subsequent delivery Wu Yanchao's wife's postpartum heat persisted for five days, producing delirium, nosebleeds and "distress in all five internal organ systems," Cheng blamed Cold invasion at the time of parturition, and sweated it out with *Chong he tang,* a harmonizing infusion laced with ginger and garlic.[31]

These case histories of gestational women show gender barriers that produced conflicts over proper management and limited the doctor's access to information. This may explain why Cheng's most vivid narratives of pregnancy told stories of his own wife, mother of at least four or five surviving children. He related in detail how her many pregnancies were dogged by nausea and aversion for cooked food until after the sixth month; how she suffered numerous miscarriages, including one that triggered a seemingly life-threatening hemorrhage; and how her recovery from childbirth depletion was always slow. Her last pregnancy evinced all these problems, and in so doing also brought Dr. Cheng as husband and as doctor face to face with the moral and health issues of abortion.

As she approached her fortieth year, suddenly her menses were one or two days late. [She] used medicines to move the menses [*tong jing*] for two or three doses, but when they produced no effect she did not dare take more. So she waited to see what the future would bring. . . . At three months her menses suddenly flowed, and [she] thought her weak body, unable to carry another child, was about to abort; fearing the difficulty of labor and delivery, miscarriage seemed like a fortunate misfortune. As matters did not go smoothly, there was no alternative to using peach kernel [*taoren*], Tibetan crocus [*honghua*], "dark *hu*" [*xuanhu*] and angelica root tail [*gui wei*] to break up Blood and abort. After one dose, the bleeding stopped. Greatly alarmed, I said, "If after these medicines

30. Cheng Congzhou, juan 2, 43b–46a.
31. Cheng Congzhou, juan 2, 45a. According to the *Jianming Zhongyi cidian,* 369, this complex formula of a dozen ingredients is designed to treat static anger and associated Fire, pain, irritability and insomnia.

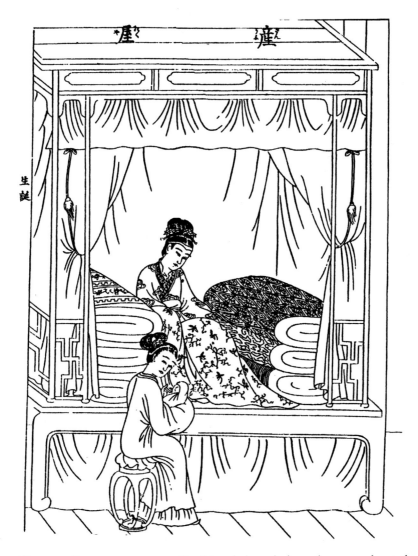

Figure 15. Postpartum recovery. Traditional obstetrical practices were observed and depicted by eighteenth-century Japanese visitors to China. Here the new mother rests upright, supported by blankets to aid postpartum discharge. From Nakagawa Tadahide, *Shinzoku kibun* (Observations of Qing Dynasty customs).

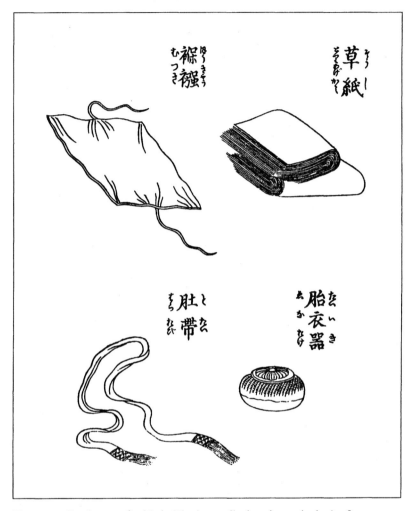

Figure 16. Equipment for birth. The items displayed are, clockwise from upper right: paper towelling to catch birth blood; container for placenta; pregnancy sash for belly support; infant's swaddling wrap. From Nakagawa Tadahide, *Shinzoku kibun* (Observations of Qing Dynasty customs).

the menstrual flow still stops, isn't it fated that this child should not perish?" She took ginseng and astragalus root and doses to stop bleeding. She bled again heavily. I said, "This [fetus] truly can't be tranquilized," and again she took peach kernel and Tibetan crocus. But then the bleeding stopped. [I] had to go back to the method of supporting the center.

Blood still flowed out dripping. After five days I reflected: with this loss of Blood, how can the fetus be so rocklike? The pulse signifies pregnancy, while the symptoms suggest it can't be so. Whether she is pregnant or not, her disorder must be treated, and quickly. So I used a strong re-plenishing formula with ginseng and *baishu* to stabilize, and after half a month she was gradually calm. At ten full months she delivered a boy, my third son, Hanbiao [Banner of Han]. All my earlier sons and daugh-ters were born prematurely; only this boy went to full term, and his constitution is extraordinary. If a mother's *qi* is depleted, her fetus ought to be weak, but here the child was full term and its body unlike the mother's. Didn't True Heaven intend this? When we doctors mistakenly use Blood-moving medicines, fetuses may perish and their families may blame the physician. From my wife's point of view this child's happy condition can't be the work of humans alone. I write this first that my fellow physicians may learn from it to avoid occasions for self-reproach, and second so that Hanbiao one day may fully know his mother's many-sided hardships, which were not only a burden of motherly toil [after birth].[32]

This narrative shows a parent's joy in a beloved late-born child and a doctor's reading of gestational labor as maternal sacrifice. It also shows a couple's tacit negotiation of the risks of reproduction. Even though this was a physician's family, his wife managed her own menstrual reg-ulating medicines, which were understood to influence the likelihood of a pregnancy's termination and were taken accordingly. Her husband's expert intervention occurred after her pregnancy was established and the situation became serious, as first he tried to save the fetus and then to protect his spouse. Menstrual regulating and Blood-breaking (*po xue*) formulas emerge as potentially dangerous yet unreliable abortifacients. Overall, the outcome owed more to fate than to human effort.

Dr. Cheng's vocational antipathy to medically assisted abortion can be seen in this light. He was not apologetic about endangering a fetus when pregnancy risked a mother's well-being—indeed, he told the story of his wife partly to teach others how to arrive at such sensitive yet pragmatic judgments. Some of his reservations had to do with the role of Heaven and fate. To assist death was deeply inauspicious. More pragmatically, the issue of abortion might be a minefield detonating

32. Cheng Congzhou, juan 2, 26b–28a. Cheng is calling attention to the toil of gestation as opposed to that of nurture. The idiom *qulao*, from the *Book of Odes*, refers to a mother's "toilsome" care for her child in the first three years of life. I owe thanks to Meng Zhang for this reference.

domestic conflict. His admonitions on the subject were born out by his story of Cheng Yangchu's wife. After eight pregnancies, she missed her period and six weeks later treated a "lump" in her stomach with peach kernel and Tibetan crocus (to break up Blood and abort), until chronic bleeding accompanied her belly's swelling. In this case family members (and unnamed other doctors) kept to a theory of "menstrual accumulations," and when Cheng diagnosed a pregnancy, the sisters-in-law opined that the "leaky fetus" must be "strange," and her husband Yangchu asked outright for an abortifacient to be administered. In the face of a family's eagerness to end a pregnancy, Cheng refused, and was proud to have brought the case to a successful conclusion by prescribing Blood-nourishing (*yang xue*) and "slippery fetus" (*hua tai*) doses to strengthen her for birth. Although he explained his strategy in terms of the risks of miscarriage to a woman's health, implicit was the fear of blame.[33] Cheng's narrative warned doctors not to risk therapies that might lead to recriminations later. When fetuses aborted for any reason, the attending doctor could be held responsible, as had happened when he failed to recognize Lu Weiyuan's kinswoman's pregnancy. While medical ethics supported abortion to protect the health of mothers, family politics might later weigh in on the side of the loss to its descent line.

Although menstrual regularity figured in textbook *fuke* as a key to overall female health and fertility, it was an insignificant feature of Cheng's casebook. One case may explain why. He expressed surprise when Lu Junxi asked for advice about his eighteen-year-old bride's irregular spotting. "Why can't she be regulated?" he wanted to know, and was told that she refused to accept medicines compounded by her new sister-in-law. Concluding from this, shrewdly enough, that the young wife must be suffering from "anger," he prescribed without visiting the patient. This prescription, rather than being a standard menstrual regulating formula, was artfully crafted to cure the angry Fire attacking the Liver system's function of Blood storage, and also to "boost Spleen, ease Liver, clear Heat, nourish Blood and make yang ascend [enhancing fertility]."[34] Here the doctor's florid diagnosis and remedy drew on theories of Ming textbook *fuke* linking menstrual irregularity, negative emotion, Liver Fire and Blood depletion. But his intervention took place because the normal home management of menstrual matters by family women themselves had broken down.

33. Cheng Congzhou, juan 1, 7a–9a.
34. Cheng Congzhou, juan 2, 4b–5b.

In sum, in all of his cases involving gestational functions, Cheng Maoxian showed himself working at some remove from the situation. His stories are of being called upon when pregnancy was in doubt or at risk, or when a postpartum woman experienced symptoms of acute illness. His most available diagnostic tool, pulse diagnosis, was recognized as unreliable concerning gestation, and could be at odds with the client's own symptomatically based understandings of pregnancy. His advice about the management of postpartum could be at odds with domestic wisdom, while the crises of miscarriage or abortion, situated at the crosscurrents of family politics of reproduction, exposed him to the risk of blame. Cheng had nothing to say in his casebook about problems of labor, delivery or lactation, nor did he report ever interacting with a midwife. The gestational body he knew best was his own wife's.

All in all, his situation was easiest when family males clearly guided the clinical encounter, as when he fielded the questions of young husbands still new to marriage, cautioned one father about the risks to his wife of abortion, or explained to another the threats a vaginal discharge posed to his daughter's fertility. This position as an expert on reproductive matters was more ambiguous when transmitted across the barriers posed by informal female authority over the management of reproductive health, or those thrown up by the standards of modesty women embraced. Ironically, these case histories show flexible interpretations of the gender boundaries of inner and outer in the conduct of daily domestic life, but from the doctor's point of view flexibility was more easily encouraged by male householders, while women themselves were the stricter guardians of their own seclusion. In sum, Cheng's narratives are a rich deconstruction of the medical "difficulty" of curing women. Clinical difficulties become problems of the social relations of healing—the barriers posed by female modesty and female authority when male doctors attended them. To cope with such difficulty, the doctor hoped to forge an alliance with family males supporting the prestige of learned medicine and the paternalist oversight of the health of family dependents.

Social Body and Gender in the Clinical Narrative

Although gender distinction was strongly embedded in the social relations of healing, Cheng Maoxian's cases constructed "separate prescriptions" narrowly, and did not imagine biologically essentialist categories of male or female. His female clients, like males, suffered from fevers and dysenteries, rashes and respiratory congestions, attacks from Wind and Cold, internal damage from food—the range of common human ills. Females and males alike experienced the humoral conditions of depletion and repletion, bodily congestion and stasis, phlegm, Damp, Heat, Wind and Cold. Humoral qualities were not translated into gendered distinctions in the manner of Galenic medical constructions of the female body as "cooler." As narratives of lives, however, Cheng's case histories give a bodily dimension to gender-specific forms of social experience, and at the same time they reveal the metaphorical resonances of the gender-laden bodily categories of yin and yang, Blood and *qi*. Social human beings are embodied, and bodily categories are read as social.

First, Cheng observed his patients' experiences of emotions, of desire, of work and rest. The stereotype that linked female emotionality with suppressed desires was an old one, going back to Sun Simiao. But negative emotion was no monopoly of Cheng's women patients. It simply appeared in gender-specific contexts: where men experienced stasis from worry over work and lawsuits and study, women experienced it in connection with conflict with in-laws and servants, grief over children, and the burdens of domestic responsibilities. When Cheng, like other doctors, treated medicine as psychoactive rather than trying to guide his clients to change behavior, he inscribed emotion as embodied and social relations as inalterable, supporting the system of cultural signs that linked natural and social worlds.

But when Cheng commented on morally blameworthy forms of unhealthful behavior in stories about sensual indulgence, he spoke of males who visited brothels, enjoyed concubines, or made themselves sick with potency medicines. Depletions from sexual license afflicted males. If women do sometimes also fall ill from erotic excitation, he said, it is because of their dreams.[35] As for excesses of the table, men and women both came to grief from rich diet, but those who washed down their meals with wine were males, while two older women were the only ones

---

35. "Yin cold syndromes don't necessarily come from bed-chamber matters; it happens that women have pathological [*xie*] dreams and fall ill this way." Cheng Congzhou, juan 1, 15b. This appears to be an indirect reference to the syndrome "dreams of intercourse with ghosts," which other doctors saw as comparable to seminal emissions in males, and which in folk medicine was understood as spirit possession.

identified as vegetarian. Alcohol appears an everyday part of late Ming upperclass social life, ambivalently criticized by the doctor, himself known as a drinker.[36] In sum, just as the doctor's bedside social rituals were respectful of female modesty, his narratives presented female bodies as naturally more continent and chaste.

Male bodies experienced the consequence of unregulated desires when they suffered from "double yin" syndromes, in the manner of Fang Tingxian. Double yin also afflicted He Zhenhua, a young itinerant doctor (*yang yi*) who had visited a brothel on his travels, and Mr. Wu, another traveller who had dined too well and then engaged in sex at an inn. In yet another case, young Xiang Zhijing, who himself was ambitious to become a doctor, feared double yin and thanked Cheng for the gentle prescription for dysentery that took into account his recent series of wet dreams. Such spontaneous seminal emissions counted as a medical problem in youth, while "bed-chamber fatigue" (*fang lao*) was a potentially serious precipitating factor in maturity.

Here Cheng's cases warned mature males of hidden weakness in seemingly vigorous individuals like Fang Tingxian, or Cheng's clan uncle whose bed-chamber-induced "inner and outer fatigue" transformed a cold (*ganmao*) into a fatal illness. Two other older men suffered apoplectic Wind-strokes when they became irate over losses at chess, and in three cases a "strange," "swollen" or "large" pulse foretold fatality for men in their fifties whom the world thought strong. In thinking of these last cases of male vulnerability, Cheng quoted an aphorism, "Tumors [*ju*] grow vigorously and old men die of vexation."[37]

On the other hand, Cheng expected women to be through with childbearing by forty, and found exceptions worthy of comment. The most remarkable of all his woman clients was a toothless common street singer who in her fifties had borne a child and whose breast-milk still flowed freely. Her vitality was an example of the sort of anomaly that made late Ming natural philosophers question the predictability of the cosmological order.[38] Those whose childbearing was done were

36. For a similar pattern in the cases of Wang Ji, see Grant 1996: chapter 4.

37. Cheng Congzhou, juan 2, 33a. One of these men died of a *yong* tumor, which Cheng implied could be an unforeseen sequel to overdosing on potency medicines. *Ju* and *yong* tumors were considered a yin yang pair: the first "cold," i.e., thick and hard to the touch, and the second "hot," producing abscesses.

38. Cheng Congzhou, juan 1, 24a–b. Cheng thought her lack of teeth particularly strange, given orthodox associations of Kidney, generative vitality, and teeth and hair.

spoken of as elderly regardless of their chronological age.[39] No woman was diagnosed with a double yin, and women's "yin Cold" patterns were identified with cold extremities spreading to the body's center and damaging digestion or respiration, not with their sexual desires. Three sedentary elderly women were diagnosed with depletions of Blood. Rheumatism (*bi*) afflicted one whose feet, though free of pain, were cold and numb past the knees, so that she moved with difficulty and one day fell down and took to her bed. Clearly Blood and *qi* were stagnant and Blood pulse was sluggish — a case of poor circulation. Cheng saw "Blood depletion of the triple yin channel" in a new widow's pains with heat spreading from her knees to her whole body, and saw a problem of storage of Blood in a an elderly vegetarian woman whose chronic rib cage pain spread to her back and spine, worse at night than in the day. In these elderly females, Blood stagnation was the mark of an inactive and confined life.

In sum, if the feebleness of age was an ungendered condition of bodily decline of both *qi* and Blood, males and females often arrived there by different paths. As stories of illness, Cheng's cases were not written to illustrate the successes of bodily self-cultivation according to the teachings on "nourishing life." Still, Cheng's chaste women were not seen as more robust in old age than his indulgent men. The variable, invisible in the discourse of nourishing life, was revealed when the bodily economies of male dissipation and female childbearing were juxtaposed. While robust males suffered hidden damage from immoderate living, females aged early through the body work of bearing children and the stasis of their social confinement. Childbearing women's burdens and older women's chronic aches and pains contrasted with the more latent vulnerabilities of seemingly vigorous males.

These stories told of social patterns of gender difference having to do with life cycles and lifestyles. The picture was a textual construction, of course, shaped by a doctor's authorial hand to foreground his personal achievements and medical pedagogy. The casebook was crafted around examples that the author thought instructive, not a sociological profile but a set of representative medical subjects — that is, types to shape clinical expectations. Each story of a case told of the bodily experience of social life, shaped by the way medicine imagined passages from youth

---

39. Fang Shunian's mother at sixty-three was the oldest sick woman discussed in the text. Five old women were in their forties, and the three widows were thirty-five, forty, and fifty-four, respectively.

to age as a bodily process and by how it moralized sexuality and health in bodies of generation and gestation.

Language and the Body
in the Clinical Narrative

On a deeper semiotic level, Cheng's stories of the bodily experience of social life were also about the social meanings of medical language that constructed the body. Stories located individual experience in a rich semantic field of named signs and sensations, relationships and qualities. Client voices as well as the voice of the doctor produced the textual reports of the agencies of disease and of the mechanisms of drug action. Among the parties to the clinical encounter, points of view could vary. The sick were represented as conservative interpreters, looking to the external environment for the sources of affliction, naming the old medical agents of Wind, Cold and poison, or the *qi* of seasons and locality. But the doctor's more internalist patterns of balance and imbalance, of depletion and repletion, of Blood and *qi* function, or of yin and yang forms of disorder were not a remote technical idiom monopolized by the expert who alone was privy to the body's hidden secrets. Language linked the intimate somatic experiences of illness to an intelligible map of the order of bodily functions and also to a range of metaphors connecting bodily and social understandings. These interrelations made medical language accessible as a common cultural property, and can be seen in Cheng's accounts of yin and yang, Blood and *qi*.

Disorders of Blood most likely involved the gestational problems of women. Fertility and fecundity were considered to be based on "ample Blood" and menstrual regulating formulas were standard to nourish yin, ease pain and avoid the depletions attendant on irregular menstrual bleeding. But menstrual stoppage called for stronger ingredients to "move Blood" which were potential abortifacients, potent enough to be risky to women's health. Medicines to "break up Blood" were commonplace, and attempts at abortion by "moving menses" were recognized and accessible expedients. On the other hand, to maintain a healthy pregnancy, it was important to keep a "tranquil fetus," and to avoid all medicines with "moving" action on *qi* to purge. Concerning birth, all parties believed that it depleted a woman's *qi* and Blood, requiring postpartum replenishment with food, medicine and rest. But Cold and Wind from outside remained recognized risks, while family members continued to take measures to cleanse "bad Blood" from the new mother's system. Whatever the deep theoretical structure of Blood as primary vitality, manifest gestational Blood was of immediate clinical concern.

Blood as a primary vitality could also appear in cold, pain and stagnations affecting circulation, showing up particularly in the body's extremities. From this point of view Blood was linked not only to rheumatic aches and cold hands and feet but to some kinds of headaches. But it also was also at work in repletions and depletions of the center, which related to Liver and Spleen system problems, that is, to functions of Blood storage and the energy systems of digestion that linked Blood to Spleen and Liver through their Five Phase relationship. Malnourished or fasting women ceased to menstruate. In all these ways, Blood was not reducible to the fluid that runs through biomedical arteries and veins. Still, Blood showed its yin nature both by its affinity with gestational and other body fluids as Water, and by affliction that was worse at night: night sweats, insomnia or periodic fevers that worsened in the evening.

Like other doctors, Chen used the phrase "Blood and *qi*" holistically, a platitude for fundamental vitalities. However, within this dyad Cheng emphasized the secondary and dependent nature of Blood, its embodiment of "the pacific, tranquil virtues of *kun,* which has *qian* to invigorate its circulation." He thought that unlike *qi* Blood was tied to the visible and material: "Isn't Blood something with form?" he asked. On the other hand, "formless *qi*" is manifest purely as motion.[40] Therefore, where stagnations of *qi* were purely functional, he expected pathologies of Blood to produce signs in swelling and congestion. In all these ways, Blood was more closely tied to tangible phenomena—not only to reproductive fluids but to the mass that congests and blocks, the volume of what is stored and the form of what flows as a liquid. Disorders involving Blood function were more frequent in women of all ages.[41]

If Blood was dependent on *qi,* how did yin relate to yang in Cheng's pattern analysis of his clients' disorders? Two particularly important issues are illustrated in the case of Fang Tingxian, who died, Cheng thought, because his doctors misread yin and yang forms of Cold Dam-

40. Cheng Congzhou, juan 2, 44a. See also 42b, 46a.
41. Cheng diagnosed Blood dysfunction alone in three females and one male. Pathologies of both Blood and *qi* afflicted seven females and two males, while *qi* syndromes were evenly divided, six and six.

age fever. Cheng explained the difference this way: in the classic yang form of such a disorder, heat blazes at the surface of the skin, including hands and feet, and pulse is "rapid" and "floating." The sufferer is red-faced and thirsty, with aching, full, chest symptoms; if in pain, the sick person is nonetheless alert and restless. Pathogenic invasion has attacked the upper, outer circulation channels of the body. In the yin form, the sufferer in spite of feverishness is torpid and unresponsive, with dark or ashen face and hands, or a countenance that if red is lifeless. The body's extremities are cold, and there may be belly pain, diarrhea and perhaps vomiting. Pulses will be "sunken" and "retarded," or "subtle" and "faint." Since here yin and yang traced the cardinal channel pathways and with them the pathological site and direction of its movement, they evoked both qualitative symptom and stages in progression. In classic Cold Damage theory, initial phases of acute fevers will be governed by the triple-yang channel "yang brightness" (*yang ming*), while at the other end of the process, governed by the triple-yin channel "extreme yin" (*jue yin*), life is in danger. In between lie the four middle channels— an intermediate ground of mixed combinations of symptoms experienced as illness evolves, such as Fang Tingxian's transitional "latent yin" situation.[42] Here the poles of yin and yang mark the contrast between the bright hectic flare-up of fever in a strong body able to resist, and the wrung-out exhaustion of one in whom an entrenched disease process has taken hold, where body heat is less important than the vulnerability of body fluids. Since they define early versus later stages of disease, case history narratives bring this out clearly, showing how yin's inner cold means a body where life may be in danger.

The unfortunate Fang Tingxian also suffered from the additional background double-yin (*jian yin*) weakness. Here yin was unpaired, standing for disorders of sexual excess, and had a special relationship with Kidney function, the seat of generative energy. Sometimes yin Cold pointed to a similar vulnerability. When Cheng's clan uncle from Min-yang suffered from bed-chamber fatigue (*nei lao*), his illness with fever-ish delirium was actually Dry-hot yin (*yin zao*), or insufficiency of Kidney Water; while the latent yin of a servant boy was a weakness of rapid

---

42. See Cheng Congzhou, juan 1, 13a–16a, for Cheng's analysis of types of Cold Damage fevers. Complications such as "latent yin" could be exacerbated by medical mismanagement, while underlying weakness from Kidney deficiency or sexual excess produced "center Cold" or "yin Cold" or even "yin Dry," where exhaustion of yin Water mimicked yang's hectic restlessness.

adolescent growth. Thus other yin syndromes also could relate to depletions of generative vitality.

In all these ways, yin disorders were understood as serious. What did Cheng have in mind when on occasion he named a disorder of yang? Once or twice he diagnosed "yang-ming repletion heat" in a fever patient. This was the early, superficial stage of a Cold Damage fever, but such disorders were not serious enough to take up much room in his casebook. He also understood yang in terms of familiar affinities with the tops of things: "The head is the first of all yang [regions]," he said in prescribing heating remedies for a man's "cold" headache.[43] At the other end of the body, whether the sufferer was a chronically cold middle-aged woman or a young girl, vaginal discharge was a sign that "true yang is inadequate." Here yang signified not only weakness above, which allowed what should be contained to drain downward, but evoked the old association in the *Inner Canon* between the head's brain marrow and reproductive Essence, presumed to be guided in its circulation by the energy along the Superintendent channel. This reasoning supported Cheng, like others, in the medical reading of *daixia* as a serious female disorder, threatening fertility.[44] Finally, one way he signaled the imminence of death was to say that "yang is lost." Yang, then, was named in the context of the superficial aspects of illness, or as a figure for life itself in the sense of primordial *qi*. It was natural, therefore, for Cheng's pattern diagnoses to name yin types of illness more often than yang ones. Yang pointed to health and recovery more readily than to the more serious types and stages of disease, and the latter were the business of the doctor.

In the bodies of Cheng's sick clients, yin and yang, Blood and *qi*, did not function simply as formally equivalent relationships of energies in dynamic balance. Nor did the ascendant phase of one simply play against the latency of the other. Embodied in a person's illness, they named concrete situations and above all they marked auspicious versus inauspicious phenomena. In the trajectory of an individual life, the body did not simply oscillate between yin and yang poles of balance and imbalance, or even between illness and health, but moved from growth to decline, from youth to age. Yang as a life principle occupied the middle

---

43. Cheng Congzhou, juan 1, 25b. The man suffered from fainting fits.

44. This reading of *daixia* implied that leaky semen was the parallel syndrome in males. But Cheng, like other doctors, also sometimes paired young men's semen loss and women's "dreams of intercourse with ghosts."

ground of health. In daily contact with the dark forces of illness, the materiality of growth and senescence, the extreme transitions of birth and death, the doctor's business was with yin.

In all these ways, yin and yang, Blood and *qi,* figured in the construction of illness as qualities and as metaphors as well as relationships patterning disease dynamics. Cheng Maoxian's practice of pattern diagnosis did not appeal to the romance of yin and yang as Water and Fire—the reading of bodily qualities popularized by Zhu Zhenheng's followers. Nor did he emphasize yin's affinity with generative Water or with the reproductive vitalities of the Kidney system. In other words, although his clients' disorders could easily have been theorized in these other ways, he did not explore the resources of the cosmological and medical vocabulary to valorize yin in its generative aspect. These may be seen merely as unspoken aspects of a whole pattern too complex to be articulated at once. But the very emphasis upon positionality that makes Chinese medical theory so flexible also privileges what is in fact named. Such naming may reflect the internal logic of medical discourse, but it will also tug at metaphorical possibilities. Words are chosen, and yet are always open to meaning more than the speaker has said.

Therefore, his narrative located yin and yang, Blood and *qi,* in the network of metaphorically resonating qualities presumed to inhere in human affairs and the natural world alike. Yang's virtue meant that life-threatening illness was figured by its absence; yin's dark qualities had an affinity with negative power. Yin and yang spoke both of dialectical relationships and of value-laden symbolizations of health as opposed to disease, vigor as opposed to decline. If identical forces of yin and yang, Blood and *qi,* were at work in the bodies of both men and women, this was testimony to their common humanity extending the generative powers of Heaven and Earth. From another aspect, yin and yang, Blood and *qi,* also inscribed onto bodies the gendered hierarchy of human social relationships. In the clinical encounter yin also named the hidden female body, the privacy of sexual matters, and the dangers attending birth and death. Blood also named the dependent and material, vulnerable yet vital reproductive function of women.

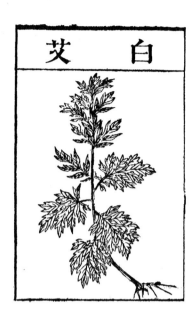

CHAPTER 8

In and Out of the Family

Ming Women as Healing Experts

In earlier chapters, women have appeared as textual subjects in male-authored medical discourses. Occasionally they have appeared indirectly as voices in narratives of the clinical encounter. These
voices of patients and family members suggest something of how the
sick understood medical learning and interacted with physicians. In
medical discourse on the gestational body, or on the management of
menstruation, it is even possible to intuit something of a distinctly female sphere of medical experience and understanding. I have argued
that women's participation in a male-dominated elite medical system
was shaped by the diffused nature of medical knowledge, and by the
fact that both sickness and healing took place at home. The medical
knowledge and practice of such women, like that of their male family
members, was a domestic skill.

However, on the fringes of my account have appeared traces of women who were healers by vocation or trade—who went out into a neighbor's or even a stranger's home to diagnose and cure, offering medicines or services in exchange for payment. They include the "child-birth doctors" (*ru yi*) of the Han through Song eras, or other midwives and birth attendants. But not all female healers were midwives. I offered glimpses of a Song woman who ran an apothecary shop and of a matron called to court to treat the illness of an empress. A look at the Ming dynasty shows that female healers like these were part of its medical landscape as well. Ironically, the Ming trend toward stricter sex segregation encouraged the demand for the services of female experts caring for the ills of other women. The roles of such women healers—their spheres of expertise, their clients, their social networks and reputations—are obviously important for rounding out any analysis of how Ming medicine was gendered.

Beyond this, the topic of female healers offers further perspective on how gender intersected with class and kinship in shaping Ming medical culture. First, the female healer contributed to medical pluralism. As the cultural ideal of the literati doctor gained ground in the Yuan and Ming dynasties, medical practitioners became a more internally stratified vocational group. Female healers, along with a variety of ritual practitioners, experts in acupuncture and moxibustion, or specialists in external medicine (*waike*), provide a lens on how class stratification of medicine shaped the diversity of medical knowledge and practice.

The female healer also highlights the role of the family in the production of medical knowledge for working physicians. If some medical men travelled to find masters and teachers with whom to apprentice, nonetheless the hereditary family practice was a standard organizing structure for the exercise of their craft. Here families performed functions that in a twentieth-century context would be thought of as public. As was the case in peasant farm families, the household mode of production made distinctions between inner and outer unlike those of the modern binary of public versus private domains. Applied to medical culture, the flexible and relational nature of Chinese inner and outer spheres produced a space for some women to function as medical workers within the family setting.[1] One preliminary survey of China's medical history before the twentieth century estimates that it preserves records on scarcely one hundred skilled female medical workers, or one-half of

---

1. For the relational nature of inner and outer and the "public" functions of families, see Ko 1994, Bray 1997.

one percent of the total number of doctors whose names are known.[2] If medically trained women were common in medical families, then, they appear to have been largely anonymous. Informal writings tell a slightly different story. In the Ming period, the many literati who complained about female healers—about their ignorance and their undue influence over their female clients—inadvertently painted a picture of a commonplace phenomenon tied to patterns of sex segregation in society at large. Where surviving texts construct female healers as either anonymous helpers or ignorant charlatans, these accounts show more than they say. Starting with the negative images in different genres of Ming literature, I explore both the power of such images to shape cultural subjects and the textual traces of alternative perspectives on female healers' lives and work.

Representing the Female Healer

In looking for the female healer, I start with the voices of suspicious scholars and physicians implying a vast gulf between reputable medicine and the nostrums proffered by women. A venerable cliché warned Ming gentlemen against visits to their women's quarters by the "three kinds of old aunties and six kinds of old grannies" (*san gu liu po*). While the three aunties were religious specialists—diviners, or Buddhist and Daoist nuns—three of the mercenary "six grannies" offered medical services: shaman healers (*shi po*), medicine sellers (*yao po*) and midwives (*wen po*).[3] Angela Leung has traced the textual history of these stereotypes back past the Yuan-era essayist Tao Zongyi (c. 1316–1402), who made the saying famous, to late Song moralists like Yuan Cai and Li Yuanbi, who wrote in support of emerging neo-Confucian ideals of female seclusion. By the fourteenth century, the classification of the three aunties and six grannies had become fixed on three groups: religious women, brokers and traders (including matchmakers), and female healers. The common ground was that all were lower class outsiders who visited gentry homes to provide services to house-bound women.[4]

2. See Zheng Jinsheng 1996.
3. Tao Zongyi, juan 10, 12a.
4. See Leung 1996. I am grateful to Angela Leung for sharing her unpublished research with me.

The stereotype of the six grannies was originally the creation of scholars and officials, not physicians. However, by the late Ming, doctors and
laymen alike appealed to it in criticizing the practices of female healers.
Take, for example, the pen portrait of "medical grannies" (*yi po, yi fu*)
by Xiao Jing, an early seventeenth-century physician from Fujian:

> There are many fools and idiots in the world who entrust the lives of
> their wives and concubines, sons and daughters, to the hands of medical
> grannies [*yi po*]. Myriads are damaged by their treatments. Even males
> who doctor for a living are often ignorant quacks. How much more is
> this the case with women whose eyes can't recognize the simplest ideo-
> graph and whose hands are ignorant of pulse diagnosis! They rely on
> artful talk, take pride in their fine skirts and jewelry, while on their middle
> finger they wear a knife[5] with which to wreck hidden damage in binding
> feet and piercing ears. How is it that everyone endures shrews like these?
>
> But they say of themselves that their medicines are efficacious for pro-
> curing abortions, so that every day matrons and wives who have lost all
> sense of decency believe in their wiles. Of dark and hidden [arts] there
> is nothing they won't do. This is why our forebears in composing house-
> hold admonitions warned that the six kinds of old grannies should not
> enter the gates.[6]

If this complaint comes from a doctor appalled by the low level of
medical practice in his native Fujian, similar opinions were voiced by
Lü Kun, an eminent scholar whose writings on statecraft were models
of late Ming official reform ideology. To hear him tell it, the medical
care of women and children was virtually monopolized by low-level
female healers, with disastrous results:

> Female doctors [*nü yi*] and female shaman healers [*shi po*] without the
> slightest iota of enlightenment all buy low-grade, worthless pills and
> powders from quack physicians, without even asking what disorders they
> cure. Sick women and children first seek out this sort of person. They
> knead here and pinch there; they apply needles and moxa at random;
> when their patients are past curing with medicines, they pull off the
> cupping jars [*huo guan*] and beat the exposed veins [*qing jin*], sending
> their ghosts off to the ancestors.[7] As for midwives ignorant of proper

---

5. Probably a sharpened fingernail used in minor surgeries. Such fingernails were
used in some cataract surgeries, and were observed on midwives by nineteenth-
century medical missionaries.

6. Xiao Jing, juan 6, 13a*n*b.

7. This describes last-ditch popular remedies. The cupping jar is for moxibustion,
and when this fails the healer beats on the exposed veins that are surface manifestations of the circulation channels.

techniques and those who treat children's poxes and feverish rashes with needles' pricking—mistreating the living and risking their lives—their crimes are particularly numerous.[8]

Another well-known official, Huang Liuhong, the seventeenth-century author of a magistrate's handbook, took particular aim at midwives, urging that gentrymen restrict their access to the inner quarters when their specific services were not needed.[9] A final example comes from Weng Zhongren, a sixteenth-century pediatric specialist from Jiangxi who scolded families for turning to women who treated pediatric Fright syndromes with massage or, worse, painful acupuncture: "I ask these evil women. . . . Who was your teacher? What tradition do you follow? They say nothing of repletion or depletion, Hot or Cold, but recklessly stick needles anywhere in the body where they will do most harm."[10]

In these complaints learned physicians were contemplating their lower class competitors; patriarchs were deploring the activities of women unbounded by family authority who had power over the reproductive bodies of their wives; officials were lamenting the toll of epidemic disease and the decline of state medical institutions since the Song. Lü Kun and Huang Liuhong took special aim at midwives, and it is easy to see how midwifery, as a medical skill essential to virtually every household, could be seen as a wedge that opened upper class doors to lower class women healers, and reproductive technologies to transgressive female uses. However, these scholarly voices were not just talking about midwives or religious ritualists. The female healer might be a pediatrician, a masseuse, one involved in cosmetic surgeries (which here includes footbinding), one skilled in acupuncture and moxibustion, or a dispenser of a wide range of ready-made medicines. Though they all insisted on her ignorance, these literati also revealed that medicine was a livelihood for her. Lü Kun spoke of the "medicine granny" as part of the extensive drug trade that linked male doctors and city shops with networks of itinerants plying the lanes and alleys of populous towns and villages. Weng Zhongren, on the other hand, portrayed a humble healer of sick children who instead of pharmacists' herbs offered cheaper alter-

8. Lü Kun, juan 2, 51*an*b.

9. Huang Liuhong, juan 31, 11. My thanks to Kenneth Pomerantz for providing this reference.

10. Weng Zhongren, juan 3, 5*an*6b. Symptoms of Fright in children ranged from mild fretfulness and crying to convulsions and high fever. Weng was concerned about misdiagnosis of early stages of smallpox.

natives, acupuncture and massage. He scolded parents for avoiding expense, claiming that quality herbal prescriptions were cheaper in the long run. All of this suggests the economic stake learned doctors had in promoting classical materia medica, as well as the collaboration of some of them in the dispensing of simpler, standard prescriptions in ready-made forms.

Female healers appeared in Ming texts, then, when gentlemen, whether scholars or doctors, considered the world of popular medicine and worried about it as cut-rate competition or as a debasement of the healing art. As a reformer hoping to revive state-supervised medical education, Lü Kun called attention to the vast bulk of local practitioners who were either marginally literate (qualified, he thought, to dispense "standard prescriptions") or totally untutored (who ought to be allowed to offer only external plasters or local fresh herbs). In calling for the education of these by means of simple texts and verses, he proposed that "men and women without distinction" be evaluated for medical literacy by a medical examiner and assigned as qualified for one of three grades of practice. But his more detailed recommendations envisioned a separate track for female healers: "Doctors should personally teach their wives about childbirth, menstruation, smallpox, [pediatric] Fright-Wind, et cetera, and their prescriptions. Female shaman healers [*shi po*] and such can receive instruction from the doctors' wives. But in difficult cases [they] must ask for advice from learned physicians. If women do not study or ask but practice medicine on their own, their husbands should be punished and the women beaten."[11] Here female healers were distributed among other itinerants, peddlers, ritualists and semiliterate purveyors of ready-made powders, pills and plasters who crowded the lower rungs of medicine as commerce. Having accepted plebeian female healers as socially essential, Lü Kun hoped to subordinate them to male authority, mediated through their female superiors in class and education—that is, wives in learned medical families.

Such female healers were represented as lower class providers of services to women and children, but not necessarily as midwives or specialists in *fuke*. But whatever functions they performed, female healers were rhetorically lumped together as grannies (*po*) or given other familiar names like "old lady" (*lao guniang*) or "old woman" (*lao wen*). Such colloquialisms named her social place as plebeian and her skills as

---

11. Lü Kun, juan 6, 62a. There is no evidence that reforms like these were ever implemented. See also Leung 1987.

rudimentary, and inasmuch as they also named her person as undignified, they denied her the respect Confucianism accords old age as well. Looking for the female healer, one first finds the stereotype of the medical "granny."

Granny or Doctor?
Traces of the Female Healer

In the late Ming opera *The Swallow's Letter,* the comic character who serves as go-between for the love affair of the hero and heroine is named Mama Meng, a medical granny whose specialty is diseases of females (*nüke yi po*). Summoned to see the heroine by her mother, Mama Meng is addressed politely as *xiansheng* (literally, teacher), while she in turn courteously asks permission to touch the girl's hand: "Miss will be angry at my forwardness, but allow me to take your pulse." Her diagnosis: "You suffer from depletion and nerves [*xu qie*], you fear Wind, in the afternoon your whole body feels hot, your affliction is Heart palpitations [*zheng chong*]."[12] Even as this diagnosis shrewdly supports the narrative theme of the heroine's lovesickness, it is classically orthodox, based on a diagnostic syndrome from the *Inner Canon.*[13] Her prescription, made up out of her medicine sack, is an infusion of three pieces of ginger and four jujube dates—a simple combination of ingredients to warm and move *qi* and to strengthen and nourish Blood. Later Mama Meng discusses the case privately with the girl's maid to ask what might lie behind the sufferer's "stasis from worry" (*si yu*), also a syndrome often associated with frustrated desires.[14] Although Mama Meng is a comic figure—fat, humpbacked, with big feet—and for Ming audiences some of the comedy may have derived from the sight of a woman parodying male medical conventions, nonetheless in the story she is shown winning male approval. The heroine's father, on returning home, sends the woman doctor (*nü yi*) a silver tael on account for future treatments.

12. Ruan Dacheng (1587–1646), 30–31.

13. *Zheng chong,* from the *Su wen,* named symptoms of rapid beating heart, with or without feelings of anxiety or fright. *Qie,* translated here as "nerves," also had medical associations with lung disease, as in *qie fei.*

14. See for example Jiang Guan, 344, where the editor warns against a superficial diagnosis of static disorder in young people lacking mates who have symptoms of hot and cold spells and "tense" readings of the pulse at the Liver position. A more subtle pulse diagnosis may reveal yin depletion heat, he says.

A more famous literary representation of a granny healer is Liu Pozi (Old Woman Liu) in the novel *Plum in the Golden Vase (Jin ping mei)*. This story of a rich rake's progress to self-destruction is enmeshed in an engrossing tapestry of late sixteenth-century city life, among prosperous merchants and low-level officials not unlike the milieu of Cheng Mao-xian's medical practice in Yangzhou. The illusion of everyday reality constructed by the anonymous author's "fine needlework and dense texture" makes the novel not only a literary masterpiece but also a guide to many aspects of late Ming social life that historical actors took for granted.[15] The hero, Ximen Qing, presides over a polygamous household where his many wives clearly prefer a healing woman to the classically trained male doctors who consort with their husband. Although Old Woman Liu is not called "doctor" (*yi*) or given any respectful title, she treats a variety of ailments of both the women and the children of the household. When a concubine, Gold Lotus, suffers from jealousy, leading to loss of appetite, headache and nausea, Liu offers a "black pill" to be taken with ginger broth at night. She is valued for her use of acupuncture for headaches. When the first wife, Moon Lady, suffers belly pain and bleeding, signalling a threatened miscarriage, she offers two "big black pills," which successfully abort the fetus.[16]

But the more complex passages show her attending a third wife's baby, Guan Ge, who is afflicted with Fright-Wind (*jingfeng*), a broad pediatric syndrome characterized by rapidly moving symptoms ranging from fretful crying and refusal to nurse to high fever with convulsions. When the infant cries all night, she prescribes an infusion of bog rush (*dengxincao*) and field mint (*bohe*), mild cooling ingredients recommended to clear the heat of children's Fright, to which she adds two doses of strongly cooling cinnabar pills (*zhusha*). Later, when the illness returns more violently, with raging heat and convulsions, she adjusts this formula to make it stronger, adding honeysuckle (*jinyinhua*) to the cooling infusion and lacing it with a Gold Foil pill (*jinbo*), a powerful mineral drug believed to "calm psyche" (*an shen*) in cases of madness and recommended for pediatric "fits" (*jing*). When this last tonic fails, reluctantly she turns to moxibustion as an emergency measure. She

15. Anon., *Jin ping mei*, 1618. There are three variant texts of this classic that circulated in manuscript among many literati in the Wanli era. Although the novel is ostensibly set in Shandong, scholars trying to date it and identify its author stress its cosmopolitan qualities and reject the notion that it is either a simple novel of manners or one bounded by regional horizons. For the phrase "fine needlework and dense texture," from the introduction to the third seventeenth-century edition, see Plaks 1987: 86.

16. *Jin ping mei*, vol. 1, 155, 428.

shows a proper appreciation of its risks, asking the senior wife, Moon Lady, to get the Master's permission before trying this. Although the novel appeals to its readership's suspicion of moxibustion—the treatment possibly "drove the pathogens within and transformed the illness into a case of slow Fright [*man jing*]"—for the time being the acute symptoms abated.[17]

Although the master of the house calls Liu an "old whore sticking needles and moxa everywhere" and threatens to haul her into court if the baby dies, in fact baby Guan Ge is doomed not by the doctors but by Gold Lotus, the malicious concubine who is jealous of her rival's fertility and provokes the child, literally frightening him to death. Old Woman Liu is not shown to be literate, but she uses pulse diagnosis as well as moxibustion and acupuncture. Moreover, her prescriptions are reasonable by Ming pediatric standards.[18] An eyebrow note suggests that Ming readers were most dubious about her use of abortifacients on Moon Lady's pregnancy, because a proper doctor's priority should be to "tranquilize the fetus" (*an tai*).[19] However, from another perspective, she put the health of the mother first, a choice that case histories like those of Cheng Maoxian show could also be made by elite male doctors.

The Plum in the Golden Vase also allows a further look at the gendering of family authority in medical matters. In the case of baby Guan Ge, the Master, Ximen Qing, faces resistance from the child's mother and other household women to his call for a "pediatric specialist," even when the illness is serious. However, he quite easily takes charge when Vase Lady, his favorite wife and baby Guan Ge's mother, fails to recover normally from her postpartum disorder, and again when she becomes seriously ill. He prefers the literati Doctor Ren, who, like Cheng Maoxian, addresses all of his questions and comments to the husband, only asking politely for permission to observe the lady's facial appearance as well as take her pulse. In this fictional world, male authority is weakest where women's ordinary illnesses and those of children are concerned, but more prestigious male doctors are looked to for emergencies.

But as Vase Lady's sickness becomes grave, Ximen Qing follows the advice of assorted friends and clients to bring into the house a succession of increasingly dubious quacks. These are all male, culminating in Dr.

17. *Jin ping mei*, vol 1, 618.
18. This and related points are discussed in Cullen 1993: 99–150.
19. This is made clear in an eyebrow note to the passage in the second Ming edition, vol. 1, 428.

Chao, described as a *fuke* specialist from "outside the city wall," who is not only unable to tell whether his client is pregnant or postpartum, but who is also portrayed as an abortionist. As death approaches, doctors of pharmacy withdraw, giving way to ritualists, and in the democracy of extremity Ximen calls for a diviner and for Daoist and Buddhist clergy, while a nun visits Vase Lady's bed-chamber. Old Woman Liu here shows herself conversant with the female shamans who perform the dance of soul summons (*tiao shen*) and is able to carry out the ritual herself.[20]

These literary narratives of female healers show women from humble backgrounds as they appeared from the point of view of elite male householders—outsiders intruding into the privileged domestic space of the gentry "inner quarters," now comical, now forward or subtly subversive. Evidence of the skills these women commanded is indirect or inadvertent. Local histories, a genre sponsored by local magistrates, also occasionally mentioned itinerant or sojourning women healers. Such narratives were also produced by literati, but they had other aims—to promote social stability and local pride by commemorating remarkable people and happenings. Here favorable comment on a female healer's abilities was not out of place.

The local history of Kunshan and Xinyang counties in seventeenth-century Jiangsu found a medical granny among the locality's chaste widows. Mistress Xu, daughter of doctors, had learned as a child to "[chant] rhymes on pulses and medicines" and was especially good at pediatrics. Widowed at twenty after two years of marriage, she survived her parents-in-law, daughter, foster daughter and adopted son-in-law and made a living in old age by selling drugs.[21] Implied in this narrative of dutiful service is that her medical skills supported these dependents. From Shaanxi comes a tale of a Mistress Han, who "travelled throughout the district practicing medical arts." Known for her skill with cases of throat blockage (*yi*), she saved the life of the magistrate's mother by removing an impediment from her throat as follows: "She boiled [numbing] pepper flower in water and had her patient rinse her mouth with this several times. She took a six-sided white stone about three inches long and marked it with a faint red line like a thread, and placed it in the patient's mouth. Telling her to swallow her saliva, with fingers she massaged the

20. *Jin ping mei*, vol. 2, chapters 54–61.

21. See *Guangxu Kun-Hsin liang xian xu xiu he zhi*, juan 38, 5a. My thanks to Ann Waltner for providing me with this reference.

outside of the throat, while with chopsticks she held the lips open and slowly pulled out a long piece of flesh wriggling like a snake." The grateful magistrate had a stone tablet carved recording her miraculous cure, and so she passed into history.[22]

A final glimpse of the Ming medical granny is supplied by scattered stories told of healers who were summoned to court to attend to palace women. Having forbidden male doctors to visit the inner quarters, the Ming emperors arranged for female healers to be selected as qualified for such service. In the early Ming, some palace maids were chosen for medical training. Shen Bang, a late Ming official who participated in selecting candidates from his district on the western edge of Beijing, left a memoir of the system as he saw it in the late sixteenth century. The three grannies—doctors (*yi po*), midwives (*wen po*) and wet nurses (*nai po*)—were selected from the local population. The wet nurses came from the families of military men posted in or near the capital, and the midwives were "experienced" local practitioners. All three groups were supervised by a palace bureau called, rather grandiosely, the Lodge of Ritual and Ceremony (*Li yi fang*). In fact, both midwives and female doctors lived and worked among the commoners of the capital city when they were not on an imperial case. Qualifications for doctors, unlike those for midwives, were thought measurable by examination. Shen reported how impressed he was with one candidate: "She was barely fifteen or sixteen years old, yet when examined on the vocation of medicine, her responses all were in good order; as good as the great specialists in prescription and pulse diagnosis." However, this young woman apparently was examined on vocational skill (*ye*), not medical learning (*xue*), while as a group the women doctors of the palace were still lumped together with midwives and baby nurses as grannies. Shen called them all "vulgar common housewives" (*chunran pifu*) and cautioned that they should be prevented from taking material advantage of their access to an exalted clientele.[23]

A bit of literary gossip about the court of the Wanli emperor shows another palace "medical woman" as just such an unscrupulous opportunist. Mistress Peng was summoned to court to treat the empress for a chronic eye ailment. Being "a great talker and wit who could tell stories of goings-on in town and courtyard," she stayed on as a palace favorite. But she was discovered by palace women to be pregnant, and when she

---

22. See the *Shaanxi tong zhi*, as reprinted in the SKQS, vol. 547:562.
23. Shen Bang, 76–77. See also Cass 1986.

gave birth the fact became known to all. The empress not only had to dismiss her but barely managed to save her from an imperial decree of execution.[24]

Finally, medical annals of curious and amazing cures occasionally praised old country women and medicine grannies (*yao po*) who showed uncanny knowledge of the therapeutic resources of field, marsh or mountain. There was the old woman drug seller (*mai yao lao wen*) who cured purulent weeping eyes with juice of wild raspberry leaves gathered by the roadside.[25] There was the village granny (*cun wen*) who concocted a toothache remedy from silk melon.[26] There was the old granny (*lao wen*) who, even though she baldly demanded money for her pains, impressed Xue Ji when she used a spindle to lance and medicate a *luoli* swelling, applying her poultice to its root twice until the tumor melted away.[27] Such tales evoke the medical granny in the archetypical form of village wise woman or witch.

The stereotype of the female medical worker as a granny constructed a common textual subject, in spite of differences in their skills, activities and clients. What was foregrounded was the gender and age of all women claiming healing expertise. But one other thing that all medical grannies had in common was physical mobility. Where fictional representations show medical women visiting rich homes as service providers, memoirs and local histories show more of their diverse lives beyond the household gates, marked by travel, economic responsibility or hardship, and even a measure of personal freedom. The skills claimed for these healers were diverse, ranging from the simple gathering of fresh herbs by a rural purveyor to the orthodox techniques of pulse-taking and prescription expected of a woman "doctor" at court.

But often a female healer attracted attention because of some work of her hands. When she practiced moxibustion and acupuncture, comment was likely to be unfavorable, showing the declining status of these techniques in late imperial society.[28] When she was praised for the minor

---

24. Shen Defu, juan 23.

25. See Jiang Guan, 202. The herb in question is *fupenzi*, identified in *bencao* as a cure for blindness and tearing of the eyes.

26. Wei Zhixiu, 433.

27. This case is from Xue Ji's volume on *waike*, as reported in He Shixi 1983: 203–4. Xue Ji commented that he thought the treatment worked because the case was not one of internal depletion. For more on *luoli* swellings, considered signs of grave illness, see below, note 56.

28. For a late Ming comment on the decline of acupuncture, see Xie Zhaozhe, juan 5, 134. See also Chao 1995: 288–91; Leung 1997.

surgeries of external medicine (*waike*) or for the treatment of eye ailments, she was also identified with manual skills[29] and with common itinerant or village sorts of practice — a domain little favored among Ming learned doctors, being less influenced by theory or canon and less bound up in the lucrative economics of pharmacy.

In sum, female healers appear to have had eclectic skills, and though their clients were usually identified as female, the range of services they offered was defined more by class than by gender. The lowest class of granny healer, then, instead of providing herbal formulas for female complaints to the wives of the gentry, more likely was someone trudging the lanes of towns and villages, peddling inexpensive remedies for the miseries of the poor. If healing herbs were the specialty of a male medical elite fastidious about physical contact, the granny's healing hands were a tactile balm, an intimate, familiar medicine of the body. If occasional narratives survive that reveal a granny's command of more prestigious techniques of pharmacy and diagnosis, nonetheless the granny image colored Ming popular constructions of female healers of all kinds, whatever their skills or experience.

Midwives

In labelling a female healer as a "granny," Ming rhetoric associated her with the quintessential granny healer, the midwife. Midwives embodied all that was transgressive and threatening about female healers in male gentry eyes: their independence and mobility, their indispensability, their knowledge of the sexual body. In the Ming, midwifery was also a skill set apart from the rest of medicine. If many midwives appear in the annals of Song medicine as simple "birth attendants," some were also called "doctor" like their male fellow healers. In Ming texts the nomenclature shifted: some female doctors were also called "granny," but no midwife was named as a kind of "doctor" like the old *ru yi*. Beyond the fragments in Chen Ziming and other works of Song *chanke,* nothing suggests that midwifery was ever taught or learned through written materials. Thus, in looking for the Ming midwife, I find her in stereotyped literary portraits or in the narratives of male doctors trying to advise clients on how to manage and use her.

In *Plum in the Golden Vase,* Old Woman Liu is an ambivalent per-

---

29. Eye specialists commonly removed cataracts with a sharpened fingernail. Mistress Peng may have had this skill.

sonage, shown in the story to be distrusted by the men but essential to the women. However, Mistress Cai, the midwife who delivers baby Guan Ge, is the object of the author's mockery. Breaking off the prose narrative of events, the author presents midwife Cai with a song:

> Here I am, Mistress Cai the midwife
> My pair of feet both quick and light
> My fancy gown of green and red
> A stylish chignon astride my head
> Flashing my bracelets filigree
> Waving my kerchief of yellow moiré
> Arriving, I deftly pocket the red-flower tip
> Sitting down, I am ready to take charge of the ship.
> Ladies fine of mansions noble—
> Yea, princesses of palace regal—
> I teach them willy-nilly the basic things a woman knows
> I make them disrobe and strip off their clothes
> For broadsided births I wield my knife dandily
> For doleful labor I massage her most handily
> As for placenta or cord just never you mind
> Breaking them off, I use hands to untwine.
> If they live we'll celebrate and I'll collect my fee
> If they die you can bet you've seen the last of me.[30]

A ditty like this could easily have served as an aria introducing a comic character in an opera. In displaying the author's well-known love of theater and gift for pastiche, it reveals some essentials of the midwife's craft—the technology of "clever hands" in massage and in manual manipulation of abnormal presentations, the crude surgeries that were sometimes resorted to. It criticizes the surgical dismemberment of fetuses in cases of "broadside" transverse presentation (*heng chan*) and shows awareness of common problems of undescended placenta or tangled umbilical cord, and of controversies over the wisdom of manual intervention at these times. It also suggests that, like Taiwanese custom through much of the twentieth century, most women's childbirth education took place in the birthing room itself, making the midwife the custodian of body knowledge preparing the rite of passage into motherhood.

The midwife's song is also a cartoon portrait of a woman who doesn't know her place: self-important, overdressed and overconfident. She may be wearing the cast-off finery of her wealthy clients that she has received

---

30. The song is omitted from the second Ming (Chongzhen) edition. See *Jin ping mei cihua*, Wanli edition, juan 30.

in payment. She is too quick on her feet to be respectably footbound, too ready with her tongue to be properly deferential. This picture of female brazenness also rhetorically alludes to her power to reduce the eroticized bodies of elegant ladies to struggling flesh given over to labor and suffering. *Plum in the Golden Vase*'s song of the midwife constructs a popular social stereotype. Doctors of the late Ming, on the other hand, continued like their Song predecessors to waver between casual accounts of midwives as fellow healers and experts in a necessary separate sphere, and didactic prose that tried to supervise and correct them from a distance. In the *fuke* of the family tradition of Wan Quan, the reliable experienced midwife was recommended as the expert, contrasted with ritualists and their prayers and prognostications on the one hand or neighborhood busybodies with their gossip and alarms on the other. "As for breach births, transverse presentations, and rear-facing heads, these are extremely dangerous. If this happens only a good midwife may be able to manage it safely; it is beyond the power of the doctors' medicine."[31] *To Benefit Yin* was content to repeat the standard advice of Chen Ziming and others concerning selection of a capable birth attendant, but Wang Qi in his eyebrow notes praised the manual techniques of good midwives, including, for example, their art in adjusting fetal position to relieve urinary blockage in late pregnancy.[32]

Xue Ji's case histories suggest that he knew and talked with midwives as fellow healers with expertise to share. He told of one who consulted him when her own daughter miscarried.[33] He passed on advice they gave on handling a retained placenta (give *yimucao* pills; try making her gag on a ball of her own hair).[34] Another of his stories, repeated by Wu Zhiwang and others, was of a midwife who confided in him about using her skill to get revenge on an overbearing employer:

A midwife told me, "I have only one daughter. Just when she was in labor with child, it happened that runners from the Attendant Censor came with a placard to summon me to his wife's lying-in. Because of her fright [at the summons] my daughter died before she was delivered. Later, when I saw the Censor, he was even more severe in his commands. His wife's labor was not a difficult one, but the child's head was turned

---

31. Wan Quan, *Wan shi furen ke*, 35.

32. *Ji yin gangmu*, Wang Qi ed., juan 9, 322–23; juan 10, 352–53, 366. Commenting on a prescription formula for "transverse presentation with hand or foot protruding," Wang Qi said, "techniques of massage are even better."

33. See Xue Ji, in ZGYXDC 5:602.

34. From a case of Xue's, quoted in *Ji yin gangmu*, Wang Qi ed., juan 11, 384.

to one side. Fearing his wrath, I did not dare use my hands, and so neither mother nor child could be saved."[35]

To Xue the moral of this story was that prudent families should cultivate the goodwill of these vital service providers. Such stories show that Ming doctors sometimes recognized midwifery as not only necessary but as a skill entitled to respect.

But such tales also call attention to the midwife's unnerving combination of informal power and low social position. The commonplace medical and literati rhetoric about the interventionist midwife was one way this tension was expressed. On the one hand, such rhetoric could be read as a matter of reasonable clinical judgment. Since male doctors were likely to be summoned to cases of childbirth, if at all, after something had gone wrong, they easily blamed difficult births on midwives' errors. Believing that the infant "turns around" to lie head downward in the womb at the last minute, doctors imagined that this natural process was interrupted if a midwife instructed her client to assume the squatting birth position and "labor" too soon. The subsequent crises were blamed on meddling hands. Clinical judgments of the midwife as rash and hasty interventionist fit comfortably with the literary representation of her as self-important hussy. Where art portrayed her as vulgar, science spoke of her aggressive management and crude technology.

This construction set the stage for additional ways in which midwives were identified with the negative and material aspects of birth, and with society's dirty work related to the physical body. Midwives had to deal with the fetal waste of miscarriages, abortions and stillbirths. They were the outsiders present when families decided a newborn should not live. As an extension of this, because midwives were normally charged with the job of disposing of the byproducts of birth, including the ritual burial of the placenta, they were presumed to be the main traffickers in these body parts, which were deemed magically potent medicines. In *Plum in the Golden Vase,* such traffic was portrayed as immoral, benefiting seekers of fertility charms while flouting ritual and injuring the persons of mother and child to whom placenta and umbilicus intimately "belonged."[36] The essayist Xie Zhaozhe associated the immorality with

35. Xue Ji, in ZGYXDC 5:599–600.

36. In *Jin ping mei* Moon Lady is given ash of umbilicus in filtered wine to expel bad Blood after her miscarriage. Later Nun Xue offers to provide her with a fertility charm that requires the placenta of a first-born child — a hard-to-find ingredient she will try to obtain from a midwife.

the folly of wealthy people who would pay as much as "a thousand *qian*" for a pill of Purple River Cart, hoping to strengthen their yang and replenish *qi* and Blood. When they bribed midwives to procure the ingredients they turned venal old women into thieves, he said. As a result, middle class and rich families "guard against midwives as they would against robbers."[37] However, since umbilical cord and Purple River Cart were valued as yang replenishers in Ming pharmacy—and were ingredients in the widely recommended Great Creation pill (*Dazao wan*) for postpartum and in "light pox" remedies for newborns, among others— the commerce in them must have been considerable. In other contexts, literati doctors like Li Shizhen, Wu Zhiwang and Wang Qi recommended such medicines.[38]

On the lowest level of society, the expertise of the midwife was called upon to deal with the abnormal and the criminal body. In the eyes of the law, they were deemed experts on the physical aspects of sex. Legal records and fictional accounts alike show court officers calling on them in rape cases, or when a woman's virginity was in question. Since midwives were the ones who determined a baby's sex at birth, they were the law's experts on genital normality and sexual identity in the rare cases when this was held to be physically in doubt. Magistrates, although responsible for supervising criminal cases, were not expected to have contact with the bodies of the dead. The matrons who assisted coroners in handling and examining female corpses were called "midwife," as were those who dealt with female prisoners.[39] In sum, a variety of stigmatized aspects of the female and sexual body were believed to be appropriately the domain of these most ambiguous of the medical "grannies." In such circumstances, it is not so surprising that midwives were often mentioned side by side with marriage brokers, or that it is said that in eighteenth-century Jiangnan, midwifery was one of the specialties of descendants of the region's Yue, its outcast "mean people."[40]

In sum, as technologists of the dangerous and dirty passages of birth,

---

37. Xie Zhaozhe, juan 5, 118–19.

38. See Li Zhizhen, *Bencao gangmu* 4:2962. Li was repulsed by the custom reported from the far south where new mothers cooked and ate their infants' fresh placentas, but he did not object to it as a dried and processed ingredient. Dried placenta is still used in Chinese medicine today, supplied by hospitals. (Zhang Jingli, personal communication.)

39. See Leung 1996: 12–13; Sommer 1994: 66–67, 72; Furth 1988: 22. The term *wen po* for a coroner's aid may have been pronounced as *ao po* (*ao* = old woman).

40. Naquin and Rawski 1987: 148.

Ming midwives were somewhat set apart from other female healers as well as from males expert in medicine. Just as the gestational body in some ways did not easily harmonize with the body of medical theory, so the midwife appeared to be something of an outsider among healers. In this light, it is easier to understand why seventeenth-century medical families might have found it difficult to take up Lü Kun's call to improve women's medical care by training the wives of elite doctors to become expert in this function. In the socially differentiated world of Ming medicine, women in medical families with access to classical skills found their niches elsewhere.

In fact, medical interest in obstetrics picked up in the eighteenth century, but took a different direction. It did not produce a movement for the learned reform of midwifery, nor did man-midwives and obstetricians begin to compete successfully with female midwives, as happened in eighteenth-century Europe. Instead, doctors and literati promoted maternal self-education, hand in hand with an increased emphasis upon natural childbirth—that is, childbirth as best experienced with a minimum of either pharmaceutical or manual intervention. Where a mid-Ming doctor like Wan Quan preferred the skilled midwife to the birthing-room ritualist, Qing medical reformers gave instructions on labor that stressed a woman's own somatic sensations as the best guide to its timing, coupled with exhortations to self-discipline and fortitude. Childbirth here was subtly moralized as a test of a woman's spiritual temper and strength of character, while self-education was to equip her (and her husband) to remain at all times the midwife's mistress. In the last years of the Ming dynasty, the learned medical innovator Zhang Jiebin anticipated the new themes, evoking traditional imagery of birth as a natural event—"when the blossom is full and the melon is round, they drop of their own accord." Counseling family supervision of birth attendants, he warned that midwives "may make heavy work of light tasks to inflate their own importance, hoping for rewards."[41] Later, in the eighteenth century, popular publishing on obstetrics became a new fashion, and these themes were echoed in printed texts addressed to literate householders, male and female alike. As gentry were exhorted to take the supervision of childbirth into their own hands, rhetoric concerning the dangers of ignorant midwifery grew even more strident.[42]

41. Zhang Jiebin, *Furen gui*, 207–8.
42. This movement began with publication of *Da sheng bian* (On Successful Childbirth) by an anonymous literatus in 1715. It was widely reprinted, and later Qing

Female Healing in Medical Lineages

What both literary and historical narratives show, as seen from inside or outside respectively, are women as medical workers crossing boundaries that normatively kept women in the domestic enclosure. Medical grannies and midwives are shown in other people's families, not their own. However, Lü Kun's proposal that doctors teach their wives to serve female clients and to instruct lower class women practitioners points back to medical families as a site of transmission of medical knowledge across gender boundaries. Such families were not only places where male healers could gain some knowledge of gestational functions from their wives, as Cheng Maoxian did. They also allowed some women healers to protect their social reputations as they harmonized domestic and public roles. Mistress Xu, the chaste widow who had learned medicine at home as a child, showed that a commoner's practice of medicine as a trade was not in principle incompatible with female virtue. While Mistress Peng, the eye doctor, caused scandal at court, a Mistress Lu, wife of a man himself in imperial medical service, had served honorably in the palace of the Yongle emperor (1403–1424) until retiring to her home district.[43] Other stories told of virtuous daughters who assisted their famous physician fathers in medical scholarship. A niece helped Yu Chang to compile his collection of case histories, completed in 1643 — a task often placed in the hands of medical disciples.[44] Zhou Rongqi's two daughters, Hu ("Blessed by Heaven") and Xi ("Blessed by the Gods"), did the colored drawings for his illustrated text on materia medica, which survives today as an example of fine Ming block printing.[45] When Wang Zhu, an eighteenth-century physician from Jiading, went blind, he apprenticed his daughter Wang Hengqi as his assistant.[46]

More significant, perhaps, than these cultured daughters seen in roles of filial service are examples of medical lineages that could have been models for Lü Kun's reforms. Here mother-in-law collaborated with

---

scholars talked of the Four Books on childbirth, all dating from the eighteenth century. See Furth 1987; Ma Dazheng 1991: 252–53.

43. Reported in the *Wuxi xian zhi*. Her husband's name was Xu Mengrong.

44. Yu Chang, *Yu Jiayan yixue san shu*. See the editor's biographical introduction to the 1984 reprint.

45. Zhou's *Bencao tupu* is held in the rare book library of the Zhongyi Yanjiuyuan in Beijing.

46. He Shixi 1991, 1:32.

daughter-in-law. One pair, from Haining county in Zhejiang, was associated with the famous Guo medical lineage, which traced its ancestry back to palace specialists in *fuke* of the Song dynasty. Like his ancestor Guo Jingzhong, who had tended palace women together with his mother, Mistress Wang, Guo Wan in the late seventeenth century practiced in collaboration with his mother, Mistress Wu, and his wife, Mistress Mao, who "were also good at pulse diagnosis and selecting medicines."[47] Earlier, in the late fifteenth century, the medical lineage established by Cheng Gongli (fl. 1464) in Xiuning, Anhui, included his son's wife, a Mistress Jiang, and *her* son's wife, Mistress Fang, to whom hundreds flocked for pediatric aid. Mistress Jiang is said to have once used surgery to save the life of an infant born without a rectal opening.[48] A saying praised Mistress Jiang and her daughter-in-law as follows: "Within they swept the courtyard clean, without they served with diagnostic skill." Other instances of the pattern of mother-in-law and daughter-in-law pairs have been noted by Zheng Jinsheng, who argues that families preferred to teach young wives instead of daughters who would marry out, perhaps taking the family medical secrets with them.[49] In sum, whether daughters, wives or mothers, these women had secure social identity within a family, to which their medical skills made an economic contribution. In this way some female healers might overcome the ambiguity of a vocational role that conflicted with the normal boundaries of neo-Confucian propriety. They were not midwives. They were not economic competitors to males but supporters of a family's productive endeavors. They may have been grandmothers, but such women were not "grannies."

Tan Yunxian:
A Female Doctor and Her Clients

These accounts of female healers in medical families tell almost nothing of what skills such women possessed or how their practice was conducted. In one case, from the mid-Ming, a woman of good family left an unusual written record of her life as a doctor.[50] Tan

---

47. Guo Aiqun 1984–87, 1:1108–9.
48. He Shixi 1991, 3:583; Liu and Gao 1982: 221.
49. Zheng Jinsheng 1996.
50. Tan Yunxian, author's preface 1511, reprinted 1585, *Nü yi zayan* (Sayings of a Female Doctor).

Yunxian (1461–1554) overcame the barriers both to learning medicine and to practicing it in her community, eventually becoming honored as a "famous doctor" (*ming yi*) and a source of pride to a gentry lineage. With a family background that included both physicians and officials, and as the author of her own collection of medical case histories, Tan was well qualified to be called a literati physician. At the same time her case history narratives of the clinical encounters between an elite woman healer and her clients show a style of practice that was quite distinct from those suggested by male-authored case history collections. (See figure 17.)

One key to Tan Yunxian's life was birth in a family that combined medicine and examination success. Her father, Tan Gang, was awarded a *jinshi* degree and became a successful official in Nanjing, and both her younger brother and nephew also eventually succeeded in the examinations and served as magistrates. However, her grandfather, Tan Fu, was a physician—a man who had entered the Wuxi medical lineage of one Huang Yuxian as an adopted son-in-law. His uxorilocal marriage to a medically accomplished physician's daughter was an example of one kind of marriage strategy in medical lineages. As Tan Gang left medicine behind for a more brilliant official career, his talented daughter studied with her grandparents, who were in charge of raising her. Tan Yunxian's recollection of this early education drew on familiar tropes about precocious brilliance in children:

> While my hair was still done up in tufts, I waited on my father. While he dined, I was ordered to sing seven-character line poems and to chant the *Classic of Filial Piety* and the teachings on female deportment. My grandfather laughed and said, "The girl is very clever, quite out of the ordinary. When she is grown she will be able to practice my medical arts." At that time I could memorize but I could not understand the import of the words. Later I studied the *Canon of Problems*, the *Canon of the Pulse*, and such day and night without rest. Then I asked Grandmother to explain the general meaning to me in her leisure moments, and suddenly I comprehended without difficulty.[51]

A second key to her life was the role of teaching and learning among women. Not only did Tan study medicine along approved literati lines, as if it were a form of classical scholarship, but the teaching passed from grandmother to granddaughter, following domestic patterns of female

51. Author's preface, dated 1511.

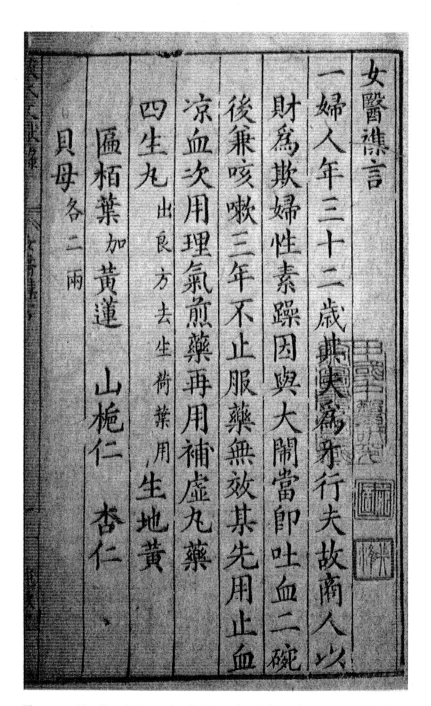

女醫譄言

一婦人年三十二歲典夫爲牙行夫故南人以

財爲欺婦性素躁因與大閙當卽吐血二碗

後兼咳嗽三年不止服藥無效其先用止血

涼血次用理氣煎藥再用補虛丸藥

四生丸 出良方去生荷葉用生地黃

區栢葉加黃連 山梔仁 杏仁

貝母各二兩

Figure 17. Tan Yunxian's casebook. Reproduced from the 1595 woodblock edition held in the rare book library of the Zhongyi Yanjiuyuan, Beijing.

education that Dorothy Ko has explored elsewhere. "Day and night they talked of nothing but medicine," recalled Tan's younger brother. The grandmother also checked Tan's diagnoses and prescriptions as she first applied her art to herself and her four children as a young mother. Through this long apprenticeship Tan moved gradually, as she said, from knowing "the import of the words" to understanding their use (*shi*) and finally to realizing the extent of medicine's efficacy (*yan*).

On the surface Tan Yunxian moved naturally from practicing medicine as a domestic skill in youth to a matronly calling of medicine as community service. However, Tan's autobiographical preface to her *Sayings of a Female Doctor* included hints of a critical moment of transition that marked her turn on an unconventional path. It coincided with her beloved grandmother's death:

> As Grandmother's end approached, she took her notebook of proven prescriptions and her apparatus for preparing medicines and personally gave them to me, saying, "Study these carefully: my eyes are dimming." Bowing, I received them, sorrowfully weeping. In the period of mourning I suffered a lingering illness for seven months. Privately, without me knowing it, my mother made financial arrangements for my death and burial. But in a confused dream Grandmother spoke to me, saying, "Your illness is not fatal. The prescription is in such and such a book on such and such a page. Follow it and in a few days you will be well. You will live to be seventy-three, and you will do great things, using my arts to save the sick without any misfortune." Affrighted, I awoke and rushed directly to prepare the prescription and was straightaway cured. Then I knew the extent of [medicine's] efficacy [*yan*].[52]

A life-threatening illness, a miraculous recovery, and a message from the spirit world beyond the grave explaining the import of this crisis — all these were signs of a special destiny awaiting her. By narrating such experiences, Tan showed how they shaped her own resolve, and, equally important, how they helped win society's acceptance. Modern anthropologists, looking at contemporary Taiwan and Korea, have traced a similar pattern of life crisis leading to supernatural visitations and blessings that empowered women to assume the identity of ritual healer in their communities.[53] Thus, although socially Tan Yunxian enjoyed high social rank (*ru ren*),[54] she claimed the legitimacy — necessity, even — of

---

52. Author's preface.

53. See Wolf 1992: 93–126; Kendall 1985: 57–61.

54. *Ru ren,* or "honored lady," was a title awarded wives and mothers of ranking civil servants.

her calling as a healer in a way that was probably familiar to women who became shamans.

It wasn't easy, then, for a woman like Tan Yunxian to become known as a doctor. Her relatively high social position helped her only after she had struggled successfully to break free in her middle years, when child-bearing was done and she was a matriarch commanding the obedience of her grown son. When she was fifty years old, her son dutifully carried out her order to publish *Sayings of a Female Doctor*, and two well con-nected kinsmen, both *jinshi*, wrote prefaces. Presented to the world as a work of charity, her book also appears as part of a campaign to estab-lish a reputation beyond question or reproach. When she died at ninety-three, people said that in her old age her cures were even more inspired than those recorded in her book. Even so, the text survived more because of a descendant's pious act of commemoration than as part of any med-ical lineage of transmission. As an author Tan was standing in for her son and grandson, whose deaths had cut off the family's ancestral al-tars.[55]

The thirty-one cases recorded in *Sayings of a Female Doctor* reveal an eclectic style of practice, mingling the pharmacy of internal medicine of the literati physician with manual technologies associated with the granny healer. Her clients, their disorders, and the social organization of her clinical work were also distinctive. She herself offered a point of departure when she said in her autobiographical preface that "family members and women friends and acquaintances, disliking to be treated by a male, came streaming to me, and over time I hit upon amazing cures, amounting to quite a number." Not only was her practice con-fined to women, but her clients came to her; she did not normally travel abroad to see the sick. Other special features of her case histories fol-lowed from this. Only one of her thirty-one cases involved a life-threatening medical emergency where a sufferer was too sick to move. None involved the sort of acute Cold Damage fevers that were the staple of Cheng Maoxian's practice and those of many other eminent male physicians. Instead, Tan Yunxian wrote about women with chronic complaints. Some had suffered for months or years from the gestational problems of *fuke:* menstrual bleeding, repeated miscarriage, barrenness,

---

55. See the postface to the second edition, dated 1585, by her great-nephew, who called himself simply "Xiu." As Xiu explained it, his great-aunt's son had died young, and her grandson had been executed for unspecified crimes (probably of a political nature). It fell to this agnatic descendant to commemorate his forebearers by pre-serving their writings.

daixia, or prolonged postpartum depletion. Here her practice fit the stereotype that female physicians were particularly well suited to deal with uniquely female complaints—a common view that the male relatives who wrote prefaces to her book showed they shared. Other chronic complaints were familiar ones: there were stagnant diarrheas (*xiexie*) from food, a case of chronic nausea (*fanwei*), and one each of chronic cough, insomnia, depletion heat, and "blocked *qi*" (*ge qi*) resulting in fatigue and loss of appetite.

But a significant number of Tan's clients suffered from skin afflictions—in China the special domain of practitioners of external medicine (*waike*). One complained of a fiery rash (*huo dan*) on her legs and thighs, another of leprous sores (*chuang lai*) all over her body; a girl's ugly enlarged "litchi nose" obviously was impairing her marriage prospects; another was wretched with an itching Wind (*feng yang*) all over her face, ears and neck. In addition to such dermatological disorders, Tan's clients suffered from internal swellings—a "tortoise lump" (*gui kuai*) or "congested lump" (*jie kuai*) in the belly, or, most ominous, the numerous small nodular *li* swellings and sores (*li chuang*) around the neck thought to be signs of potentially grave illness.[56] In treating complaints like these Tan offered, in addition to the prescription tonics of internal medicine, topical treatments—often medicinal pastes and washes, but above all the penetrating heat of moxibustion. If she had a distinctive therapeutic signature, it was as an expert in this medical art of the hands, deployed in eleven of her cases.[57]

Tan Yunxian's casebook, then, offers a glimpse of one of the oldest of Chinese medical arts, which, like its more famous counterpart, acupuncture, was declining in prestige in the Ming dynasty. Moxibustion

56. Tan's descriptions of these neck lesions resemble some in textbook accounts of *luoli,* even though she called them simply *li chuang.* Biomedical clinicians sometimes identify *luoli* as tubercular lymphoma or lupus. Today the latter syndrome is far more common in females than in males, particularly young adult women. See Kiple 1993: 848–51. Ming physicians and laypeople alike took the appearance of skin lesions in a string along the neck as a sign of a life-threatening illness. A sixteenth-century official described his sister's disease this way: "The swellings gathered below her neck. The pharmacy texts say that in places where there is much *qi* and little Blood it is hard to effect a cure. People say that if there is one knot, one will die in a year; if there are many knots, one will die in as many years. Sister had one or two knots." See Li Kaixian, 2:418–19. My thanks to Ann Waltner for this reference.

57. *Fuke* (eleven cases) and *waike* (nine cases) were the largest categories in Tan's casebook. The breakdown of the *fuke* cases was as follows: two menstruation, two miscarriage, two other illness in pregnancy, three postpartum, one barrenness, one abortion. The *waike* divided into five cases of body rashes and four of *li* lumps or knots around the neck.

was not divorced from the older mainstream of medical theory: like the acupuncturist's needle, moxa stimulated qi circulation when applied at the classically approved sites of the invisible aperture points connecting the body surface to the network of channels within. The moxa, an aromatic preparation of dried artemisia burnt on the skin (with or without the assistance of a cupping jar), transmitted a deep if sometimes painful heat, reducing swelling, easing aches and soreness, and opening up blocked paths of circulation. Song and Yuan medical authorities had attempted to standardize the number and location of the body's apertures, and their links to the body's cardinal and other channels; they had also argued over whether moxibustion worked by replenishing depletion or by draining pathogens out of the body, or both. Tan's case narratives reported the loci selected, the number of applications, and whether the moxa was to burn actively or not—but offered no views on such points of theory.[58]

Tan Yunxian's moxibustion treatments cured four cases of *li* sores and swellings, and two cases of abdominal swellings. But she also used it for chronic digestive malfunction, for a chronic cough, and on a woman who was barren. In selecting the proper apertures for treatment in each case, Tan focused on a localized pathological site rather than relying primarily on a holistic strategy of action at a distance. The young women with *li* swellings received moxa at the base of the neck, behind the ears, and along the shoulders as well as along the circulation channel that runs through the back of the elbow. Sufferers from indigestion had heat applied to three points down the center of the chest, along the Conception channel. A young mother with a chronic cough and fatigue got treatments along the Superintendent channel of the upper back and adjacent to the shoulder blade, as well as along the circulation channel that ran behind the knee, while the barren wife had heat applied to her lower cinnabar field below the navel. Only a few laconic remarks hinted of Tan's understanding of moxa's efficacy: it drove out Wind and Damp from a boatwoman's hands that were numb from gripping the tiller; it counteracted the "depletion Damp" of a stagnant diarrhea; the "power of the Fire" (*huo li*) penetrated a client's vital center to revive her appetite for food. Tan spoke of moxibustion as warming and drying, efficacious against the old pathogenic agents of Wind, Damp and Cold. While Cheng Maoxian recommended moxibustion only in extreme situations

58. For history of moxibustion see Needham and Lu 1980: 170–84; Fu Weikang 1990: 257–60, 345–48.

when herbal tonics could not reach a patient too sick to swallow, Tan wrote of its broader efficacy. "Such chronic illness is not curable by medicines alone," she said of a young woman's congested lumps (*jie kuai*) in her belly, showing her confidence in this as a sovereign remedy. She used it to warm a woman's "Cold womb," quoting with approval the classic saying, "Needle and she will become barren; give moxa three times and she will be fertile."[59]

However, Tan Yunxian did not neglect herbal prescriptions, which she always prescribed as a complement to moxibustion, and which she relied on exclusively in a majority of the cases she wrote about. Her shorthand reports on her own prescriptions suggest that she followed an eclectic strategy, adjusting and modifying existing standard formulas rather than creating her own signature combinations of ingredients. She named a number of pharmacy texts as sources: these included collections identified with Zhu Zhenheng and Li Gao, but also the famous compendium of standard prescriptions from the Song state medical bureau; a fourteenth-century work by Li Heng, *Prescription Treasures from the Sleeve* (*Xiu zhen fang*);[60] and an unidentified *Marvelous Prescriptions* (*Zhaixuan fang*).

In her *fuke* cases Tan followed a middle path, adherent of no particular school of thought. In a case of chronic irregular menstrual bleeding caused by overwork, she started out with "Replenish center and boost *qi*" infusion, directed at strengthening digestive function, to be followed later by Zhu Zhenheng's Replenish Yin pill to protect fluids. For threatened miscarriage she used the old fetal tranquilizer Purple Thyme infusion as a foundation, supplemented by skullcap to cool maternal Fire and *baishu* to replenish center and aid digestion. For a woman weakened by multiple pregnancies followed by a self-induced abortion, she offered a standard formula from the Song medical bureau for digestion, and then balanced Blood-nourishing Four Ingredients infusion with supplements to restore vitality by stimulating *qi*: bastard cardamom (*sharen*),

59. Tan said she was quoting a text called *Ming tang zhen jiu* (Bright Hall of Acupuncture and Moxibustion), which evokes old generic titles for illustrated works on acupuncture and moxibustion. The dangers of acupuncture as opposed to moxibustion for female reproductive function are supported by the clinical view, still common today in TCM, that needling a woman on the *shi men* point (on the Conception channel below the navel, often identified with the Cinnabar Field) will cause her to abort or render her infertile.

60. Li Heng was a physician from Hofei, Anhui, whose *Xiuzhen fang,* completed in 1390, was reprinted several times in the fifteenth and early sixteenth centuries. Since sleeves were commonly used as pockets, the title suggests a handbook.

bitter orange (*zhishi*), and nutgrass (*xiangfu*). Broadly speaking, she balanced attention to strengthening digestive function with concern for nourishing Blood and fluids, and for warming with *qi*-moving aromatics. She drew on both old Song standard formulas and those of later masters. She did not explain her strategies with reference to theories of pattern diagnosis, yin yang, or the Five Phases. At most she followed Zhu Zhenheng's model of the relationship between Fire, emotion and generative vitality, as in her account of the following case of menstrual irregularity:

> A woman of fifty-three. Because her menses were irregular her primordial *qi* was extremely weak, afflicting her with symptoms of depletion of both Blood and *qi*. I took her pulse several times: the pulse at the Heart position was strongly floating and rebounding, six beats to the breath.[61] This woman had overworked to the point of damaging her Heart. The Heart is the body's ruler; when Heart Fire moves, the menstrual period is not on time, and when it comes it increases depletion and weakness.[62]

In this case the centerpiece of Tan's therapy was Angelica and Amber pill (*Gui-po wan*) — combining angelica (*danggui*) for Blood with amber (*hupo*), which acts on *qi* and regulates Heart energy. Heart Fire, easily aroused by anger, is responsible for miscarriages, she explained to another client.

As a diagnostician, Tan reported the results of a pulse examination only four times, a striking contrast with the case histories of male doctors. If other physicians had been previously consulted by her clients, she scarcely mentioned any, nor did family members intrude with comments, criticisms or opinion. At the center of most of her case narratives was a dialogue like the following one between healer and client:

> A thirty-eight-year-old woman. She was afflicted with a vaginal flux of Blood [*xuebeng*] that went on continuously for three months. It changed into a dripping discharge of Blood [*xuelin*] that lasted three years. No medicines helped. I inquired as to the reason. She said, "My household runs a kiln for a living. When my husband is gone I personally move bricks and tiles all day long. It is the second watch [at night] before I stop. I happened to have my menstrual period and it's brought about this illness." I said, "You work too hard." I gave her "Replenish center and boost *qi*" infusion, taken from Danxi's [Zhu Zhenheng's] formulas . . . [and] later Replenish Yin pill.[63]

61. Physicians commonly measured the rate of pulse against their own breathing.
62. Tan Yunxian, 13b–14b.
63. Tan Yunxian, 2*an*b.

"Inquiring as to the reason" for the illness, Tan listened and noted down what her clients told her. A boatman's wife, like the brick-maker's wife, was a poor woman who told her about work: "Spring and fall, night and day, in wind and rain, in fair weather or foul, every day I ply this boat, and it has given me this disorder [numb hands]." More prosperous clients spoke of family problems. Suffering from a malarial fever with dysentery while pregnant, a young woman explained, "I happened to eat chicken with noodles and my parents[-in-law] scolded me, and as a result I got this illness." Bedridden for a year and coughing bloody sputum, a middle-aged woman explained, "First my daughter died, and I suffered damage from weeping; then not half a year later my husband also died, and more weeping damaged me further." Four women spoke of wayward spouses. "My husband is rich and took a concubine and I have to bear it." Another saw the concubine as the result of her own repeated miscarriages: "[I] don't plan to oppose it, but the sorrow is too hard to bear; household affairs are complicated, and in addition I am unable to get pregnant. . . ." However, the barren wife blamed her failure on her husband's frequent visits to prostitutes: "Because of this my menstrual periods have become very troublesome, adding up to much loss of Blood, and as a consequence I have a white discharge and my lower belly is cold and aching." Sometimes Tan heard about an illness from a female relative, like the weeping mother-in-law who asked her to save her sick daughter-in-law, who was unable to eat from a throat blockage, or the mother whose daughter's health was "ruined" from the aftermath of a self-induced abortion.

Tan sympathized with complaints like these in her diagnostic comments. To two poor women who gave birth in wretched cottages she explained that their postpartum illnesses came from premature labor, plus exposure to Wind and sun. To a worn-out servant girl she explained she had gone back to work too soon after a Cold Damage fever. Two women who miscarried had hidden their anger, so that Fire turned within and destabilized the fetus. Perhaps Tan's silence about her clients' sexual lives was out of respect for their modesty, but a diagnosis of overwork was her standard explanation for the causes of their misery. When they suffered damage from negative emotions it was because of the toll exacted by the need to remain stoical, or because of burdens too great to bear. In sum, Tan told stories of suffering linked to hard labor, repressed resentments, overwhelming grief and gestational damage. In these narratives the doctor was represented as a sympathetic listener and as a healer sharing a common vocabulary and language of the body with those she treated.

Tan's narratives assumed that disorders of women, like those of men, would respond to therapies focused on metabolic functioning of digestion, or on the *qi*-moving warmth of moxibustion or aromatic herbs. Skin problems had no special affinity for females, and she left no clue, as a biomedical expert might expect, that she or others thought of *li* swellings as typically a female affliction. Emotion was an important factor in the etiology of her clients' ailments, but she saw them worried by money troubles, family illness and work as well as by the specifically female problems of too many children or too few, or of wayward husbands who visited prostitutes or took a concubine.

Nonetheless, like Cheng Maoxian, she wrote about many cases of gestational disorders among her clients, confirming that these loomed large among the female clients in a practice. These cases evoked a gestational body subject to damage by a host of threats. Overworking during the menstrual period, for example, weakened women and led to irregularity and depletion, and this depletion if unchecked compromised primordial *qi*. Postpartum was a time of vulnerability, when failure to rest or exposure to Wind and Cold could undermine later health. Like miscarriage, abortion was a serious crisis that endangers long-term vitality. The negative emotions aroused by a husband taking a concubine because of his wife's failure to produce an heir made successful pregnancy more difficult. A husband who visited prostitutes might trigger his wife's venereal illness. Here a woman doctor and her clients talked about the gestational body in an idiom that both echoes Chen Ziming's holistic *fuke* and evokes concerns that late-twentieth-century health professionals working on women's health still find expressed today.[64]

Gender, Class, and Medical Pluralism

Based on the record of her life in her casebook, Tan Yunxian was an exceptional individual. She may have emerged from the ranks of women healers in medical lineages, but she certainly cannot be taken as typical of them. Nonetheless, something can be learned of female physicians (*nü yi*) and their clients by placing Tan against the stereotype of the granny healer on the one hand and the male literati phy-

64. See Johnson 1975; Furth and Chen 1992.

sician as represented by Cheng Maoxian on the other. Socially Tan Yunxian's family far outranked Cheng Maoxian's, and her authority in the eyes of her clients appears less subject to question. Her clients, like his, included both rich and poor,[65] but she gave them neither name nor title, so that her narratives construct a democracy of female suffering in which the doctor-patient relationship is personal and the doctor's authority is unchallenged. As stories of woman-to-woman interaction, her narratives reveal less clinical conflict and a less complex social field than a doctor like Cheng Maoxian reported, but suggest a more secure clinical hierarchy of power.

Yet, paradoxically, much in her cases also suggests a more popular style of medical practice than his. In diagnosis she relied on looking and listening more than on pulse. She addressed symptoms directly, and her explanations of etiology avoided pattern diagnosis. Most often she named the perennial environmental agents of disease, Wind, Cold, Damp and Heat, to which she sometimes added Poison, while internally she saw straightforward dysfunctions of digestion or depletions of Blood and *qi*, triggered by the wear and tear of emotions or hard work or reproductive labor. In prescribing she followed no school but selected eclectically from both Song and Ming models, often relying on standard formulas as a foundation. Above all, her emphasis upon external medicine, chronic afflictions and the technology of moxibustion all set her practice apart from the more typical male pattern I have explored through the cases of Cheng Maoxian. Cheng's cases show male learned medicine as focused on crisis management and on internal medicine (*neike*), especially epidemic disease and acute fevers, and favoring herbal technologies over all others. Tan Yunxian's narrative of her practice as a female physician may show us traces of popular medicine as practiced by healers of both sexes and used by both women and poorer sufferers.[66]

Nonetheless, these popular fields of expertise were also associated with the socially inferior granny healer. Zheng Jinsheng's survey found

65. Tan's narrative identified seven clients as poor, ten as rich, and one as from an official family. Thirteen cases were socially unidentifiable.

66. Similar popular styles of healing have been found in the *fuke* traditions of the Bamboo Forest Temple (Zhulin si) of Xiaoshan county, Zhejiang. This was a religious lineage of practitioners who claimed origins in the Southern Song, but whose surviving writings date from the Qing dynasty. They did not take pulses and craft prescriptions but simply asked about symptoms and offered ready-made formulas. Since their clients were laboring women, they stressed strong *qi*-moving ingredients. In the eighteenth and nineteenth centuries they were famous for a line of patent medicines. See Liao Yuqun 1986: 159–61. See Yi-Li Wu 1998 for the Xiaoshan tradition in Qing *fuke*.

female healers clustered in the specialties of pediatrics and external medicine, in addition to *fuke*.[67] While not a pediatrician, Tan Yunxian also
was expert in a medicine of hands on flesh, like Mistress Peng the eye
doctor, Mistress Han who cured a throat obstruction, or the unnamed
surgeon of *luoli* swellings admired by Xue Ji. Like the masseuse or surgeon, the moxibustionist's work required a physical intimacy of bodily
contact that Ming women could not easily seek from a male. Could it
be that a Ming feminization of moxibustion went hand in hand with its
decline in prestige, just as the rising prestige of the literati-physician
model of elite practice was linked to its ritualized code of limited physical
contact between healers and the sick? Without knowing more about
how and when the services of moxibustion were provided to Ming
males, I cannot carry this line of questioning very far. What is clear is
that even outside the sphere of *fuke*, the commonalities between Tan
Yunxian's practice and those glimpsed among granny healers suggest
that Ming female healing was not only socially more plebeian and culturally more popular but more likely to offer technologies that involved
a hands-on medicine of bodily contact. Their clinical styles therefore
constructed a more material corporeality than the Yellow Emperor's
body.

In Tan Yunxian, a rare woman was helped by her high social rank to
achieve the status of a literati doctor, gaining local fame for classical
skills applied as a humanitarian art. But even Tan Yunxian employed
distinctive approaches to therapy resembling those that other female
healers shared with more plebeian practitioners. This intersection of
class and gender in the practice of female healers is what made the
"granny" model of their work so rhetorically powerful. A woman found
it easiest to escape the granny trap if she functioned as wife, mother or
daughter-in-law within a healing family. A positive side of this was that
the family need not function simply as a restrictive institution of patriarchal control; it also fostered access to medical skills and was a platform
from which women working as healers were producing contributors to
the family unit. As such they were vital intermediaries for the transmission of clinical knowledge and practice across gender boundaries. However, whatever their informal authority, the respectability of female doctors depended upon the presumption that patriarchal family authority
guided them.

Finally, gender appears to have defined a female healer by her clients

67. Zheng Jinsheng 1996.

even more than by her clients' disorders. In this context, the rhetorical trope of the "six kinds of old grannies" not only inscribed male superiority for physicians as experts as well as for literati as household heads, but it may have also complicated the gender and class relationships among female healers themselves. In textual representation, the archetype of the granny healer was the midwife. I do not know whether healers identified as medical grannies (*yi po, yi fu*) ever attended births. Nor can I be sure that every woman labeled a midwife (*wen po, zuo po*, etc.) in fact had birthing skills and no others. But midwives, who may have been very numerous,[68] practiced a socially marginal crisis medicine that took them into others' houses at all hours of the day or night to assist in the dangerous and sullying passages of birth. Here female healers seeking respectability faced a paradox. On the one hand, their niches in the world of medical practice depended upon the system of sex segregation that made women as sufferers seek out one of their own for advice. On the other hand, there were strong social incentives for female healers with the greatest resources—those from medical families—to distance themselves from a specialty that, however essential to most women, lacked the dignity to which medicine aspired. Thus the "granny" label may have worked rhetorically to establish not just class boundaries but a vocational boundary between midwives and other kinds of female healers as well.

Narrative Voices and the Culturally Constructed Body

From the narratives of Tan Yunxian's clinical encounters we can now look back over the earlier chapters of this book and begin to sum up the journey they trace. On one level my account has moved from more abstract discourse about the medical body in general to narratives of individuals' experience. The history of learned medicine gradually unpacks the things one needs to know in order to understand the physicians' accounts of individual cases recorded here. Nonetheless, the

---

68. By extrapolation, the twentieth-century public health reformer Marion Yang estimated in 1930 that there were 200,000 old-style midwives needing retraining. In 1958, Communist reformers claimed to have retrained 774,983 midwives, while reporting the total number of doctors of TCM as a more modest 487,000. See Banister 1987: 58–59, and Yang 1930: 428–31.

cases of Tan Yunxian and Cheng Maoxian do not reveal practice as opposed to theory; rather they complete my analysis of how the medical body was constituted in the clinical dialogue and came to be known in the social and semantic field of the clinical encounter. These brief narratives of what clients told and what doctors said to educate and persuade are where we best see the language they had in common and the kind of body that language animated.

Although Cheng Maoxian was more engaged in learned discourse than Tan Yunxian, neither made much clinical use of the formal categories of symbolic correlations. Occasionally Cheng tried to explain the course of an illness by referring to a sequence of the Five Phases, but unless he was talking specifically about Cold Damage fevers, he did not identify the path of disease along the cardinal or other specific channels. Tan Yunxian represented the circulation channels simply via points on the body surface where the heat of moxa could penetrate. Most often both spoke of a more general circulation of vitalities of Blood and *qi* that might be static and blocked, or overagitated and given to wayward motion. The five *zang* organ systems were important as centers of broadly defined functions, but their modes of interaction were left unspecified. Here the formal correspondences of correlative cosmology translated into a phenomenology of bodily consciousness. As a healer sensitive to the emotional lives of her clients, Tan paid special attention to Heart's capacity for psychic arousal, whether to fright or worry or longing. Cheng's stories also evoked Liver's anger, Spleen's calm equilibrium, Kidney's reservoirs of potency and resolve.

Cheng used pattern analysis of the roots of disorder more than Tan did, most notably to distinguish types and stages of Cold Damage fever as yang, requiring the doctor to reduce heat or yin, calling for him to safeguard fluids. As categories of early and later stages of illness, yin and yang were elusive, occasioning confusion in doctor and clients alike. By contrast, patterns of internal Hot and Cold readily evoked bodily sensations, while repletion and depletion translated into bodily somatics of being full or empty, drained of vitality or swollen with some palpable excess. Thus, while these binary patterns could name the deeper roots of pathology, diagnoses and drug actions explained them in words that brought doctor and client together in a common idiom linking body awareness and medical doctrine. Although cases reported patient voices through the doctor's interpretation, most of the time indirectly, the clinical dialogues show the key role sick people played in grounding medical discourse in the suffering of which they alone were the subjects.

Both sets of case narratives show the extent to which patients and doctors returned over and over again to a popular etiological vocabulary that stressed external agency over internal root patterns of disorder, and found common ground in a symptom-based approach to diagnosis and cure. Even more than Cheng, Tan reported her clients as struck by the old familiar climatic excesses — Wind, Cold, Heat and Damp — to which was added Phlegm, the humor of the moist south. Occasionally a virulent corruption invaded as Poison. Tan found these categories adequate to explain her therapeutic strategies of driving out Wind, drying Damp or cleansing Poison. Nonetheless, external pathological agents and internal humoral imbalances were named in an overlapping vocabulary that left interpretation open.

As for the language of bodily gender in these narratives, the pair Blood and *qi* were everyday terms for the primary vitalities of the body. In the case history context, the term Essence referred to semen, not to higher levels of creative vitality. When Tan and Cheng spoke of Blood and *qi* separately, they called attention to the asymmetries between them. Not only did *qi* lead Blood, but life itself depended upon primordial *qi* (*yuan qi*). Blood was something more material that circulated, identified with fluids, and with the transformations of reproductive Blood that were particularly important to women. If yin and yang were confusing as markers of an acute fever's progress — the technical idiom of Cold Damage theory — yin was incorporated into the everyday names of drug formulas aiding Water and generative vitality, associated with sexuality. Even though the leadership of Blood as a pharmaceutical strategy was relatively unimportant to them, gender ideology continued to inform their understandings of the Blood-*qi* relationship.

These medical case narratives paid only limited attention to the complex yin yang Five Phase system of the Yellow Emperor's body, with its network of circulation channels and associated organ systems. In Ming case histories, medical theory appeared as linguistic fragments in a clinical dialogue resonating with the semantic play of formal, somatic and metaphorical meanings, and integrated into a drama of bodily gesture and social performance. Nonetheless, even as fragments, theory made an essential contribution, assuring all parties to the clinical encounter that the bodies in question, in sickness and in health, were intelligible as part of an overarching natural and cosmological order.

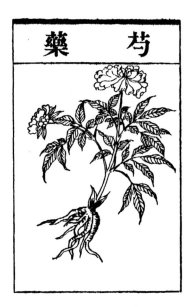

CHAPTER 9

Conclusion

In taking up the study of China's medical history from a position on its feminist margins, I have been led down three paths. The first path, of history, has followed over time the trajectory of *fuke* as a learned discourse. *Fuke* was part of medicine as a science and the institutions and practices that supported it, shaped by the patterns of change over a seven-hundred-year span of China's medical history. On the one hand this has led me to focus on the recorded teachings of learned physicians seeking doctrinal underpinnings for their clinical reasoning. On the other hand, my search for women as patients and healers has fostered a broader shift of perspective on medical history, away from experts at the center to focus on the interaction of healers and their clients and on the dialogical nature of the medical language through which the body was known.

The second path has been that of gender ideology in medicine. In Chinese cosmology yin and yang were not attributes of sexed bodies but themselves the foundation of gendered meanings diffused in bodies and in the world at large. Accordingly, the normative medical body of the Yellow Emperor, incorporating both yin and yang relationships, was androgynous. Even though this human (rather than the sexed) body was considered the proper subject of medical inquiry, physicians believed in the need for "separate prescriptions" for women and accommodated their practice to the gendered spheres of inner and outer social space. Narratives of separate prescriptions reveal tensions between the androgynous body of generation and a female gestational body, while narratives of the clinical encounter show how social rituals to negotiate inner and outer space were an integral part of the experience of sickness and cure.

My final path has been to explore the cultural constructions of the body in China's medical history in order to ask some interpretive questions about the project of body history itself. Here I have aimed to expose, if not to settle, epistemological issues that arise the minute one takes up such a topic. Ultimately these may be undecidable by appeals to the forms of local knowledge that history explores, but they bear on the meanings we can give to both body and gender.

History

Fuke was never at the center of the medical culture of imperial China, but nevertheless learned medicine for women was shaped by the institutional and intellectual vicissitudes of that center. *Fuke* matured as a distinct division of medical knowledge as part of the Song dynasty movement to establish practice based on a public medical canon sponsored by the imperial state and communicated through print. It became one of the disciplines mastered by the new "literati" physicians—men whose claims to knowledge were based on scholarship in the classics, as distinct from personal, lineage-based modes of transmission. In the thirteenth and fourteenth centuries, when the agenda of such learned physicians was to rethink the etiology of febrile disorders, they applied their revisionist doctrines and clinical strategies to *fuke* as well.

Song *fuke* doctrine stressed "the leadership of Blood" in women, calling attention to female difference. Using pattern diagnosis, physicians identified a wide variety of internal illnesses in women as disorders of Blood function, and theorized menstruation as a holistic process whose regulation was important to women's general health as well as their fertility. "Separate prescriptions" acting directly on Blood function, presuming the dominance of Blood over *qi* in females, were popular as applications of holistic theory. But by the late Ming authorities generally preferred to limit separate prescriptions to a narrower range of gestational and fertility disorders—a strategy that reflected doctrinal shifts linking circulation channel functions more tightly to organ physiology, and bodily processes more firmly to material structures. As Ming physicians followed the tenets of neo-Confucian ethical thought to stress the importance of sexual and appetitive continence in the management of health, women's bodies, like men's, also appeared in learned discourse to be more intertwined with a morality of personal responsibility.

If these changes reflected a gradual rationalization of medical thought within the framework of an abiding model of bodily androgyny, the challenge of female difference was reflected in tension between constructions of generation and of gestation. Having both generative and gestational functions, menstruation was central to holistic interpretations of the generative body in women, and the accompanying pharmacy of "menstrual regulation" contributed to Ming medicine's highly literary refinement of the prescription art. However, the management of gestation and birth itself remained an eclectic sphere where male physicians were largely outsiders, and where scholarly interpretation of underlying patterns was not well integrated into clinical strategies. The decline of ritual obstetrics, new theories of sexual differentiation in the womb, and the medicalization of beliefs about the pollution of childbirth were Ming markers of this eclecticism.

However, in spite of its secondary importance from the point of view of medical doctrine, the substantial historical record on separate prescriptions for women remains testimony to a serious medical mission. As early as the seventh century C.E., Sun Simiao had spoken of the importance of women and children to life. The parallel between *fuke* and the simultaneous development of pediatrics by elite physicians in the Song dynasty and after shows how these specialties had a common raison d'être in safeguarding family descent lines, mandating paternalistic oversight of the interconnected bodies of women and children.

The story of *fuke* shifts interpretation of the history of medicine from an expert-centered to a client-centered perspective. Looking for women as patients and as healers leads to the home, the setting of most illness experience, and to self-care and family care as the primary forms of healing practice. If medicine as a domestic skill was important to many private gentlemen who studied it in order to fulfill their filial duties, some of their wives and mothers also participated in medical practice this way. When male healers entered the home to treat the sick they had to negotiate the social networks of domestic relationships, including those giving older women authority over younger women and children, or those improvised when senior males sickened. Female healers, while variable in status, emerge as an eclectic group skilled in a variety of hands-on technologies as well as pharmacy, whose client base was protected by the separation of the sexes. All of these things were part of the social patterns that fostered the diffusion of medical knowledge and expertise, and limited the authority of even literati physicians in their relationships with their gentry clients. The intensification of sex segregation in Ming dynasty China made male physicians particularly dependent upon patriarchal authority in gentry families if they were to treat women successfully, while simultaneously giving women in those families incentive to shelter a separate female sphere. Domestic gender boundaries both limited elite practice of *fuke* and protected this female sphere.

Finally, *fuke* throws light on the nature of medical textuality in relation to hierarchies of clinical practice. Domestic and lineage-based modes of medical learning were based on oral and handwritten forms of transmission and on practical and instrumental forms of recordkeeping. The print culture that facilitated the codification of medical classics did not erase these older and perennial technologies of communication, nor did it ensure a continuous, cumulative transmission of much in the medical archive.

When the case history emerged as the most important new genre of medical writing in the Ming, it called attention to the limitations of the codified canon as opposed to the clinical dialogue as the epistemological foundation of medical knowledge. Through case histories it is possible to hear patient voices shaping nosological categories out of their reported experiences of illness, and to grasp the metaphorical resonances of the fragments of theory that were articulated at the bedside. Patients, both male and female, often differed with their doctors' constructions of their problems, were knowledgeable about drug actions, and wanted therapies to address symptoms directly. Explanations of illness etiology—whether pathogenic environmental *qi*, conduct, emotions or the toll of bodily labor—called attention to the everyday business of living. The diffused nature of medical authority, the domestic setting of practice, and the dialogical basis of diagnosis all fostered a medical culture where the idiom of illness was a shared property, not cut off from the language of everyday experience.

The print culture that facilitated the textual transmission of medical knowledge helped establish the cultural ideal of the literati physician as it emerged in the Song. By the early Ming, such physicians were taking their place at the top of a more stratified hierarchy of practitioners within and without medical lineages without eliminating medical pluralism below. Printed medical works multiplied and diversified, exposing through their textual instability the more fundamental dependence of medical knowledge upon practice. Nonetheless, the cultural hegemony of print further robbed religious healing of prestige, and many kinds of female healers, along with midwives, were left even more on the margins than they had been before. Class and gender hierarchies reinforced each other as hands-on medical technologies like acupuncture, external medicine, and moxibustion became more identified with lower class and female practitioners.

Gender

An apparent paradox has presented a problem for the interpretation of gender in late imperial China. On the one hand, inner and outer spheres established social hierarchy and shaped the divisions of labor, space and movement organizing daily life. These, together with the gendered moral precepts summarized as the "three bonds and five relationships," were hegemonic social norms ordering the status of parents and children, husbands and wives. By contrast, the boundaries of gender constructed in bodily accounts of yin and yang, Blood and *qi*, were flexible and shifting ones, sharing in the emphasis on transmutation and change characteristic of the underlying cosmology of yin yang and the Five Phases. This potential for transformation and change was seen as one of the fundamental, inherent powers of the human body, recognized by both medicine and religion.

How are we to understand such apparently conflicting and contradictory accounts, where bodily gender was based on a plastic androgyny while social gender was based on fixed hierarchy? While it is a mistake to argue that any cultural system must necessarily exhibit congruence between all of its parts, as in a functionalist model, we still have to deal with the fact that Chinese natural philosophy was holistic, teaching the unity of Heaven, Earth, and Humanity, and that classical Chinese thought did not easily imagine a bifurcation of nature and culture.

This being true, medicine and the body did in fact become a site where conflicting ideas of nature were contested. These conflicts appeared in *fuke* when physicians found that a holistic model of the Yellow Emperor's body was more easily adapted to functions of generation than to those of gestation. In the Song, physicians accommodated ritual obstetrics, in effect accepting entrenched folk and religious beliefs about the pollution of childbirth that essentialized female gender as unclean. They also tried to interpret pregnancy and birth as a cosmological process of "completion" based on yin yang and the Five Phases. Their search for clinical strategies based on learned medical theory for the management of gestational processes bore fruit in an elaborate medicalization of menstruation as a bodily marker of female fertility, health and generative power. With the decline of ritual obstetrics in the Ming they reinterpreted the problems of postpartum, emphasizing depletion over pollution. However, repressed pollution beliefs resurfaced in pediatrics to be inscribed on the bodies of infants and children going through inevitable bouts of pediatric disease. Pregnancy and postpartum remained primarily the domain of a symptom-based pharmacy, of female family management, and of the midwife. Where generativity was the attribute of the androgynous body, uniting human males and females in the creative act of begetting new life replicating cosmic pattern, gestation was the attribute of a more material female body entangled in the negative and defiling passages of birth and death. Moreover, this body was ritually hidden from men.

Nonetheless, Chinese medical thought never abandoned the vision of bodily androgyny, but with twists and turns returned to it again and again. If Blood and *qi* spoke of the gendered relations of hierarchy in that body, yin and yang spoke of relations of equality. Whether imagined as benign or inimical, yin's power to match yang spoke of gender equivalence — of ways men and women were alike in the capacity to create new life, and in the democracy of death. The symbolic resources of the body, like those of the world at large, were polysemic. As a language of power, yin and yang, Blood and *qi,* spoke both of a necessary subordination of women to men in society and of their interdependence in the collective structures of kinship at the foundation of social life. Within such collective structures, the shifting nature of yin yang positionality taught that one's social relationships of inferiority and superiority inevitably shifted over time from youth to age, even as Blood's incorporation into *qi* by the process of encompassment always reestablished cosmic gender hierarchy at ever-ascending levels. Where views of female bodily inferiority associated with gestation naturalized male antagonism or fear in the social relations of men and women, androgyny naturalized gender harmony as a social basis of the family.

The body, then, spoke of parenthood, and called attention to how the functions of generation and gestation related to the social transitions of kinship identity involved in becoming a mother or a father. What role did the bodily function of maternity play in the social construction we call motherhood? In the commonplace Confucian moral tales of filial piety and exemplary womanhood, the ideal mother was usually represented as a matriarch owed filial service by grown children, not as a young mother of nurslings at the breast. Legitimate wives who became mothers gained status as ancestors-to-be that supported their social prestige in the family as they aged. Such ritually based relationships gave social motherhood priority over bodily maternity and empowered elite wives at the expense of their families' concubines and bondmaids.[1] Moreover, male literati in late imperial China, who were devoted chroniclers of their mothers' sufferings, often honored such "formal mothers" (*dimu*) for the instruction, discipline and sacrificial labor that constituted proper motherly teaching.

But didactic discourse spoke of care (*yang*) as well as teaching (*jiao*). The doctor Cheng Maoxian had this in mind when he wrote the history of his wife's miscarriages for their son, suggesting that children needed extra reminders of their debt owed for the maternal bodily labor of pregnancy and birth. It was from mothers—and some fathers—that sons must have learned the narratives of bodily caring that embellished their written recollections of childhood—the drain of breast-feeding or of weaning with premasticated food (*ru bu*), the depletions of maternal illness, the toll of nursing the young child through smallpox or other pediatric crises.[2] Although not all such nursing was done by biological mothers (wet-nursing was common), what counts here is the importance of such details about bodily care in narratives men learned from the women who reared them. As against formal didactic literature, sons' accounts of the more intimate side of motherhood brought attention back to the bodily tie. Such accounts reinforce the anthropologist Margery Wolf's view that a "uterine" mother-son dyad operated within, and sometimes at odds with, the Chinese patrilineal family group.

Confucian philosophy itself was not entirely silent on these issues. The ritual obligation of a son to mourn his father and mother for the

1. Waltner 1990 discusses the power of first wives formally to adopt their husbands' sons by concubines, a power that Bray 1997 interprets in the context of competition among women within elite families to control reproductive resources.

2. Hsiung P'ing-chen 1995: 87–117, discusses mother-son relationships based upon biographical and autobiographical narratives of over eight hundred Qing-period men.

three years that he had depended upon parental care in infancy was measured by the maternal body—the length of time between conception and weaning.[3] Such a Confucian mourning practice can be compared to the even more dramatic popular Buddhist rituals of atonement performed by a son at his mother's funeral. By drinking the red fluid that represented the blood of childbirth, the son took upon himself the burden of pollution that his mother otherwise would have to expiate in the "Bloody Pond" of Buddhist purgatory.[4] These were rituals built around moral stories of maternal bodily sacrifice and bodily stigma.

Such stories show the religious basis of accounts of both female weakness and female uncleanness. But neither did androgyny offer a stable vision of bodily health for women. While representing male and female as homologous, the Ming discourse on generation and nourishing life taught a women that her menstrual cycle was the female equivalent of male seminal vitality, and that the labor of gestating and giving birth cost her a disproportionate measure of generative vitality compared with males. Together with the medicalization of pollution beliefs, this left women with the possibility of interpreting their functions of gestation as a negative bodily power or as a sacrificial labor resulting in a socially acceptable weakness. It was through these bodily powers and liabilities that women as wives and mothers were both threatening and essential to the solidarity of the patrilineal kinship unit.

How did bodily paternity compare with maternity? On one level, for a Ming dynasty Chinese father, far more than for a mother, parenthood was bound up in the ritual foundations of agnatic kinship as constructed in neo-Confucian *Daoxue*. Descent relationships were not understood as biological in the biomedical sense of the term but were transmitted by ancestral *qi* linking agnatic ancestors and descendants. Accordingly, physicians taught that the natural process of inheritance—the parental endowment to a child through the union of yin and yang—transmitted the generic human bodily form, not individual or social characteristics.[5] The notion of individual biological inheritance among modern Europeans has been profoundly shaped by a bilateral kinship system biologized as blood. In the agnatic kinship system of Ming China, by contrast, paternity passed via *qi* as a purely male endowment residing in a family patriline. Wives were ritually encompassed by their husbands'

---

3. This insight comes from a conversation with Hsiung Ping-chen.
4. For the Bloody Pond ceremony, see Seaman 1981 and Beata Grant 1989.
5. For further discussion see Furth 1994.

lineages, tied to sons and not daughters, becoming ritual outsiders to their natal families. The children of concubines were ritually equivalent to those of primary wives. There were several ways for fathers to substitute an adoptive child for a natural one, to name an heir rather than beget him. But in this context the ability of women to adopt—to become social mothers—was itself dependent upon the adoptive child's recognition by its social or natural father. Other forms of adoption were mere fostering, outside of the significant kinship collective.

If agnatic kinship lay in a patrilineal name, materialized as an ancestral *qi* not identifiable with modern biological meanings, this does not mean that the kinship of males around a common name had no bodily basis. When lineages preferred agnatic adoption over all other forms, when they excluded daughters from inheritance or from ritual roles in the ancestral cults of their natal families, they increased the responsibility that fell on male bodies alone to constitute kinship. At least one form of ancestral ritual spelled this out in the gender symbolism assigned to the bodies of the dead. The *qi* of ancestors transmitted to descendants became embodied in the south Chinese customs surrounding dual burial. The yin flesh of the deceased was encouraged to rot away underground soon after death, allowing the yang bones to be reinterred as the ritually correct form of corporeality for the ancestral graveyard. This regional ritual illustrates a more general principle that the collective body of the ancestors, both male and female, is yang.[6]

Here bodily paternity is linked to the ancestral spirits, and bodily maternity, by contrast, is a sacrifice to those spirits. The association of paternal body and spiritual achievement was expressed not only in the ancestor cult but in the bodily self-cultivation of the inner alchemist. Imagined as the attribute of a male body of power, generative Essence had the potential to nourish the male body of longevity. When adepts sought immortality by fashioning an immortal embryo, the repressed image of the maternal gestational body returned in myth, realizing the ideal androgyny of the sage.

Theory

Today's feminist theories of the cultural construction of gender are shaped by an ideological commitment to understand bodily

---

6. This Cantonese ritual complex is discussed in Watson 1982: 179–82.

gender difference as a Foucauldian discourse of science as biopower. Our scholarly interpretations of the gender system of traditional China are set against the sharp cultural break that occurred as the nineteenth-century European colonial powers introduced Western science and social thought and precipitated the collapse of the Confucian episteme. In the twentieth century, the "woman question" became part of a discourse of nationalism and modernization, making women a recognized public group in emerging civic debate, while a sexualized new femininity was increasingly understood in terms of bioscience and mass consumer culture. Both of these can be seen as features of the colonial modernity of the late Qing treaty ports and the Westernized urban centers of the Republican era (1911–1949).[7] By historical contrast, it has been attractive to paint traditional culture as rejecting all essentialized gender identities, evoking the ideal of an older "Orient" free of modern pathologies.

However, biological essentialism as a critical category is also culturally specific to a time and place. It emerged out of the crisis of European Enlightenment in the eighteenth century as both an ambiguous accommodation to democratic social creeds and a challenge to Christian natural philosophy. When discourse located gender difference in a scientifically authoritative body, it insulated gender hierarchy from new equalitarian social ideologies. But such essentialism is not the only way that gender difference can be philosophically naturalized in the body. In late imperial China, both body and society were part of a system of signs linked to a larger cosmological order. This organicism precluded understanding nature as separate from culture, or bifurcating bodily and social gender. Yin and yang's very multivalence produced a view of nature as suffused with gendered attributes that did not depend upon the body alone for their point of reference.

At the same time, as attributes of nature yin and yang taught lessons about the body as well. Through yin and yang, a teleology of reproduction shaped the deepest bodily meanings. Some features of the Confucian family ethic appear to resemble the procreative imperative of Catholic Christian doctrines on sex and marriage. Nonetheless, yin and yang moralized the erotic domain in ways profoundly unfamiliar to European tradition. Rather than being fleshly appetites marking a fallen human nature, the generative body functions that males and females share gave the sexual an aura of the sacred. Wisely managed, these were creative capacities by which universal life was continued through the generations and the foundation of human society was assured.

7. Barlow 1994; Dikötter 1995.

Looking at all of this suggests how far we in late twentieth-century Europe and North America have come to naturalize the divorce of sex and reproduction. Today we are close to considering a sexual culture disassociated from family-based social organization — one that is hard to imagine without radically new reproductive technologies — as expressing the truth about gender. This separation of sexuality and reproduction constructs modern sexual androgyny — gender identity sameness — around the erotic experiences sexual partners share (whether these are experienced in same-sex or heterosexual pairs). When our discourse marginalizes gestational capacities as insignificant for bodily gender, we sustain androgyny by making the erotic the center of sexual identity, repressing maternity and paternity as well. By comparison, the Chinese medical bodies discussed here were imagined in a cultural context in which the common project of parenthood constituted the cultural meaning of androgyny, and the generative and the gestational forms of embodiment remained connected.

In today's Euro-American sexual culture, the erasure of reproductive meanings from the sexual body is a basis for sexual equality between males and females and for the discursive equivalence between homosexual and heterosexual modes of intimacy. Though the Chinese discourse on bodily androgyny was based on a diametrically opposed view of the body's deepest purposes, the men who constructed it also wrote as if the shared erotic domain told the most pleasing stories of gender homology or complementarity. Their effort to extend that complementarity from generation to gestation was imperfect, and at times broke down. Nonetheless, medicine taught males that eros could not be imagined independent of masculine powers of generation, even as it taught women more ambiguously that through generation and gestation their bodily natures would come to completion.

The resulting vision of bodily androgyny valorized gender interdependence in a familistic social order. Its body of yin and yang claimed the high ground as a metaphorical representation of the dynamic organicism of a cosmos uniting Heaven, Earth, and Humanity. But the implication that bodies belong not to oneself but to some larger order of significance is recognizable as a foundation of the Confucian patriarchal kinship system. As such it subordinated women to men and both to the ancestors, prefiguring, perhaps ominously, today's nationalist appropriations of the fertile bodies of women and men to serve state reproductive agendas.

Finally, the strength of discourse analysis is that it shows the production of bodies as a cultural work of language, bodily gesture and social performance. Its weakness, however, is an inability to find boundaries outside of discourse itself. My project here has been to lead readers into an imaginative engagement with unfamiliar cultural bodies both as aspects of Chinese history and as examples of alternative ways of constructing gender. If my readers have been able to enter this imaginative domain, I maintain that it is because other bodies become intelligible to us through a process of learning. At some level that learning is a kind of recognition. Philosophically, this implies prior points of reference in the realm of bodies to which our various discourses or languages of experience can refer and find translations pointing to common ground. Without such translations the multiplicity of languages of the body may all too easily construct attributes of groups divided from each other by the discursive politics of mutually exclusive identities. By asserting that there are limits to what is culturally constructed in discourse, we are able to reclaim for human bodies a common humanity.

Bibliography

Primary Sources

Anon. *Chan bao zhufang* 產寶諸方 (Prescriptions from the Birth Treasury). 1 juan. Preface by Wang Qingyue 王卿月, 1167. Edition: Ding Bing, ed., *Danggui caotang yixue congshu*, ce 8. 1878.

Anon. *Chanru beiyao* 產乳備要 (Essentials for Childbirth Readiness). Probably eleventh or twelfth century. Edition: Ding Bing, ed., *Danggui caotang yixue congshu*, ce 7. 1878.

Anon. *Chanyu baoqing ji* 產育保慶集 (Collection for Safeguarding the Blessed Event). n.d. Manuscript held in the East Asian Collection of the Library of Congress.

Anon. *Da sheng bian* 達生編 (On Successful Childbirth). 1715. "Jizhai jushi" 亟齋居士 (pseud.), comp. 1 juan. Edition: First edition held in the rare book library of the Zhongyi Yanjiuyuan in Beijing.

Anon. *Huangdi neijing* 黃帝內經 (The Yellow Emperor's Inner Canon). Probably first century B.C.E. Edition: Ren Yingqiu 任應秋, ed., *Huangdi neijing zhangju suoyin* 黃帝內經章句索引 (The Yellow Emperor's Inner Canon, by Chapter and Section, with Concordance). Beijing: Renmin weisheng chubanshe, 1986. Includes *Su wen* 素問 (Basic Questions) and *Ling shu* 靈樞 (Divine Pivot).

Anon. *Jiang hu yishu michuan* 江湖醫術秘傳 (Secretly Transmitted Medical Arts from the "Rivers and Lakes" [itinerant healers]). Undated; probably early twentieth century. 4 juan. Edition: Held in the Library of Congress.

Anon. *Jin ping mei cihua* 金瓶梅詞話 (The Song-story of the Plum in the Golden Vase). 100 chapters. Wanli ed.

Anon. *Jin ping mei* 金瓶梅 (The Plum in the Golden Vase). 100 chapters. Edition: Reprint of the second edition (originally published sometime between 1628 and 1640). Hong Kong: Sanlian, 1990. 2 vols.

Anon. *Kun yuan shi bao* 坤元是保 (True Protection of the Female Origin). n.d. Edition: Manuscript held in the rare book library of the Zhongyi Yanjiuyuan in Beijing.

Anon. *Nanjing* 難經 (The Canon of Problems). Probably second century C.E. Edition: Paul Unschuld, *Nanjing: The Classic of Difficult Issues* (Berkeley: University of California Press, 1986). Contains Chinese text and translation into English.

Anon. *Shengyu xiang jie* 聖諭像解 (Sacred Edict Illustrated and Explained). 1879. Edition: Jiangsu wushu, 1980. 2 vols.

Anon. *Yi yuan* 醫苑 (Medical Browsings). 1875. Anonymous manuscript anthology. Contains a *Zhujie tai chan dadonglun* 注解胎產大通論 (Annotated Obstetrical Survey) purported to be by Yang Zijian 楊子健 with a preface by Zhang Shengdao 張聲道, dated 1025. Held in the rare book library of the Zhongyi Yanjiuyuan in Beijing.

Cao Bingzhang 曹炳章, ed. 1936. *Zhongguo yixue dacheng* 中國醫學大成 (Encyclopedia of Chinese Medicine). Edition: 1990 reprint of the original Yuelu shushe edition. 6 vols. Abbreviated as ZGYXDC.

Chao Yingchun 趙應春, comp. 1556. *Danxi xiansheng zhifa xinyao* 丹溪先生治法心要 (Essentials of Mr. Danxi's Methods of Treatment). 8 juan. Edition: Photolithographed reprint. Taipei: Xinwenfeng, 1982. 2 vols.

Chao Yuanfang 巢元方. [Fl. 605–616]. *Zhubing yuanhou lun* 諸病源候論 (On the Origins and Symptoms of Disease). 50 juan. Edition: ZGYXDC, vol. 2.

Chen Ziming 陳自明, comp. 1237; rev. 1284. *Furen ta quan liang fang* 婦人大全良方 (All-Inclusive Good Prescriptions for Women). 24 juan. Edition: Recension of Yu Ying'ao 余瀛鰲, et al. Beijing: Renmin weisheng chubanshe, 1985. This text is based upon the Yuan dynasty Qinyoushutang 勤有書堂 *jiao pian* edition, supplemented by the Ming Zhengde edition edited by Xiong Zongli 態宗立, the 1548 edition by Xue Ji 薛己, and the SKQS.

Cheng Congzhou 程從周 (Cheng Maoxian 程茂先). Preface 1633. *Cheng Maoxian yi'an* 程茂先醫案 (Medical Cases of Cheng Maoxian). 2 juan. Edition: Photolithographed reprint of the first edition. Shanghai: Shanghai guji shudian, 1979.

Chu Cheng 褚澄. [Fl. 483 C.E.]. *Chu shi yi shu* 褚氏遺書 (Bequeathed Writings of Master Chu). Edition: SKQS, vol. 734. The text reprinted in juan 74 of the *Shuo fu* 說郛, the Ming anthology compiled by Tao Zongyi 陶宗儀, is identical except for the absence of section titles.

Ding Bing 丁丙, ed. 1878. *Danggui caotang yixue congshu* 當歸草堂醫學叢書 (Medical Collection from Angelica Cottage). 10 vols. Available in the rare book library of the Zhongyi Yanjiuyuan, Beijing.

Fang Guang 方廣, comp. Preface 1536. *Danxi xinfa fuyu* 丹溪心法附餘 (Essential Arts of Danxi, with Supplementary Additions). 24 juan. Edition: Photolithographed reprint. Taipei: Xinwenfeng chuban gongsi, 1974. 5 vols.

Fu Shan 傅山. n.d. "Duan hong long" 斷紅龍 (Beheading the Red Dragon). Appendix to *Shang cheng xiu Dao mishu sizhong* 上乘修道秘書四種 (Four Secret Volumes on Cultivating the Dao Conveyed from on High). Edition: Xiao Tianshi, comp., *Daozang jinghua* 道藏精華 (Quintessence of the Daoist Canon), series 12, no. 2. Taipei, 1965.

Guo Jizhong 郭稽中 and Li Shisheng 李師聖. 1131. *Chanyu baoqing ji [fang]* 產育寶慶集 [方] (Childbirth Treasury Collection [of Prescriptions]). 2 juan. Editions: Reprinted in Ding Bing, ed., *Danggui caotang yixue congshu*, 1878, and in Zhu Duanzhang, *Weishengjia bao chanke beiyao*, 1887. Both of these editions add a second juan of prescriptions to a first juan composed of twenty-one topics.

Hong Mai 洪邁 [1123–1202]. *Yijian zhi* 夷堅志 (A Record of the Listener). 207 juan. Edition: *Tushu jicheng* 圖書集成 (Reader's Complete Library), series 76, vols. 28–43.

Huang Liuhong 黃六鴻. Preface 1694. *Fu hui quanshu* 福惠全書 (Complete Book of Happiness and Benevolence). Edition: Yamane Yukio, ed. Kyoto: Fukekei Zensho, 1974.

Huizong 徽宗. Original preface 1118. *Sheng ji jing* 聖濟經 (Canon of Sagely Benefaction). 10 juan. Edition: Reprint edited by Liu Shuqing 劉淑清. Beijing: Renmin weisheng chubanshe, 1990. This edition is based on Lu Xinyuan's 陸心源 1887 recension, which in turn was based on manuscripts annotated by Wu Ti 吳褆 in the Southern Song.

Jiang Guan 江瓘. 1552. *Ming yi lei an* 名醫類案 (Case Histories from Famous Doctors). 20 juan. Edition: Fascimile reprint of the Zhibuzuzhai congshu edition of 1770. Beijing: Renmin weisheng chubanshe, 1957, 1982.

Kou Zongshi 寇宗奭. First published 1116. *Bencao yanyi* 本草衍義 (An Exposition of Materia Medica). 20 juan. Edition: ZGYXDC, vol. 2.

Li Kaixian 李開先. [1502–1568]. *Li Kaixian ji* 李開先集 (Collected Works of Li Kaixian). Edition: Shanghai: Zhonghua shuju, 1959. 3 vols.

Li Shizhen 李時珍. First published 1596. *Bencao gangmu* 本草綱目 (Systematic Materia Medica). 52 juan. Editions: 1896 illustrated woodblock edition by Weiguzhai; Beijing: Renmin weisheng chubanshe, 1975. 4 vols.

Li Yu 李漁. 1671. *Xian qing ouji* 閒情偶寄 (Casual Expressions of Idle Feelings). Edition: Zhejiang guji chubanshe, 1985.

Li Zhongzi 李中梓. 1642. *Shanbu yisheng wei lun* 刪補頤生微論 (Subtle Discourse on Nurturing Life: Revised Version). 4 juan. Edition: Woodblock edition held in the Gest Library, Princeton University.

Lin Zhihan 林之翰. 1723. *Si zhen juewei* 四診抉微 (The Subtleties of Diagnosis). 8 juan. Edition: Beijing: Renmin weisheng chubanshe, 1957, 1983.

Ling shu. See Huangdi neijing

Liu Fang 劉昉. 1150. *You you xin shu* 幼幼新書 (New Book on Caring for the Young). 40 juan. Edition: Ma Jixing 馬繼興 et al., eds. Beijing: Renmin weisheng chubanshe, 1987.

Lü Kun 呂坤. 1598. "Shi zheng lu" 實政錄 (Record of Practical Administration). Edition: Vol. 19, juan 2 of *Lü zi yi shu* 呂子遺書 (Bequeathed Writings of Master Lü), 1827.

Maijing. See Wang Shuhe.

Nakagawa Tadahide 中川忠英. 1800. *Shinzoku kibun* 清俗紀聞 (Observations of Qing Dynasty Customs). Edition: Tokyo: Heibonsha, 1966.

Ouyang Xiu 歐陽修. Eleventh century. "Zou shi lu" 奏事錄 (Record of Things Memorialized). Edition: Juan 219 of *Ouyang Wenzhong gong quanji* 歐陽文忠公全集 (Complete Works of Ouyang Xiu), 1819.

Qi Zhongfu 齊仲甫. Original preface 1220. *Nüke baiwen* 女科百問 (One Hundred Questions on Medicine for Females). 2 juan. Edition: Facsimile reprint of the Zongbutang edition of 1735. Shanghai: Shanghai guji shudian, 1983.

———. N.d. *Chan bao baiwen* 產寶百問 (One Hundred Question Birth Treasury). 5 juan. Edition: Held in the rare book library of the Zhongyi Yanjiuyuan in Beijing.

Qian Yi 錢乙. Eleventh century. *Xiaoer yaozheng zhenjue* 小兒藥証真訣 (Veracious Instructions for Diagnosing and Treating Children). Edition: Shanghai: Weisheng chubanshe, 1958.

Ruan Dacheng 阮大鋮. Early seventeenth century. *Yanzi jian* 燕子箋 (The Swallow's Letter). Edition: Beijing Zhonghua shuju, 1988.

SKQS. See *Siku quanshu*

Shen Bang 沈榜. 1593. *Wan shu zaji* 宛署雜記 (Jottings on a Posting at Wan[ping]). Edition: Beijing chubanshe, 1961.

Shen Defu 沈德符. [1578–1642]. *Wanli yehuo bian* 萬歷野獲編 (Private Gleanings of the Wanli Reign). 30 juan. Edition: Taipei: Wei-wen, 1976. 5 vols.

Siku quanshu 四庫全書 (The Complete Collection of the Four Treasuries). 1,500 vols. Edition: Taipei: Taiwan shangwu yinshuguan reprint of Wenyuange edition, 1983. Abbreviated as SKQS.

Su wen. See *Huangdi neijing*

Sun Simiao 孫思邈. Completed c. 652 C.E. *Beiji qianjin yaofang* 備急千金要方 (Prescriptions Worth a Thousand for Every Emergency). 30 juan. Edition: Beijing: Renmin weisheng chubanshe, 1955, 1994.

———. Completed c. 682 C.E. *Qianjin yi fang* 千金翼方 (Supplementary Prescriptions Worth a Thousand). 30 juan. Edition: Beijing: Renmin weisheng chubanshe, n.d.

Sun Yikui 孫一奎. 1584. *Chi shui xuan zhu quanji* 赤水玄珠全集 (Pearls of Wisdom [transmitted] from Red River). 30 juan. Edition: Ling Tianyi 凌天翼, ed. Beijing: Renmin weisheng chubanshe, 1986.

Taiping sheng hui fang. See Wang Huaiyin

Tamba Yasuyori 丹波康賴. Completed 982 C.E. *Ishinpo* 醫心方 (Prescriptions at the Heart of Medicine). Edition: Fascimile of 1854 edition by Taki Genkin. Beijing: Renmin weisheng chubanshe, 1955. 2 vols.

Tan Yunxian 談允賢. 1511, 1585. *Nü yi zayan* 女醫雜言 (Sayings of a Female Doctor). Edition: Copy of the second (1585) edition held in the rare book library of the Zhongyi Yanjiuyuan in Beijing.

Tao Xinyuan 陶心源, comp. 1876. *Shiwanjuan lou congshu* 十萬卷樓叢書 (Collection from the Tower of a Myriad Volumes). 8 vols.

Tao Zongyi 陶宗儀. Fourteenth century. *Chuo geng lu* 輟耕錄 (Recorded When Ploughing Is Done). Edition: Mao Jin 毛晉, ed. *Jindai mishu* 津逮秘書 (Secret Volumes Ferried to Shore), vol. 121. Shanghai: Poguzhai, 1922.

Wan Quan 萬全. N.d. *Douzhen "ge zhi" yaolun* 痘疹格至要論 (Basic Discourse on "Natural Knowledge" of Smallpox). Edition: Ming edition held in the Gest Library, Princeton University.

———. Author's prefaces 1549, 1579. *Wan shi jia chuan douzhen xinfa* 萬氏家傳痘疹心法 (Essentials of the Wan Family Tradition [concerning] Smallpox).

23 juan. Edition: Collated by the Lotian County Health Bureau and published by the Hubei renmin chubanshe, 1985.

——. Preface 1645. *Wan shi jia chuan yang sheng si yao* 萬氏家傳養生四要 (The Wan Family's Four Essentials for Nourishing Life). 5 juan. Edition: Collated by the Lotian County Health Bureau and published by the Hubei renmin chubanshe, 1984.

——. Prefaces 1654, 1667. *Wan shi furen ke* 萬氏婦人科 (Mister Wan's Medicine for Women). 3 juan. Edition: Collated by the Lotian County Health Bureau and published by the Hubei renmin chubanshe, 1983.

——. Prefaces 1654, 1667. *Wan shi jia chuan guang si jiyao* 萬氏家傳廣嗣紀要 (The Wan Family's Essential Record on Multiplying Descendants). 16 juan. Edition: Collated by the Lotian County Health Bureau and published by the Hubei renmin chubanshe, 1986.

——. 1712. *Wan Mizhai quanshu* 萬密齋全書 (Complete Works of Wan Mizhai). 10 vols. Edition: Shifutang. Held in the Gest Library, Princeton University.

Wang Chong 王充. [27 C.E.–100]. "Si wei pian" 四違篇 (On the Four Taboos). Juan 23 of *Lun heng* 論衡 (Contrarian Essays). Edition: Shanghai: Renmin chubanshe, 1974.

Wang Huaiyin 王懷隱 et al., comp. 978–992. *Taiping sheng hui fang* 太平聖惠方 (Imperial Grace Formulary). Edition: Beijing: Renmin weisheng chubanshe, 1958. 2 vols.

Wang Kentang 王肯堂. 1602. *Yi lun* 醫論 (Medical Discourses). 3 juan. Edition: Beijing: Renmin weisheng chubanshe, 1993.

——. 1608. *Nüke zheng zhi zhunsheng* 女科證治準繩 (Guideline for the Treatment of Female Disorders). 5 juan. Edition: Beijing: Renmin weisheng chubanshe, 1993. Vol. 6 of Wang's collected works.

Wang Shuhe 王叔和. c. 280 C.E. *Maijing* 脈經 (Canon of the Pulse). 10 juan. Edition: ZGYXDC, vol. 1.

Wang Xi 王熹, comp. 752 C.E. *Wai tai mi yao* 外台秘要 (Essential Secrets of the Palace Library). 40 juan. Edition: Fascimile reprint of 1657 edition. Beijing: Renmin weisheng chubanshe, 1955, 1982.

Wei Zhixiu 魏之琇. 1770. *Xu ming yi lei an* 續名醫類案 (More Cases from Famous Doctors). 36 juan. Edition: Fascimile reprint of the Xinshutang blocks. Beijing: Renmin weisheng chubanshe, 1957, 1982.

Weng Zhongren 翁仲仁. 1579. *Douzhen jinjing lu* 痘疹金鏡錄 (On the Golden Mirror of Smallpox). 4 juan. Edition: First edition held in the rare book library of the Zhongyi Yanjiuyuan, Beijing.

Wu Qian 吳謙 et al. 1742. *Yi zong jinjian* 醫宗金鑑 (Golden Mirror of Medicine). Imperially sponsored encyclopedia in 90 juan. Edition: Beijing: Renmin weisheng chubanshe, 1963, 1973, 1981. 5 vols.

Wu Zhiwang 武之望. 1620, 1621. *Ji yin gangmu* 濟陰綱目 (To Benefit Yin: A Comprehensive Guide). 5 juan. Edition: First edition held in the rare book library of the Zhongyi Yanjiuyuan, Beijing.

——. 1626. *Ji yang gangmu* 濟陽綱目 (To Benefit Yang: A Comprehensive Guide). 108 juan. Edition: 1856 woodblock edition compiled by Zhang Nan 張楠 et al.

——. Edited by Wang Qi 汪淇. 1665. *Ji yin gangmu* 濟陰綱目 (To Benefit Yin: A Comprehensive Guide). 14 juan, plus appendix "Bao sheng suishi" 保生碎事 (Trivia for Safeguarding Life). Editions: First editions held in the rare book library of the Zhongyi Yanjiuyuan, Beijing; and in the Cabinet Library, Tokyo; reprint of 1958, Shanghai: Keji weisheng chubanshe.

Xiao Jing 肖京. 1644. *Xian qi jiu zheng lun* 軒岐救正論 (On Seeking Truth in the Medical Arts). 6 juan. Edition: Photolithographed reproduction of the first edition. Beijing: Guji chubanshe, 1983.

Xiao Xun 蕭壎. First published 1684. *Nüke jing lun* 女科經論 (Medicine for Females According to the Classics). 8 juan. Edition: ZGYXDC, vol. 5.

Xie Zhaozhe 謝肇淛. [1567–1624]. *Wu zazu* 五雜組 (Five-Part Miscellany). 16 juan. Edition: Taipei: Weiwen chubanshe, 1977.

Xue Ji 薛己. 1547. *Jiaozhu furen liang fang* 校註婦人良方 (Revised Good Prescriptions for Women). 24 juan. Edition: ZGYXDC, vol. 5.

Yin Zhenren 尹眞人. 1615. *Xingming gui zhi* 性命圭旨 (Leading to the Core of Life). Edition: Held in the library of the Needham Research Institute, Cambridge, England.

Yu Chang 喻昌. 1661. *Yu Jiayan yixue san shu* 喻嘉言醫學三書 (The Medical Learning of Yu Jiayan [Yu Chang] in Three Volumes). Edition: Reprint by Kiangxi renmin chubanshe, 1984.

Yu Chong 虞沇. 1140. *Bei chan ji yong fang* 備產急用方 (Useful Prescriptions Ready-Made to Assist in Birth). Edition: Zhu Duanzhang, ed., *Weishengjia bao chanke beiyao* (1184), juan 6; reprinted in Tao Xinyuan, ed., *Shiwanjuan lou congshu*, 1887.

Yu Qiao 俞橋. 1544. *Guang si yaoyu* 廣嗣要語 (Essential Words on Propagating Descendants). 1 juan. Edition: *Zhenben yishu jicheng* 珍本醫書集成 (Anthology of Rare Medical Books), vol. 14. Shanghai: Kexue jishu chubanshe, 1986.

Yuan Hao 袁顥. Fifteenth century. "Yuan shi jiaxun" 袁氏家訓 (Yuan Family Instructions). In *Yuan shi congshu* 袁氏叢書 (Collected Writings of the Yuan Family), vol. 1. Edition: Ming edition in the Naikaku Bunko, Tokyo.

Yuan Huang 袁黃. 1591. *Qi si zhenquan* 祈嗣眞詮 (Veracious Explanation of the Blessing of Heirs). 1 juan. Edition: *Congshu jicheng* 叢書集成 (Complete [classical] Library), vol. 2986.

——. 1591. *She sheng san yao* 攝生三要 (Three Essentials for Furthering Life). 1 juan. Edition: *Daozang jinghua lu* 道藏精華錄 (Records of the Quintessence of the Daoist Canon), vol. 1. Hangzhou: Zhejiang guji chubanshe, 1989.

Yue Fujia 岳甫嘉. 1635. *Miaoyizhai yixue zhengyin zhongzi bian* 妙一齋醫學正印種子編 (Orthodox Medical Learning from the Studio of Wondrous Unity: On Begetting Heirs). Edition: Beijing: Zhongyi guji chubanshe, 1986.

Zan Yin 咎殷. [Fl. 897]. *Chan bao* 產寶 (Birth Treasury). 3 juan. Edition: ZGYXDC, vol. 5.

ZGYXDC. *See* Cao Bingzhang

Zhang Gao 張杲. Completed 1224. *Yi shuo* 醫說 (Talks About Medicine). 10 juan. Edition: Shanghai Zhongyi xueyuan shuguan. 1933; reprint 1984. 2 vols.

Zhang Ji 張機 (Zhang Zhongjing 張仲景). [Eastern Han 25 C.E.–220]. *Jin gui yaolüe lunzhu* 金匱要略論註 (Essentials of the Golden Casket, annotated). Edition: SKQS, vol. 734.

Zhang Jiebin 張介賓. Preface 1624. *Furen gui* 婦人規 (Regulations for Women). 2 juan. Edition: Guangzhou: Guangdong keji chubanshe, 1984, 1986.

Zhou Rongqi 周榮起. 1630. *Bencao tupu* 本草圖譜 (Illustrated Materia Medica). Edition: Ming edition held in the rare book library of the Zhongyi Yanjiuyuan in Beijing.

Zhu Duanzhang 朱端章. 1184. *Weishengjia bao chanke beiyao* 衛生家寶產科備要 (Essentials on Childbirth Preparedness from the Treasury of the House of Good Health). Medical anthology in 8 juan. Edition: 1887 reprint in Tao Xinyuan, comp., *Shiwanjuan lou congshu*. Held in the rare book library of the Zhongyi Yanjiuyuan in Beijing.

Zhu Huiming 朱惠明. First published 1594. *Douzhen chuan xinlu* 痘疹傳心錄 (Transmitted Essentials on Pox Disorders). 16 juan. Edition: 1786 edition held by the Gest Library, Princeton University.

Zhu Xi 朱熹. 1270. *Zhuzi xingli yulei* 朱子性理語類 (Conversations of Zhu Xi on Nature and Principle, Classified by Topic). Edition: Shanghai: Guji chubanshe, 1992, reprinted from the SKQS.

Zhu Zhenheng 朱震亨. Preface 1347. *Ge zhi yu lun* 格致餘類 (More on the "Natural Knowledge" of Phenomena). Edition: SKQS, vol. 746.

———. Preface 1347. *Ju fang fahui* 局方發揮 (Exposé of Official Prescriptions). Edition: SKQS, vol. 746.

———. 1993. *Danxi yi ji* 丹溪醫集 (Collected Medical Writings of Danxi [Zhu Zhenheng]). Edited by the Zhejiang sheng Zhongyi yao yanjiuyuan wenxian yanjiuso.

Secondary Sources

Ahern, Emily M. 1975. "The Power and Pollution of Chinese Women." In *Women in Chinese Society*, ed. Margery Wolf and Roxane Witke, 193–214. Stanford, Calif.: Stanford University Press.

Baldrian-Hussein, Farzeon. 1989–90. "Inner Alchemy: Notes on the Origin and Use of the Term *Neidan*." *Cahiers d'Extrême-Asia* 5: 163–90.

Banister, Judith. 1987. *China's Changing Population*. Stanford, Calif.: Stanford University Press.

Baoning si Mingdai shui lu hua 寶宁寺明代水陸畫 (Ming Dynasty Wall Murals from the Baoning Temple). 1988, 1995. Beijing: Wenwu chubanshe.

Barlow, Tani E. 1994. "Theorizing Woman: *Funü, Guojia, Jiating* (Chinese Woman, Chinese State, Chinese Family)." In *Body, Subject and Power in China*, ed. Angela Zito and Tani E. Barlow, 253–89. Chicago: University of Chicago Press.

Birge, Bettine. 1995. "Levirate Marriage and the Revival of Widow Chastity in Yuan China." *Asia Major*, 8.2.

———. Forthcoming. *Women, Property and Confucian Reaction in Sung and Yuan China (960–1368)*. Cambridge, England: Cambridge University Press.

Bol, Peter K. 1992. *This Culture of Ours—Intellectual Transitions in T'ang and Sung China*. Stanford, Calif.: Stanford University Press.

Bossler, Beverly. 1996. "Woman's Literacy in Song Dynasty China: Preliminary Inquiries." Paper delivered to the Conference on Women in Confucian Cultures in Pre-Modern China, Korea and Japan. University of California, San Diego, June 28–July 1, 1996.

———. Forthcoming. *Powerful Relations: Kinship, Status and the State in Sung China (960–1279)*. Cambridge, Mass.: Harvard Council on East Asian Studies.

Bray, Francesca. 1995. "A Deathly Disorder: Understanding Women's Health in Late Imperial China." In *Knowledge and the Scholarly Medical Traditions*, ed. Don Bates, 235–50. Cambridge, England: Cambridge University Press.

———. 1997. *Technology and Gender: Fabrics of Power in Late Imperial China*. Berkeley: University of California Press.

Brokaw, Cynthia. 1991. *The Ledgers of Merit and Demerit: Social Change and Moral Order in Late Imperial China*. Princeton, N.J.: Princeton University Press.

Butler, Judith. 1990. *Gender Trouble: Feminism and the Subversion of Identity*. New York: Routledge.

———. 1993. *Bodies That Matter: On the Discursive Limits of Sex*. New York: Routledge.

Cao Bingzhang 曹炳章. 1936. *Zhongguo yixue dacheng zongmu tiyao* 中國醫學大成總目提要 (Analytical Bibliography of the Encyclopedia of Chinese Medical Learning). Original bibliographical volume to ZGYXDC, not reprinted.

Carlitz, Katherine. 1991. "Social Uses of Female Virtue in Late Ming Editions of *Lienü zhuan*." *Late Imperial China* 12.2:117–48.

———. 1997. "Shrines, Governing-Class Identity, and the Cult of Widow Fidelity in Mid-Ming Jiangnan." *Journal of Asian Studies* 56.3:612–40.

Cass, Victoria. 1986. "Female Healers in the Ming and the Lodge of Ritual and Ceremony." *Journal of the American Oriental Society* 106.1:233–40.

Chan, Wing-tsit. 1963. *A Source Book in Chinese Philosophy*. Princeton, N.J.: Princeton University Press.

Chang, Chia-feng. 1996. *Aspects of Smallpox and Its Significance in Chinese History*. Ph.D. diss., University of London School of Oriental and African Studies.

Chao, Yuanling. 1995. *Medicine and Society in Late Imperial China: Physicians in Suzhou*. Ph.D. diss., University of California, Los Angeles.

Chen Bangxian 陳邦賢. 1982 (preface 1964). *Ershiliu shi yixue shiliao huibian* 二十六史醫學史料滙編 (Collected Historical Materials on Medicine from the Twenty-Six Dynastic Histories). Beijing: Zhongyi Yanjiuyuan, Zhongguo Yishi Wenxian Yanjiuso.

Chen Menglei 陳夢雷 et al., comp. *Gujin tushu jicheng: Yibu quanlu* 古今圖書集成醫部全錄 (Complete Medical Sections from the Imperial Encyclopedia [juan 501–20]). Edition: Beijing, 1962: Renmin weisheng chubanshe. 12 vols.

Chen Yuan-peng 陳元朋. 1995. "Song dai de 'ru yi'—jian ping Robert P.

Hymes youguan Song-Yuan yizhe diwei de lundian" 宋代的儒醫——兼評 Robert P. Hymes 有關宋元醫者地位的論點 ("Literati Doctors" of the Song Dynasty—with Comment on Robert P. Hymes' "Doctors in Song and Yuan"). *Xin shi xue* 新史學 (New History) 6.1 (March): 179–203.

——. 1997. *Liang Song de "shang yi shiren" yu "ru yi"—jian lun qi zai Jin-Yuan de liubian* 兩宋的尚醫士人與儒醫——兼論其在金元的流變 (Song "Gentleman Admirers of Medicine" and the Literati Physician—Together with a Discussion of Their Jin-Yuan Evolution). Taipei: Guoli Taiwan Daxue wenshi congkan.

Cherniack, Susan. 1994. "Book Culture and Textual Transmission in Sung China." *Harvard Journal of Asiatic Studies* 54.1:5–125.

Chia, Lucille. 1996. "The Development of the Jianyang Book Trade, Song-Yuan." *Late Imperial China* 17.1:10–48.

Chung, Priscilla Ching. 1981. *Palace Women in the Northern Song: 960–1126.* Leiden: E. J. Brill.

Corbin, Alain. 1986. *The Foul and the Fragrant.* Cambridge, Mass.: Harvard University Press.

Cullen, Christopher. 1993. "Patients and Healers in Late Imperial China: Evidence from the *Jinpingmei.*" *History of Science* 31:99–150.

Despeux, Catherine. 1990. *Immortelles de la Chine ancienne: Taoism et alchemie féminine.* Paris: Pardes.

——. Forthcoming. "Le *wuyun liuqi* et l'innovation en medécine sous les Song." In *Innovation in Chinese Medicine,* ed. Elisabeth Hsu. Cambridge, England: Needham Research Institute Monograph Series, Cambridge University Press.

DeWoskin, Kenneth J. 1983. *Doctors, Diviners and Magicians of Ancient China: Biographies of Fang-shih.* New York: Columbia University Press.

Dikötter, Frank. 1995. *Sex, Culture and Modernity in China.* Honolulu: University of Hawai'i Press.

Ding Ling. Tani E. Barlow and Gary Bjorge, eds. 1989. *I Myself Am a Woman: Selected Works of Ding Ling.* Boston: Beacon Press.

Dong Guangdong 董光東 and Liu Huiling 劉惠玲. 1995. "Ming-Qing shiqi Xin'an yaodian ji qi yiyaoxue zuoyong." 明清時期新安葯店及其醫葯學作用 (Ming-Qing Pharmacy Shops in Xin'an and their Role in Medical Learning). *Zhonghua yishi zazhi* 中華醫史雜志 (Journal of China's Medical History) 25.1.1:30–34.

Duden, Barbara. 1991. *The Woman Beneath the Skin: A Doctor's Patients in Eighteenth-Century Germany.* Cambridge, Mass.: Harvard University Press.

——. 1993. *Disembodying Women: Perspectives on Pregnancy and the Unborn.* Cambridge, Mass.: Harvard University Press.

Ebrey, Patricia Buckley. 1993. *The Inner Quarters: Marriage and the Lives of Chinese Women in the Sung Period.* Berkeley: University of California Press.

——. 1995. "Marriage among the Song Elite." In *Chinese Historical Micro-Demography*, ed. Stevan Harrell, 21–47. Berkeley, Calif.: University of California Press.

Elvin, Mark. 1984. "Female Virtue and the State in China." *Past and Present* 104 (August): 111–52.

———. 1989. "Tales of *Shen* and *Xin*: Body-Person and Heart-Mind in China During the Last One Hundred and Fifty Years." In *Fragments for a History of the Human Body, Part Two*, eds. Michel Feher et al., 267–349. Zone Press; distributed by MIT Press, Cambridge, Mass.

Fan Xingzhun 范行准. 1961, 1985. *Zhongguo yixue shilüe* 中國醫學史略 (Brief History of Chinese Medicine). Beijing: Zhongyi guqi chubanshe.

Farquhar, Judith. 1994. *Knowing Practice: The Clinical Encounter of Chinese Medicine*. Boulder, Colorado: Westview Press.

———. 1996. "'Medicine and the Changes Are One': An Essay in Divination Healing with Commentary." *Chinese Science* 13:107–34.

Foucault, Michel. 1973. *The Birth of the Clinic: Archeology of Medical Perception*. New York: Sheridan Smith.

———. 1978, 1985, 1986. *The History of Sexuality. Volume 1, An Introduction; volume 2, The Use of Pleasure; volume 3, The Care of the Self*. New York: Pantheon.

Fu Weikang 傅維康 et al. 1990. *Zhongguo yixue shi* 中國醫學史 (History of China's Medical Learning). Shanghai: Zhongyi xueyuan chubanshe.

Fung, Yu-lan. 1952. *History of Chinese Philosophy* . Translated by Derk Bodde. 2 vols. Princeton, N.J.: Princeton University Press.

Furth, Charlotte. 1987. "Concepts of Pregnancy, Childbirth and Infancy in Qing Dynasty China." *Journal of Asian Studies* 46.1:7–35.

———. 1988. "Androgynous Males and Deficient Females: Biology and Gender Boundaries in Sixteenth and Seventeenth Century China." *Late Imperial China* 9.2:1–31.

———. 1994. "Rethinking Van Gulik: Sexuality and Reproduction in Traditional Chinese Medicine." In *Engendering China: Women, Culture and the State*, ed. Christina K. Gilmartin, Gail Hershatter, et al., 125–46. Cambridge, Mass.: Harvard University Press.

———. 1995. "From Birth to Birth: The Growing Body in Chinese Medicine." In *Chinese Views of Childhood*, ed. Anne Behnke Kinney, 157–91. Honolulu: University of Hawai'i Press.

Furth, Charlotte, and Chen Shu-yueh. 1992. "Chinese Medicine and the Anthropology of Menstruation in Contemporary Taiwan." *Medical Anthropology Quarterly*, n. s., 6.1: 27–48.

Good, Bryan. 1994. *Medicine, Rationality and Experience: An Anthropological Perspective*. Cambridge, England: Cambridge University Press.

Grant, Beata. 1989. "The Spiritual Saga of Woman Huang: From Pollution to Purification." In *Ritual Opera, Operatic Ritual: Mu-lien Rescues His Mother in Chinese Popular Culture*, ed. David Johnson, 224–311. The Chinese Popular Culture Project. Distributed by the University of California, Berkeley, Institute of East Asian Studies.

Grant, Joanna. 1996. *Wang Ji's "Shishan yi'an": Aspects of Gender and Culture in Ming Dynasty Medical Case Histories*. Ph.D. diss., University of London.

Guo Aiqun 郭靄春, ed. 1984–87. *Zhongguo fensheng yi jikao* 中國分省醫籍考 (Evidential Scholarship on Medicine Organized by China's Provinces). 2 vols. Tianjin: Tianjin Zhongyi xueyuan.

Guo Licheng 郭立誠. 1979. *Zhongguo shengyu lisu kao* 中國生育禮俗考

(Investigation of Chinese Childbirth Rituals and Customs). Taipei: Wenshizhe chubanshe.

Hanson, Marta. 1995. "Merchants of Medicine: Huizhou Mercantile Consciousness, Morality and Medical Patronage in Seventeenth-Century China." In *East Asian Science: Tradition and Beyond*, 207–14. Osaka: Kansai University Press.

———. 1997. *Inventing a Tradition in Chinese Medicine: From Universal Canon to Local Medicine in South China, The Seventeenth to the Nineteenth Century.* Ph.D. diss., University of Pennsylvania.

Harrell, Stevan. 1985. "The Rich Get Children: Segmentation, Stratification, and Population in Three Chekiang Lineages, 1550–1850." In *Family and Population in East Asian History*, ed. Susan Hanley and Arthur P. Wolf, 81–109. Berkeley: University of California Press.

He Shixi 何時希. 1983. *Lidai wuming yijia yan an* 歷代無名醫家驗案 (Historical Cases of Effective Treatment by Anonymous Doctors). Shanghai: Xuelin chubanshe.

———, comp. 1984. *Zhenben nüke yishu ji yi bazhong* 珍本女科醫書輯佚八種 (A Precious Compilation of Eight Lost Medical Books on Female Disorders). Eight anonymous texts, reconstructed from fragments of Tang and pre-Tang works. Shanghai: Xuelin chubanshe.

———. 1991. *Zhongguo lidai yijia zhuan lu* 中國歷代醫家傳錄 (Biographical Records on Physicians in Chinese History). 3 vols. Beijing: Renmin weisheng chubanshe.

Henderson, John B. 1984. *The Development and Decline of Chinese Cosmology.* New York: Columbia University Press.

Hollander, Anne. 1978. *Seeing Through Clothes.* New York: Avon.

Holmgren, Jennifer. 1985. "The Economic Foundations of Virtue: Widow Remarriage in Early and Modern China." *Australian Journal of Chinese Affairs* 13:1–27.

Hsiung Ping-chen. 1994. "Constructed Emotions: The Bond between Mothers and Sons in Late Imperial China." *Late Imperial China* 15.1:87–117.

Hsiung Ping-chen 熊秉真 (Xiong Bingzhen). 1995. *You you: Chuantong Zhongguo de qiangbao zhi dao* 幼幼: 傳統中國的襁褓之道 (Caring for the Young: The Newborn's Path in Traditional China). Taipei: Lianjing chuban shiye gongsi.

———. Forthcoming. "More or Less: Cultural and Medical Factors Behind Marital Fertility in Late Imperial China." In *Abortion, Infanticide and Reproductive Culture in East Asia, Past and Present*, ed. James Z. Lee and Saito Osamu. Oxford, England: Oxford University Press.

Hu Wenkai 胡文楷. 1985. *Lidai funü zhuzuo kao* 歷代婦女著作考 (An Examination of Women's Writing through the Dynasties). Shanghai: Shanghai guji chubanshe.

Hymes, Robert P. 1987. "Not Quite Gentlemen? Doctors in Song and Yuan." *Chinese Science* 8:9–76.

Jiang Yazhou 姜亞洲 and Li Minglian 李明廉. 1988. "'Ji yin gangmu' kaoshu" 濟陰綱目考述 (Critical Inquiry into *Ji yin gangmu*). *Zhonghua yishi zazhi* 中華醫史雜志 (Journal of China's Medical History) 18.2: 115–118.

Jianming Zhongyi cidian 簡明中醫辭典 (Concise Dictionary of Chinese Medicine). 1979, 1982. Compiled by the Editorial Committee of the Dictionary of Chinese Medicine. Beijing: Renmin weisheng chubanshe.

Johnson, Elizabeth. 1975. "Women and Childbearing in Kwan Mun Hau Village." In *Women in Chinese Society*, ed. Margery Wolf and Roxane Witke, 215–41. Stanford, Calif.: Stanford University Press.

Kendall, Laurel. 1985. *Shamans, Housewives and Other Restless Spirits: Women in Korean Ritual Life*. Honolulu: University of Hawai'i Press.

Kiple, Kenneth F., ed. 1993. *The Cambridge World History of Human Disease*. Cambridge, England: Cambridge University Press.

Kleinman, Arthur. 1980. *Patients and Healers in the Context of Culture: An Exploration of the Borderland between Anthropology, Medicine, and Psychiatry*. Berkeley: University of California Press.

Ko, Dorothy. 1994. *Teachers of the Inner Chambers: Women and Culture in Seventeenth-Century China*. Stanford, Calif.: Stanford University Press.

———. 1997. "The Body as Attire: The Shifting Meanings of Footbinding in Seventeenth-Century China." *Journal of Women's History* 18.4 (Winter): 8–27.

Kuriyama, Shigehisa. 1994. "The Imagination of Winds and the Development of the Chinese Conception of the Body." In *Body, Subject and Power in China*, ed. Angela Zito and Tani E. Barlow, 23–41. Chicago: University of Chicago Press.

LaFleur, William R. 1992. *Liquid Life: Buddhism and Abortion in Japan*. Princeton, N.J.: Princeton University Press.

Laqueur, Thomas. 1990. *Making Sex: Body and Gender from the Greeks to Freud*. Cambridge, Mass.: Harvard University Press.

Late Imperial China. 1992. Special issue: "Symposium on Poetry and Women's Culture in Late Imperial China." Vol. 13.1 (June).

Lee, James Z., and Cameron D. Campbell. 1997. *Fate and Fortune in Rural China: Social Organization and Population Behavior in Liaoning, 1774–1873*. Cambridge, England: Cambridge University Press.

Lee, James Z., and Saito Osamu, eds. Forthcoming. *Abortion, Infanticide and Reproductive Culture in East Asia, Past and Present*. Oxford, England: Oxford University Press.

Lee Jen-der 李貞德 (Li Zhende). 1996. "Han-Tang zhijian yi shu zhong de shengchan zhi dao" 漢唐之間醫書中的生產之道 (Childbirth in the Medical Writings of Late Antiquity and Early Medieval China). *Zhongyang yanjiuyuan lishi yuyan yanjiuso jikan* 中央研究院歷史語言研究所集刊 (Bulletin of the Institute of History and Philology, Academia Sinica) 67.3:533–654.

———. 1997. "Han-Tang zhi jian qiu zi yifang shitan—jian lun fuke lanshang yu xingbie lunshu" 漢唐之間求子醫方試探—兼論婦科濫觴與性別論述 (Reproductive Medicine in Late Antiquity and Early Medieval China: Gender Discourse and the Birth of Gynecology). *Bulletin of the Institute of History and Philology: Academia Sinica* 68.2:283–367.

Lee, T'ao (Li Tao). 1950. "The Doctor in Chinese Drama." *Chinese Medical Journal* 68:34–43.

Leung, Angela Ki Che. 1987. "Organized Medicine in Ming-Qing China:

State and Private Medical Institutions in the Lower Yangzi Region." *Late Imperial China* 8.1:134–66.

——. 1996. "Women Practicing Medicine in Pre-modern China." Paper presented at the workshop on New Directions in the Study of Chinese Women 1000–1800, Leiden University, Netherlands, Sept. 11–13, 1996.

——. 1997. "Transmission of Medical Knowledge from the Sung to the Ming." Paper presented at the Conference on the Sung-Yuan-Ming Transition, Lake Arrowhead, California, June 5–11, 1997.

Li Jingwei 李經緯. 1990. "Bei Song huangdi yu yixue" 北宋皇帝與醫學 (Northern Song Emperors and Medicine). *Zhongguo keji shiliao* 中國科技史料 (China Historical Materials of Science and Technology) 10.3:3–20.

Li Jingwei 李經緯 et al. 1988. *Zhongyi renwu cidian* 中醫人物詞典 (Biographical Dictionary of Chinese Medicine). Shanghai: Cishu chubanshe.

Li, Tao (Lee, T'ao). 1958. "A Brief History of Obstetrics and Gynecology in China from Ancient Times to Before the Opium War." *Chinese Medical Journal* 77 (November): 477–86.

Li Yun 李云, ed. 1988. *Zhongyi renmin cidian* 中醫人民辭典 (Biographical Dictionary of Chinese Medicine). Beijing: Guoji wenhua chubangongsi.

Liang Jun 梁峻. 1995. *Zhongguo gudai yizheng shilüe* 中國古代醫政史略 (Brief History of Medicine and the State in Ancient China). Urumqi: Nei Menggu renmin chubanshe.

Liao Junchuan 廖濬泉. 1981. "'Zhouyi' yu Zhongyixue lilun de guanxi" 周易與中醫學理論的關系 (The Relationship between the *Book of Changes* and the Study of Chinese Medical Theory). *Yunnan Zhongyi zazhi* 雲南中醫雜誌 (Yunnan Journal of Chinese Medicine) 5:181–88.

Liao Yuqun 廖育群. 1986. "Xiao shan Zhulin si nüke kaolüe" 蕭山竹林寺女科考略 (Study of Medicine for Females from the Bamboo Forest Temple of Xiao Mountain). *Zhonghua yishi zazhi* 中華醫史雜誌 (Journal of China's Medical History) 16.3:159–61.

Liu Haipo 劉海波 and Gao Chang 高暢. 1982. "Wo guo gudai nü yishi" 我國古代女醫師 (Our Nation's Female Physicians of Olden Times). *Zhonghua yishi zazhi* 中華醫史雜誌 (Journal of China's Medical History) 12.4:221.

Liu Jingzhen 劉靜貞. 1995. "Cong sun zi huai tai de baoying chuanshuo kan Song dai funü de shengyü wenti" 從損子壞胎的報應傳說看宋代婦女的生育問題 (The Question of Childbearing in the Song dynasty from the Perspective of Tales of Retribution from Aborted Fetuses and Dead Infants). *Dalu zazhi* 大陸雜誌 (Continental Journal) 90.1:25–38.

Liu Shijue 劉時覺. 1995. "'Danxi xinfa' ji Zhu shi xiangguan zhuzuo kao" 丹溪心法及朱氏相關著作考 (A Correlation of Texts of *Essential Arts of Danxi* in Relationship to Master Zhu's Authorship). *Zhonghua yishi zazhi* 中華醫史雜誌 (Journal of China's Medical History) 25.2:111–13.

Liu, Ts'ui-jung. 1995a. "A Comparison of Lineage Populations in South China, ca. 1300–1900." In *Chinese Historical Micro-Demography*, ed. Stevan Harrell, 94–120. Berkeley: University of California Press.

——. 1995b. "Demographic Constraint and Family Structure in Traditional Chinese Lineages, ca. 1200–1900." In *Chinese Historical Micro-Demography*, ed. Stevan Harrell, 121–40. Berkeley: University of California Press.

Liu, Ts'un-yan. 1970. "Taoist Self-Cultivation in Ming Thought." In *Self and Society in Ming Thought*, ed. Wm. Theodore de Bary et al., 291–330. New York: Columbia University Press.

Lock, Margaret. 1993. *Encounters with Aging: Mythologies of Menopause in Japan and North America*. Berkeley: University of California Press.

———. 1995. "Cultures of Biomedicine." *Items: Newsletter of the Social Science Research Council* 49.1 (March).

Ma Dazheng 馬大正. 1991. *Zhongguo fuchanke fazhan shi* 中國婦產科發展史 (A History of the Development of Gynecology and Obstetrics in China). Xi'an: Shaanxi kexue jiaoyu chubanshe.

Ma Jixing 馬繼興. 1990. *Zhongyi wenxian xue* 中醫文獻學 (The Study of Chinese Medical Literature). Shanghai: Shanghai kexue jishu.

Ma, Kan-wen. 1983. "Obstetrics in Ancient China." In *Proceedings of the Seventh International Symposium on the Comparative History of Medicine—East and West*, 145–73. Tokyo.

Mann, Susan. 1997. *Precious Records: Women in China's Long Eighteenth Century*. Stanford, Calif.: Stanford University Press.

Martin, Emily. 1988. "Gender and Ideological Differences in Representations of Life and Death." In *Death Ritual in Late Imperial and Modern China,* ed. James L. Watson and Evelyn S. Rawski, 164–79. Berkeley: University of California Press.

Mawangdui Han mu bo shu: Tai chan shu 馬王堆漢墓帛書: 胎產書. (Manuscripts on Silk from the Han Dynasty Tombs at Mawangdui: Book of Gestation and Birth). 1985, Beijing: Wenwu chubanshe. Vol. 4.

Miyasita Saburo 宮下三郎. 1982. "Hung-ch'ien, Red Lead, an Elixir of Life in the Ming Dynasty." In *Explorations in the History of Science and Technology in China: A Special Number of the "Collections of Essays on Chinese Literature and History,"* ed. Li Guohao, Zhang Mengwen, et al., 583–85. Shanghai: Classics Publishing House.

Naquin, Susan, and Evelyn Rawski. 1987. *Chinese Society in the Eighteenth Century*. New Haven, Conn.: Yale University Press.

Needham, Joseph. 1954— . *Science and Civilization in China*. Seventeen volumes to date. Cambridge, England: Cambridge University Press. Abbreviated as SCC.

———. 1962. With the assistance of Wang Ling. *History of Scientific Thought*. Vol. 2 of *Science and Civilization in China*. Cambridge, England: Cambridge University Press.

———, et al. 1970. *Clerks and Craftsmen in China and the West*. Cambridge, England: Cambridge University Press.

Needham, Joseph, and Lu Gwei-djen. 1980. *Celestial Lancets: A History and Rationale of Acupuncture and Moxa*. Cambridge, England: Cambridge University Press.

———. 1983. *Spagyrical Discovery and Invention: Physiological Alchemy*. Vol. 5, part 5 of *Science and Civilization in China*. Cambridge, England: Cambridge University Press.

Okanishi Tameto 岡西爲人. 1948. *Song yiqian yi jikao* 宋以前醫籍考 (The Study of Medical Books of the Song Dynasty and Earlier). Shengyuan.

Ots, Thomas. 1994. "The Silenced Body—The Expressive *Leib:* On the Dialectic of Mind and Life in Chinese Cathartic Healing." In *Embodiment and Experience: The Existential Ground of Culture and the Self*, ed. Thomas Csordas, 116–36. Cambridge Studies in Medical Anthropology. Cambridge, England: Cambridge University Press.

Overmyer, Daniel L. 1985. "Values in Chinese Sectarian Literature: Ming and Ch'ing *Pao-chuan.*" In *Popular Culture in Late Imperial China*, ed. David Johnson, Andrew Nathan, et al., 219–54. Berkeley: University of California Press.

Peterson, Willard J. 1979. *Bitter Gourd: Fang I-chih and the Impetus for Intellectual Change*. New Haven, Conn.: Yale University Press.

Plaks, Andrew. 1987. *Four Masterworks of the Ming Novel*. Princeton, N.J.: Princeton University Press.

Pomata, Gianna. 1984. "Menstruation and Bloodletting in Seventeenth-Century Bologna." Paper presented at the Berkshire Conference on Women's History.

Porkert, Manfred. 1974. *Theoretical Foundations of Chinese Medicine: Systems of Correspondence*. East Asian Science Series 3. Cambridge, Mass.: MIT Press.

Porter, Roy, ed. 1985. *Patients and Practitioners: Lay Perceptions of Medicine in Pre-Industrial Societies*. Cambridge, England: Cambridge University Press.

Qian Xinzhong 錢信忠, ed. 1987. *Zhongguo yixue baike quanshu: yixue shi* 中國醫學百科全書: 醫學史 (Encyclopedia of Chinese Medicine: Medical History). Shanghai: Shanghai kexue jishu chubanshe.

Ren Yingqiu 任應秋. 1980, 1983. *Zhongyi gejia xueshuo* 中醫各家學說 (Study of the Schools of Thought in Chinese Medicine). Shanghai: Kexue zhishu chubanshe.

Robinet, Isabelle. 1989. "Original Contributions of *Neidan* to Taoism and Chinese Thought." In *Taoist Meditation and Longevity Techniques*, ed. Livia Kohn with Yoshinobu Sakade, 297–330. Ann Arbor, Mich.: Center for Chinese Studies, University of Michigan.

Rosenberg, Charles E., and Janet Golden, eds. 1992. *Framing Disease: Studies in Cultural History*. New York: Rutgers University Press.

Scarry, Elaine. 1985. *The Body in Pain: The Making and Unmaking of the World*. Oxford, England: Oxford University Press.

Scheper-Hughes, Nancy, and Margaret Lock. 1989. "The Mindful Body: A Prolegomenon to Future Work in Medical Anthropology." *Medical Anthropology Quarterly* 3:6–41.

Schipper, Kristofer. 1993. *The Taoist Body*. Translated from the French by Karen Duval. Berkeley: University of California Press.

Schwartz, Benjamin. 1985. *The World of Thought in Ancient China*. Cambridge, Mass.: Harvard University Press.

Scott, Joan W. 1986. "Gender: A Useful Category of Historical Analysis." *American Historical Review* 91:1053–75.

Seaman, Gary. 1981. "The Sexual Politics of Karmic Retribution." In *The Anthropology of Taiwanese Society*, ed. Emily Martin and Hill Gates, 381–96. Stanford, Calif.: Stanford University Press.

Seidel, Anna. 1970. "A Taoist Immortal of the Ming Dynasty: Chang San-feng."

In *Self and Society in Ming Thought*, ed. Wm. Theodore de Bary et al. 483–531. New York: Columbia University Press.

Sivin, Nathan. 1987. *Traditional Medicine in Contemporary China: A Partial Translation of "Revised Outline of Chinese Medicine" (1972) with an Introductory Study on Change in Present-Day and Early Medicine*. Ann Arbor, Mich.: Center for Chinese Studies, University of Michigan.

——. 1993. "Huang ti nei ching." In *Early Chinese Texts*, ed. Michael Loewe, 196–215. Berkeley: University of California, Berkeley Society for the Study of Early China.

——. 1995a. "State, Cosmos and the Body in the Last Three Centuries B.C." *Harvard Journal of Asiatic Studies* 55.1:5–37.

——. 1995b. "Text and Experience in Classical Chinese Medicine." In *Knowledge and the Scholarly Medical Traditions*, ed. Don Bates, 177–204. Cambridge, England: Cambridge University Press.

——. 1995c. *Science in Ancient China: Researches and Reflections*. Brookfield, Vermont, and Aldershot, Hampshire: Variorum.

Sommer, Matthew Harvey. 1994. *Sex, Law and Society in Late Imperial China*. Ph.D. diss., University of California, Los Angeles.

Song Shugong 宋書功. 1991. *Zhongguo gudai fangshi yangsheng jiyao* 中國古代房室養生集要 (Essentials on Nourishing Life in the Bed-Chamber in Ancient China). Beijing: Xinhua shudian.

Souliere, Ellen. 1986. *Palace Women of the Ming Dynasty*. Ph.D. diss., Princeton University.

Stafford, Barbara Maria. 1991. *Body Criticism: Imaging the Unseen in Enlightenment Art and Medicine*. Cambridge, Mass.: MIT Press.

Tamba no Mototane 丹波元胤. 1956. *Zhongguo yiji kao* 中國醫籍考 (Studies of China's Medical Books). Reprint of 1831 original. Beijing: Renmin weisheng chubanshe.

Tao Yuanfeng 陶御風 et al. 1988. *Lidai biji yishi bielu* 歷代筆記醫事別錄 (An Informal Record of Medical Matters from the Historical Anecdotal Literature). Tianjin: Tianjin kexue zhishu chubanshe.

T'ien, Ju-k'ang. 1988. *Male Anxiety and Female Chastity: A Comparative Study of Chinese Ethical Values in Ming-Ch'ing Times*. Leiden: E. J. Brill.

Unschuld, Paul. 1979. *Medical Ethics in Imperial China: A Study in Historical Anthropology*. Berkeley: University of California Press.

——. 1986. *Medicine in China: A History of Pharmaceutics*. Berkeley: University of California Press.

Van Gulik, R. H. 1974. *Sexual Life in Ancient China*. Leiden: E. J. Brill.

Waltner, Ann. 1990. *Getting an Heir: Adoption and the Construction of Kinship in Late Imperial China*. Honolulu: University of Hawai'i Press.

Wang Dapeng 王大鵬. 1981. "Shilun 'Zhouyi' dui zuguo yixue de yingxiang" 試論周易對祖國醫學的影響 (Inquiry into the Influence of the *Book of Changes* on the Fatherland's Medical Learning). *Zhejiang Zhongyi zazhi* 浙江中醫雜誌 (Zhejiang Journal of Chinese Medicine) 6:242–44.

Watson, James. 1982. "Of Flesh and Bones: The Management of Death Pollution in Cantonese Society." In *Death and the Regeneration of Life*, eds.

Maurice Bloch and Jonathan Parry, 155–86. Cambridge, England: Cambridge University Press.

Weeks, Jeffrey. 1986. *Sexuality*. New York: Tavistock.

Widmer, Ellen. 1989. "The Epistolary World of Female Talent in Seventeenth-Century China." *Late Imperial China* 10.2:1–43.

———. 1996. "The Huanduzhai of Hangzhou and Suzhou: A Study in Seventeenth-Century Publishing." *Harvard Journal of Asiatic Studies* 56.1:77–122.

Widmer, Ellen, and Kang-I Sun Chang, eds. 1997. *Writing Women in Late Imperial China*. Stanford, Calif.: Stanford University Press.

Wile, Douglas. 1992. *Art of the Bedchamber: The Chinese Sexual Yoga Classics Including Women's Solo Meditation Texts*. Albany: State University of New York Press.

Wolf, Margery. 1992. *A Thrice-Told Tale: Feminism, Postmodernism and Ethnographic Responsibility*. Stanford, Calif.: Stanford University Press.

Wu Baoqi 吳寶琪. 1989. "Song dai chanyu zhi fengsu yanjiu" 宋代產育之風俗研究 (Research on Song Dynasty Childbirth Customs). *Henan daxue xuebao* 河南大學學報 (Henan University Journal) 1:39–45.

Wu, Yi-Li. 1998. *Transmitted Secrets: The Doctors of the Lower Yangzi Region and Popular Gynecology in Late Imperial China*. Ph.D. diss., Yale University.

Wu, Yiyi. 1993–94. "A Medical Line of Many Masters: A Prosopographical Study of Liu Wansu and His Disciples from the Jin to the Early Ming." *Chinese Science* 11:36–65.

Xue Qinglu 薛清錄 et al., comp. 1991. *Quanguo Zhongyi tushu lianhe mulu* 全國中醫圖書關合目錄 (Combined Catalogue of the Nation's Library [holdings] on Chinese Medicine). Zhongyi Yanjiuyuan Tushuguan 中醫研究院圖書館. Beijing: Zhongyi guji chubanshe.

Yang, Marion. 1930. "Control of Practicing Midwives in China." *Chinese Medical Journal* 44.5:428–31.

Yongle Gong pihua 永樂宮壁畫 (Wall Paintings from the Yongle Palace). 1981. Kyoto: Bi no bi.

Zhang Songgeng 張松耕. 1957. "Bu xu liang yao ziheche" 補虛良葯紫河車 (Purple River Cart: A Good Medicine for Replenishing Depletion). *Zhejiang Zhongyi zazhi* 浙江中醫雜誌 (Zhejiang Journal of Chinese Medicine) 5:211.

Zheng, Jinsheng. 1996. "Female Medical Workers in Ancient China." Paper presented at the Eighth International Conference on the History of Science in East Asia, Seoul, Korea, 26–31 August 1996.

Zhong yao da cidian 中藥大辭典 (Encyclopedic Dictionary of Chinese Materia Medica). 1975. Shanghai: Renmin chubanshe. 2 vols.

Zhongwen da cidian 中文大辭典 (Encyclopedic Dictionary of the Chinese Language). 1968. 40 vols. Ed. Chang Chi-yun 張其勻. Taipei: Institute for Advanced Chinese Studies, in cooperation with the National War College.

Zhu Bangxian 朱邦賢, ed. 1991. *Zhongyi bingzheng xiao fang cidian* 中醫病証小方辭典 (Dictionary of Prescription Formulas in Chinese Medicine by Syndrome). Tianjin: Kexue zhishu chubanshe.

Zito, Angela, and Tani E. Barlow., eds. 1994. *Body, Subject and Power in China*. Chicago: University of Chicago Press.

Character Glossary

† Materia medica and prescription formula

an lu fa　安廬法
an shen　安神
an tai　安胎

ba gang　八綱
ba yi　八益
bai mai heju　百脈和聚
bai mai qi dao　百脈齊到
†baifuling　白茯苓
†baishao [yao]　白芍 [藥]
†baishu　白術
†baizhi　白芷
†banxia　半夏
bao　胞
bao leng　胞冷
bao nang　胞囊
"Bao sheng suishi"　保生碎事
Baopuzi　抱樸子
Baoshou cuihe guan　保壽粹和館
Bei chan ji yong fang　備產急用方
Beiji qianjin yaofang　備急千金要
　方

ben　本
bencao　本草
bi　痺
bian　變
bian zheng　辨證
†biandou　扁豆
Bianque　扁鵲
biao　表
bichen　嬖臣
bie fang　別方
biji　筆記
bing　病
bing ming　稟命
†binlang　檳榔
†bohe　薄荷
bu　補
bu xue　補血
bu zhong yi qi　補中益氣

canyue　參閱
†canzhi　蠶紙
Cha Wang　查望

†chaihu　柴胡

chan　產

Chan bao　產寶

Chan bao baiwen　產寶百問

Chan bao baoqing ji　產寶保慶集

Chan bao fang　產寶方

Chan bao zalu　產寶雜錄

Chan bao zhufang　產寶諸方

chan fa　產法

Chan jia yaojue　產家要訣

Chan shu　產書

chan tu　產圖

chang　常

Chanjing　產經

chanke　產科

Chanru beiyao　產乳備要

Chanyu baiwen　產育百問

Chanyu baoqing ji　產育寶慶集

Chanyu baoqing ji[fang]　產育寶慶
集方

Chao Yuanfang　巢元方

chen　臣

Chen Chuliang　陳楚良

Chen Wenzhong　陳文中

Chen Yan　陳言

Chen Yi [Chen Jingfu]　陳沂 [陳靜復]

Chen Ziming　陳自明

Cheng Congzhou [Cheng Maoxian]
程從周 [程茂先]

cheng fang　成方

Cheng Gongli　程公禮

Cheng Maoxian [Cheng Congzhou]
程茂先 [程從周]

†*Cheng qi tang*　承氣湯

†chishao　赤芍

†*Chong he tang*　衝和湯

chong mai　衝脈

Chu Cheng　褚澄

Chu shi yi shu　褚氏遺書

chuang　瘡

chuang lai　瘡癩

†chuanxiong　川芎

chun wen　春溫

"chunran pifu"　蠢然匹婦

cui chan li　催產禮

cui sheng　催生

cun shen　存神

cun wen[ao]　村媼

Da sheng bian　達生篇

†dahuang　大黃

dai　帶

Dai Liang　戴良

dai mai　帶脈

daixia　帶下

daixia yi　帶下醫

dan　丹

dan jing　丹經

dan tian　丹田

†danggui　當歸

Daoshi　道士

Daoxue　道學

Daozang　道藏

†*Dazao wan*　大造丸

†dengxincao　燈心草

di zhi　地支

†digupi　地骨皮

†dihuang　地黃

dian　癲

die　胅

dimu　嫡母

ding　鼎

dou　豆

dou chuang　豆瘡

douzhen　痘疹

du　毒

du mai　督脈

duan chan　斷產

duan hong long　斷紅龍
†duzhong　杜仲

e lu　惡露
erke　兒科

fa biao　發表
fan men　煩悶
Fan Zhongyan　范仲淹
fang lao　房勞
fang shi　方士
fang shu　房術 (art of bedchamber)
fang shu　房書 (bedchamber books)
fang wei　方位
"Fang zhong bu yi"　房中補益
fanwei　翻胃
"fei nan fei nü"　非男非女
fen　分
feng　風
feng yang　風癢
fenghan　風寒
fenmen　憤悶
Fo fa ling shou danfang　佛法靈壽
　丹方
†Foshou　佛手
fu　婦 (woman)
fu　腑 (organ system)
fu　符 (charm)
Fu Shan　傳山
fuke　婦科
†fuling　茯苓
†fupenzi　覆盆子
Furen da quan liang fang　婦人大全
　良方
"furen yi xue wei zhu"　婦人以血爲主
†fuzi　附子

gan　疳 (malnutrition)
gan　肝 (liver)

gan bing　感病
gan jing　趕經
gan ying　感應
†gancao　甘草
ganhuo　肝火
ganmao　感冒
gao　膏
†gaoben　藁本
ge qi　隔氣
Ge zhi yu lun　格至余論
gengnian qi　更年期
Gong Tingxian　龔廷賢
gong xia　攻下
gu qi　谷氣
gu tai　周胎
gu tong　骨通
Gu Yanwu　顧炎武
gu zheng　骨蒸
guan yuan　關元
guang si　廣嗣
Guang si yaolüe　廣嗣要略
Guang si yaoyu　廣嗣要語
Guangling　廣陵
gui　桂
gui kuai　龜塊
gui pi　歸脾
"gui shen"　鬼神
†Gui-po wan　歸珀丸
†gui-shao　歸芍
†gui-wei　歸尾
guniang　姑娘
Guo Jingzhong　郭敬仲
Guo Jizhong　郭稽中
Guo Maoxun　郭茂恂
Guo Wan　郭琬
Guo Zhaoqian　郭昭乾

han　寒
†Hei shen san　黑神散

†heiganjiang　黑乾姜
heng chan　橫產
Hong lou meng　紅樓夢
†honghua　紅花
†hongqian　紅鉛
houtian　後天
houtian yuan qi　後天元氣
hua tai　滑胎
Hua Tuo　華佗
hua zhi　化滯
Huainanzi　淮南字
huan dan　還丹
Huanduzhai　還讀齋
Huang ting jing　黃庭經
Huang Yuxian　黃遇仙
Huangdi neijing　黃帝內經
†huanglian　黃連
†huangqi　黃芪
†huangqin　黃芩
†hugu　虎骨
Huizhou　徽州
Huizong　徽宗
hun　魂
hun tong　魂童
huo　火
huo dan　火丹
huo guan　火罐
huo li　火力
huo xue　活血
huoluan　霍亂
†hupo　琥珀

Ji sheng fang　濟生方
Ji yang gangmu　濟陽綱目
Ji yin gangmu　濟陰綱目
jia　瘕
jia ren　家人
jian yin　兼陰
Jiang Guan　江瓘

jianshi　箋釋
jiao　敎
†jiaoai　膠艾
jiaoqi　腳氣
Jiaozhu furen liang fang　校註婦人
　　良方
ji'e　忌惡
jie biao　解表
jie kuai　結塊
jie wei　借位
jiji　既濟
jijia　積瘕
jiju　積聚
jin dan　金丹
Jin Hanfeng　金閶風
Jin gui yaolüe　金匱要略
Jin ping mei　金瓶梅
†jinbo　金箔
jing　精 (essence)
jing　痙 (fit)
jing　驚 (fright)
jing　經 (classic, channel)
jing qi　精氣
jing wang　精旺
jing xue　精血
jingfeng　驚風
jingluo　經絡
jingmai　經脈
jingshen　精神
"Jingshen xun"　精神訓
Jinjing　禁經
jinshi　進士
†jinyingzi　金櫻子
†jinyinhua　金銀花
"Jizhai jushi"　巫齋居士
ju　疽
ju fang　局方
Ju fang fahui　局方發揮
ju jia　舉家

ju jing　居經
juan　卷
jue　厥
jue yin　厥陰
jun　君
jun huo　君火

kan　坎
kan sheng　看生
kan sheng ren　看生人
kan shengchan　看生產
ke　渴 (thirst)
ke　科 (discipline)
"ke xiazhi"　可下之
Kou Zongshi　寇宗奭
ku jiao　苦交
kuang　狂
kun　坤

lao guniang　老姑娘
lao wen　老媼
li　離 (trigram)
li　痢 (dysentery)
li　癧 (swelling)
li chuang　癧瘡
Li Dongyuan [Li Gao]　李東垣
　[李杲]
Li Heng　李恒
Li Shisheng　李師聖
Li Shizhen　李時珍
Li Yan　李梴
Li yi fang　禮義房
Li Yu　李漁
Li Yuanbi　李元弼
li zhong　理中
†Li zhong wan　理中丸
Li Zhongzi　李中梓
†lian dan　楝丹
†lianhua　蓮花

Liji　禮記
lin　淋
ling　靈
Ling shu　靈樞
†ling-lian　苓連
Liu Fang　劉昉
†Liu he tang　六和湯
liu qi　流氣
Liu Wansu　劉完素
lu　爐
Lü Kun　呂坤
Luan Gong　欒公
lun　論
Lunheng　論衡
luo　絡
luoli　瘰癧
†lurong　鹿茸
Luxing jing　顱顖經

Ma Fu　馬服
Ma Yiqing　馬益卿
†mahuang　麻黃
mai　脈
mai yao lao wen[ao]　賣藥老媼
†maidong [maimendong]　麥冬
　[麥門冬]
Maijing　脈經
man jing　慢驚
men　門
†mengchong　蝱蟲
mi fang　密方
†mianqu　麵麴
Min Qiji　閔齊伋
Min Sheng　閔聲
ming men　命門
ming tang　明堂
Ming tang zhen jiu　明堂針灸
ming yi　名醫
Ming yi lei an　名醫類案

†mudan pi　牡丹皮
†muxiang　木香

nai po　奶婆
nan　男
Nanjing　難經
nanke　男科
nei　內
nei dan　內丹
nei lao　內勞
nei ren　內人
neike　內科
†niuxi　牛膝
niwan　泥丸
nong　膿
nu　怒 (anger)
nü　女 (female)
nü gong　女工 (紅)
nü jin dan　女金丹
nü yi　女醫
Nü yi zayan　女醫雜言
Nüke baiwen　女科百問
Nüke yaozhi　女科要旨
nüke yi po　女科醫婆

Pang Anshi　龐安時
pei　胚
pi　脾 (spleen)
pi　痞 (blockage)
po　魄 (material soul)
po　婆 (granny)
po xue　破血

qi　氣
qi feng　臍風
qi jing　奇經
Qi si zhenquan　祈嗣眞詮
qi sun　七損
Qi Zhongfu　齊仲甫
qi ziling　臍姿靈

qian　乾
Qian Yi　錢乙
qian yin　前陰
Qibo　岐伯
qie　怯 (fearful)
qie　切 (pulse)
qie fei　怯肺
qing　情
qing jin　青筋
qing re　清熱
qingyu　情欲 (desires)
qingyu　情慾 (passion)
Qiu si quanshu　求嗣全書
qiu zao　秋燥
†qiushi　秋石
qu feng　祛風
†queluan　雀卵
qulao　劬勞

ran　染
re　熱
"re ru xueshi"　熱入血室
ren　人 (humanity)
ren　任 (channel)
ren mai　任脈
†renshen　人參
†rougui　肉桂
ru　乳 (breast)
ru　儒 (literati)
ru bu　乳哺
ru ren　儒人
ru yi　乳醫 (childbirth doctor)
ru yi　蓐醫 (childbirth doctor)
ru yi　儒醫 (literati physician)

"san gu liu po"　三姑六婆
san jiao　三焦
San yin fang　三因方
se　色
shan　疝

†shancha 山查
shang feng 傷風
shang yi shiren 尚醫士人
shanghan 傷寒
Shanghan lun 傷寒論
†sharen 沙仁
she sheng 攝生
She sheng san yao 攝生三要
shen 腎 (kidney)
shen 神 (psyche/spirit/consciousness)
shen 身 (body)
Shen Gua 沈括
†Shen jia wujisan 沈家五集散
shen silü 神思慮
†sheng dihuang 生地黃
Sheng ji jing 聖濟經
Sheng ji zonglu 聖濟總錄
†Sheng jin yuan 勝金圓
†Sheng mai san 生脈散
"sheng sheng bu xi" 生生不息
shenti 身體
shi 始 (origin)
shi 使 (envoy)
shi 實 (repletion)
shi 試 (use)
shi 勢 (timing/circumstances)
shi 濕 (damp)
"Shi chan lun" 十產論
shi kan chan 師看產
shi men 石門
shi po 師婆
shi re 濕熱
Shi yi 十翼 (Ten Wings)
shi yi 世醫 (medical lineage)
Shiji 史記
†shilianzi 石蓮子
shisan sha shen 十三煞神
Shishan yi'an 石山醫案
shou sheng 收生

shou tai 瘦胎
shou xing 收形
shoujueyin 手厥陰
shoushaoyang 手少陽
shoushaoyin 手少陰
shousheng zhi ren 收生之人
shoutaiyang 手太陽
shoutaiyin 手太陰
shouyangming 手陽明
shu 數 (number)
shu 署 (summer heat)
shu fa 術法
shu re 署熱
†shuiyin 水銀
†shuizhi 水蛭
Shuo fu 說郛
shuyuan 書院
si dajia 四大家
†Si junzi tang 四君子湯
si yu 思郁
Siku quanshu 四庫全書
Sima Qian 司馬遷
†Siwu tang 四物湯
su fang 素方
Su wen 素問
sui 歲
Sun Simiao 孫思邈
Sun Yikui 孫一奎
sun zi 損子

tai 胎
tai du 胎毒
tai jiao 胎教
tai shen 胎神
Tai shi ju 太史局
Tai su 太素
tai xin 胎心
Taiji 太極
Taiping sheng hui fang 太平聖惠方
Taiyi 太醫

Taiyi ju　大醫局

tan　痰

Tan Fu　談復

Tan Gang　談綱

Tan Yunxian　談允賢

Tao Hongjing　陶弘景

Tao Hua　陶華

Tao Zongyi　陶宗儀

†taoren　桃仁

Ti Xuanzi　體玄子

tian gan　天干

tian shui　天水

tiangui　天癸

tiangui zhi　天癸至

†tianlinggao　天靈高

tiao jing　調經

tiao shen　跳神

tong fang　通方

tong jing　通經

tong li　通利

tong xue　通血

tong yong　通用

Tongshu　通書

†Tu nao cui sheng wan　兔腦催生丸

†tusi　菟絲

wai　外

wai dan　外丹

Wai tai mi yao　外台秘要

waike　外科

Wan bing hui chun　萬病回春

wan chengzhe　晚成者

Wan jin fang　萬金方

Wan Quan　萬全

Wang Chong　王充

Wang furen　王婦人

Wang Hengqi　王恆其

Wang Huaiyin　王懷隱

Wang Ji　汪機

Wang Jingyue　王卿月

Wang Kentang　王肯堂

Wang Qi　汪淇

Wang Xi [Tao]　王熹

Wang Yangming　王陽明

Wang Zhu　王珠

wei　味 (flavor)

wei　衛 (defensive channel)

Wei Zhixiu　魏之琇

wen　文 (literary)

wen　溫 (warm)

wen bu　溫補

wen po [ao po]　媼婆

wen po　穩婆

wen, wang, wen, qie　問, 望, 聞, 切

Weng Zhongren　翁仲仁

wenyi　瘟疫

wu　武 (military)

wu　靈 (shaman)

Wu Muxi　吳慕溪

Wu Qian　吳謙

Wu Ti　吳禔

wu wei　五味

wu xing　五行 (five phases)

wu xing　五性 (human feelings)

wu yun liu qi　五連六氣

Wu Zhiwang　武之望

Wulin Chen shi jiazhuan xian fang
　武林陳氏家傳仙方

†wulingzhi　五靈脂

†wuweizi　五味子

xi dou　希痘

xi er hui　洗兒會

Xi Wang Mu nüxiu zhengtu shi ze
　西王母女修正途十則

xia　下

xian dao　仙道

Xian qi jiu zheng lun　軒岐救正論

xiang　象

xiang huo　相火

†xiangfu　香附

†xiangru　香薷

xiansheng　先生

xiantian　先天

"xiantian huanghuang huhu"　先天
恍恍惚惚

"xiantian zhen yi zhi ling qi"　先天
眞一之靈氣

Xiao Jing　蕭京

Xiao pin fang　小品方

xie　邪

xie guimei　邪鬼魅

xie meng　邪夢

xie xia　瀉下

Xie Zhaozhe　謝肇淛

xiexie　泄瀉

xin　信

xin jing　心驚

"xin zhong fenmen"　心中憤悶

Xin'an　新安

xing　性 (nature)

xing　形 (physical form)

xing nian　姓年

Xiu zhen fang　袖珍方

xu　虛

Xu Chunfu　徐春甫

Xu Gu　許穀

Xu Ke　徐珂

xu qie　虛怯

xu re　虛熱

Xu Wenyi　許文懿

xuan men　玄門

xuan pin zhi men　玄牝之門

†xuanhu　玄胡

xue　學 (learning)

xue　血 (blood)

xue fen　血分

xue hai　血海

Xue Ji　薛己

Xue Xian　薛軒

xuebeng　血崩

xuefeng　血風

xuelin　血淋

xuepai　學派

xulao　虛勞

xusun　虛損

yamen　衙門

yan　驗

yan si　燕私

Yan Yonghe　嚴用和

yang　陽 (partner of yin)

yang　養 (to nourish, care for)

"Yang chang you yu, yin chang bu zu"
陽常有餘, 陰常不足

yang lao　養老

yang ming　陽明

Yang Shangshan　楊上善

yang sheng　養生

Yang Shiying　楊士瀛

yang xue　養血

yang yi　瘍醫

Yang Zijian　楊子建

yanhu [suo]　延胡 [索]

Yanzi jian　燕子箋

yao　藥

yao po　藥婆

ye　業

Ye Shaoyuan　葉紹袁

Ye Xiaoluan　葉小鸞

yi　噎 (throat blockage)

yi　疫 (epidemic fever)

yi　議 (opinion)

yi　醫 (doctor)

yi fu　醫婦

yi gong　醫工

yi guan chanke　醫官產科

yi po　醫婆

yi qi　一氣

"yi ren bu ren"　以人補人

Yijing　易經

†yimucao　益母草

yin　陰

yin chu　陰處

yin han　陰寒

yin hu　陰戶

yin qi　陰氣

yin qi　陰器 (genitals)

yin xu yang bo　陰虛陽搏

yin xue　陰血

yin zao　陰燥

yin zhong　陰中

ying　營

yinzhen　癮疹

Yixue ru men　醫學入門

yong　癰

yong yi　庸醫

you tai sha　遊胎殺

You you xin shu　幼幼新書

yu　喻 (oral instructions)

yu　郁 (stasis)

yu　瘀 (congestion)

Yu Chang [Yu Jiayan]　喻昌 [喻嘉言]

Yu Chong　虞沆

Yu Qiao　俞橋

Yu zang　禹藏

yuan　元

Yuan Cai　袁采

"Yuan dou"　原痘

Yuan Hao　袁顥

Yuan Huang [Yuan Liaofan]　袁黃 [袁了凡]

yuan pan　院判

yuan qi　元氣

yuan shen　元神

yue　月

yue shui　月水

yuejing　月經

yujie　郁結

yunu　郁怒

za bing　雜病

Zan Yin　昝殷

zang　臟

zao　燥

zao hua　造化

Zhaixuan fang　摘玄方

zhan chi long　斬赤龍

Zhang Congzheng [Zhang Ziho]　張從正 [張子和]

Zhang Gao　張杲

Zhang Ji [Zhang Zhongjing]　張機 [張仲景]

Zhang Jiebin [Zhang Jingyue]　張介賓 [張景岳]

Zhang Sanfeng　張三豐

Zhang Yuansu [Zhang Jiegu]　張元素 [張潔古]

zhen　疹

Zhen jiu jiayi jing　針灸甲乙經

zhen qi　眞氣

zhen yin　眞陰

zheng　症

zheng chong　怔忡

zhi　脂 (fat)

zhi　治 (cure)

Zhi yi lu　質疑錄

†zhike　枳殼

†zhimu　知母

†zhishi　枳實

zhixia　滯下

zhong bing　眾病

zhong ji　眾疾

zhong zi　種子

zhongfeng　中風

Zhou Dunyi　周敦頤

Zhou Hu　周祜

Zhou Rongqi　周榮起

Zhou Ting　周頲

Zhou Xi　周禧

zhu　疰

Zhu Zhenheng [Zhu Danxi]　朱震亨 [朱丹溪]

Zhubing yuanhou lun　諸病源侯論

Zhulin si　竹林寺

†zhusha　朱砂

zhuyou fa　祝由法

Zhuzi yulei　朱子語類

zi　子

†ziheche　紫河車

†zisu　紫蘇

†Zisu tang　紫蘇湯

zou zhu　走注

zu qi　祖氣

zujueyin　足厥陰

zuo　佐

zuo po　坐婆

zuo yue　坐月 (作月)

zushaoyang　足少陽

zushaoyin　足少陰

zutaiyang　足太陽

zutaiyin　足太陰

zuyangming　足陽明

Index